# Initial Management of Injuries

To our wives, Victoria and Anne
and our children, Tara, Julie, Ronnie, Lindsey, Kelly,
Sabrina, Luke, Jack, Grace, and Tim for their devotion
and patience.

# Initial Management of Injuries
## An evidence based approach

Edited by

**Ronald F Sing**
*Clinical Assistant Professor of Surgery, School of Medicine, University of North Carolina at Chapel Hill and Faculty, Department of Surgery, Carolinas Medical Center, Charlotte, North Carolina, USA*

**Patrick M Reilly**
*Assistant Professor of Surgery, University of Pennsylvania Medical Center and School of Medicine, Division of Trauma and Surgical Critical Care, Philadelphia, Pennsylvania, USA*

and

**W Joseph Messick**
*Late of the Department of Surgery, Carolinas Medical Center and Clinical Associate Professor of Surgery, School of Medicine, University of North Carolina at Chapel Hill, Chapel Hill, North Carolina, USA*

© BMJ Books 2001
BMJ Books is an imprint of the BMJ Publishing Group

First published in 2001
by BMJ Books, BMA House, Tavistock Square,
London WC1H 9JR

www.bmjbooks.com

**British Library Cataloguing in Publication Data**

A catalogue record for this book is available from the British Library

ISBN 0-7279-1477-4

Cover design by Landmark Design, Croydon, Surrey
Typeset by Academic and Technical Typesetting, Bristol
Printed and bound by J W Arrowsmith Ltd, Bristol

# Contents

## In memorium

We mourn the loss of our friend, mentor, and colleague, W Joseph Messick MD, who died during the production of *Initial Management of Injuries: An evidence based approach*.

This book is dedicated to the memory of Joe and to his family.

# Contributors

**Ronnie S Benoit** Assistant Chief for Pediatric Trauma, Inova Fairfax Hospital, Falls Church, VA, USA; Clinical Assistant Professor of Surgery, Georgetown University, Washington, DC, USA

**Karen J Brasel** Assistant Professor of Surgery, Medical College of Wisconsin Department of Surgery, Division of Trauma/Critical Care, Milwaukee, WI, USA

**L D Britt** Brickhouse Professor and Chairman of Surgery, Department of Surgery, Eastern Virginia Medical School, Norfolk, VA, USA

**Eddy H Carrillo** Associate Professor of Surgery, Department of Surgery, University of Louisville School of Medicine and Director of Trauma Services at University of Louisville Hospital, Louisville, KY, USA

**David L Ciraulo** University of Tennessee College of Medicine, Chattanooga Unit, Chattanooga, TN, USA

**Thomas V Clancy** Medical Director, Trauma Service, New Hanover Regional Medical Center, Wilmington, NC, USA; Professor of Surgery, University of North Carolina at Chapel Hill, Chapel Hill, NC, USA

**Frederic Cole** Assistant Professor of Surgery, Department of Surgery, Eastern Virginia Medical School, Norfolk, VA, USA

**Edward E Cornwell** Associate Professor of Surgery, Chief, Adult Trauma Services, Johns Hopkins University School of Medicine, Baltimore, MD, USA

**Bernard J Costello** Chief Resident of Oral and Maxillofacial Surgery at the University of Pennsylvania Medical Center, the Children's Hospital of Philadelphia, and the University of Pennsylvania School of Dental Medicine, Philadelphia, PA, USA

**Edward T Dickinson** Director of EMS Field Operations, Assistant Professor, Department of Emergency Medicine, University of Pennsylvania, Philadelphia, PA, USA

**J Christopher DiGiacomo** Associate Professor of Surgery, SUNY Stoneybrook; Associate Director of Trauma, The Long Island Comprehensive Trauma Center, Nassau County Medical Center, East Meadow, NY, USA

**Kenneth A Egol** NYU Hospital for Joint Diseases, Department of Orthopedic Surgery, New York, NY, USA

**Samir M Fakhry** Chief, Trauma Services, Inova Fairfax Hospital, Falls Church, VA, USA; Clinical Professor of Surgery, Georgetown University, Washington, DC, USA

**Marsha Ford** Assistant Chairman and Director of Toxicology, Department of Emergency Medicine; Director, Carolinas Poison Center, Carolinas Medical Center, Charlotte, NC, USA; Associate Clinical Professor of Emergency Medicine, University of North Carolina at Chapel Hill, Chapel Hill, NC, USA

**Steven L Frick** Pediatric Orthopedics, Assistant Residency Program Director, Department of Orthopedic Surgery, Carolinas Medical Center, Charlotte, NC, USA

**Thomas Genuit** Fellow, Trauma and Surgical Critical Care, University of Maryland Medical Center, R Adams Cowley Shock Trauma Center; Clinical Instructor of Surgery, University of Maryland School of Medicine, Baltimore, MD, USA

**Michael A Gibbs** Residency Program Director, Department of Emergency Medicine, Carolinas Medical Center, Charlotte, NC, USA; Medical Director, MedCenter Air; Associate Professor of Emergency Medicine, University of North Carolina at Chapel Hill, Chapel Hill, NC, USA

**Vicente H Gracias** Assistant Professor of Surgery, University of Pennsylvania, Medical Center and School of Medicine, Division of Trauma and Surgical Critical Care, Philadelphia, PA, USA

**Michael D Grossman** Assistant Professor of Surgery, University of Pennsylvania; Chief, Trauma and Surgical Critical Care, St Luke Hospital, Bethlehem, PA, USA

**Barbara M Guise** Mid-Atlantic Emergency Medical Associates, Charlotte, NC, USA

**William S Hoff** Assistant Professor of Surgery, University of Pennsylvania, Philadelphia, PA, USA; Chairman, Department of Traumatology, Brandywine Hospital, Coatesville, PA, USA

**Toan Huynh** Director, Surgical Intensive Care Unit, Trauma, Critical Care Services, Department of Surgery, Carolinas Medical Center, Charlotte, NC, USA

**David G Jacobs** Associate Trauma Director, Trauma Service, Carolinas Medical Center, Charlotte, NC, USA

**Madhav A Karunakar** Orthopedic Surgery, The University of Michigan, Ann Arbor, MI, USA

**Lewis J Kaplan** Assistant Professor of Surgery, MCP Hahnemann University, Department of Surgery, Philadelphia, PA, USA

**James F Kellam** The Orthopedic Trauma Service, Carolinas Medical Center, Charlotte, NC, USA

**W Joseph Messick** Late of the Department of Surgery, Carolinas Medical Center and Clinical Associate Professor of Surgery, University of North Carolina at Chapel Hill, School of Medicine, Chapel Hill, NC, USA

**William S Miles** Director, Surgical Critical Care, Department of Surgery, Carolinas Medical Center, Charlotte, NC, USA; Clinical Assistant Professor of Surgery, University of North Carolina at Chapel Hill, Chapel Hill, NC, USA

**Douglas McGee** Associate Director, Emergency Medicine Residency Program, Albert Einstein Medical Center, Philadelphia, PA, USA

**Lena M Napolitano** Division Chief and Program Director, Surgical Critical Care, University of Maryland Medical Center and R Adams Cowley Shock Trauma Center; Associate Professor of Surgery, University of Maryland School of Medicine, Baltimore, MD, USA

**Brent L Norris** Division Chief, Orthopaedic Trauma, Department of Orthopaedic Surgery, University of Tennessee College of Medicine, Chattanooga Unit, Chattanooga, TN, USA

**Peter J Nowotarski** Division Chief, Orthopaedic Trauma, Department of Orthopaedic Surgery, University of Tennessee College of Medicine, Chattanooga Unit, Chattanooga, TN, USA

**Alvin Ong** Orthopaedic Trauma Fellow, Department of Orthopaedic Surgery, Carolinas Medical Center, Charlotte, NC, USA

**Roger N Passmore** Chief Resident, Department of Orthopaedic Surgery, University of Tennessee College of Medicine, Chattanooga Unit, Chattanooga, TN, USA

**Andrew D Perron** Assistant Professor, Emergency Medicine and Sports Medicine, University of Virginia, Charlottesville, VA, USA

**Patrick M Reilly** Assistant Professor of Surgery at the University of Pennsylvania Medical Center and School of Medicine, Division of Trauma and Surgical Critical Care, Philadelphia, PA, USA

**J David Richardson** Professor and Vice-Chairman, Department of Surgery, University of Louisville School of Medicine, Trauma Program in Surgery, University of Louisville Hospital, Louisville, KY, USA

**Aurelio Rodriguez** Associate Director of Trauma, R Adams Cowley Shock Trauma Center; Professor of Surgery, University of Maryland School of Medicine, Baltimore, MD, USA

**Edmund J Rutherford** Associate Professor of Surgery, Chief, Surgical Critical Care, University of North Carolina at Chapel Hill, Chapel Hill, NC, USA

**Thomas A Santora** Associate Professor of Surgery, MCP Hahnemann University, Department of Surgery, Philadelphia, PA, USA

**Jennifer Sarafin** Trauma Nurse Case Manager, Carolinas Medical Center, Charlotte, NC, USA

**Glenn K Schemmer** Associate Director, Maternal–Fetal Medicine, Department of Obstetrics and Gynecology, Carolinas Medical Center, Charlotte, NC, USA

**Gerald W Shaftan** Chairman, Department of Surgery, Nassau County Medical Center, East Meadow, NY, USA; Professor of Surgery, State University of New York, Stoneybrook, NY, USA

**Keith Silverstein** Assistant Professor of Oral and Maxillofacial Surgery at the University of Pennsylvania Medical Center, the Children's Hospital of Philadelphia; University of Pennsylvania School of Dental Medicine, Philadelphia, PA, USA

**Ronald F Sing** Clinical Assistant Professor of Surgery, School of Medicine, University of North Carolina at Chapel Hill, Chapel Hill, NC, USA; Faculty, Department of Surgery, Carolinas Medical Center, Charlotte, NC, USA

**Philip W Smith** University of Tennessee College of Medicine, Chattanooga Unit, Chattanooga, TN, USA

**Michael H Thomason** Co-chair, Department of Surgery; Director, Trauma Services, Carolinas Medical Center, Charlotte, NC, USA; Clinical Professor of Surgery, School of Medicine, University of North Carolina at Chapel Hill, Chapel Hill, NC, USA

**Glen H Tinkoff** Director, Trauma Program, Christiana Hospital; Clinical Assistant Professor, Thomas Jefferson University, Newark, DE, USA

**Christian Tomaszewski** Department of Emergency Medicine, Carolinas Medical Center, Charlotte, NC, USA

**Stanley Z Trooskin** Professor of Surgery, MCP Hahnemann University, Department of Surgery, Philadelphia, PA, USA

**Philip A Visser** Department of Surgery, Carolinas Medical Center, Charlotte, NC, USA

**Ron M Walls** Chair, Department of Emergency Medicine, Brigham & Women's Hospital; Associate Professor of Medicine, Division of Emergency Medicine, Harvard Medical School, Boston, MA, USA

**Christopher D Wohltmann** Chief of Trauma and Surgical Critical Care, William Beaumont Army Medical Center, El Paso, TX, USA

# Foreword

It is an honor to introduce this new textbook. Having known and personally worked with the editors and many of the authors, I am especially pleased because this is a timely contribution unique in format, contemporary, and clinically relevant. The book's content is immediately applicable for the student, physician, and surgeon called to care for critically injured people.

Drs Sing and Reilly draw on their strong backgrounds as clinical educators in trauma surgery and have selected many of the more difficult clinical problems we experience in the trauma resuscitation bay and operating room. Besides the expertise they bring to the content, the editors have selected some of the United States's leading surgeons and physicians as authors. The chapters deal with a number of "hot" topics as they relate to the initial diagnosis and management of extreme injuries such as complex pelvic fracture presenting with exsanguination, the mangled extremity, blunt aortic injury, and gunshot injury to difficult anatomical regions such as the back and flank, mediastinum, and gluteal area. Simultaneously, the book addresses several issues common to busy trauma centers but usually not as well covered in texts of this nature. These include reviews of maxillofacial trauma, hematuria, hypothermia, drowning, mass casualty, and evaluation of the sexually assaulted patient. These reviews are written to provide concise, pragmatic information for the physician at the bedside.

Each subject is explored and presented as a clinical problem. The problem is developed with a concise description of its clinical relevance and difficulty, and is followed by an outline of the most important literature on the subject. Each citation includes a summary of that paper's design, results, conclusions, and clinical application to the problem. Citations are classified according to an evidence-based hierarchy. Lastly, the authors present what is, based on their review of the topic and literature, a practical algorithm for the diagnosis or management of each topic. These have been styled as simple diagrams that are easy to read. Each provides a safe pathway when navigating the clinical fray of patients with complex injuries and situations that need rapid solutions. They are applicable, accurate, and based on the best science in the literature for the problem.

The trilogy of text, annotated bibliography, and algorithm is strengthened by insisting that the literature be classified according to the quality of the evidence presented. The reader has the advantage of a literature review weighted by scientific merit. Combined with an expert's interpretation, this novel approach makes the book very important for the field of traumatology and emergency care.

C. William Schwab MD, FACS
Professor of Surgery
Division of Traumatology and Surgical Critical Care
Department of Surgery
University of Pennsylvania School of Medicine
Philadelphia, PA
USA

# Introduction

Many textbooks have been written regarding the care of the injured patient, however, most deal with the treatment of known injuries or disease processes. The challenge of trauma care involves not only the diagnosis and treatment of injuries, but the decisions that must be made in the setting of shock. These challenges are rarely addressed in textbooks dealing with trauma. Even the treatment of a known condition or injury may take differing paths depending on other more life-threatening injuries or the hemodynamic status of the patient. Again, information regarding these clinical decisions are often absent from current texts.

*Initial Management of Injuries: An evidence based approach*, tackles the decisions faced by the physician early in the presentation of the injured patient. Our purpose is not to discuss the techniques of treating a specific injury or disease process, but to give the clinician a framework to help in rapidly initiating diagnostic and therapeutic decisions – evidence based algorithms. The algorithms in this book have been developed by experts in the field of trauma care, many of whom have published extensively in their respective fields. These algorithms are based on extensive literature review and the references are annotated and classified according to their level of evidence:

Class I    well-designed prospective, randomized, controlled trials
Class II   Prospective studies and large retrospective analyses based on reliable data
Class III  Small, retrospective studies, case series, and expert opinion.

This textbook will be useful to surgeons, emergency physicians, orthopaedic surgeons, neurosurgeons, and all physicians who encounter the injured patient. The real challenges faced by the providers of trauma care are those decisions encountered when competing algorithms intersect in the multiply injured patient. No algorithm is possible for this, only clinical experience. Although it is impossible to develop an algorithm to address the complexity of the many potential scenarios (for example, multisystem injuries), this book will greatly assist in the systematic approach to the initial management of injuries.

# 1 Trauma triage

*Edward T Dickinson*

## Introduction

Appropriate trauma triage by prehospital providers is a crucial component of an effective trauma system. The ultimate goal is to deliver the "right patient to the right hospital at the right time". Inherent in trauma triage by emergency medical technicians and paramedics are the phenomena of overtriage and undertriage of injured patients. It is accepted that some degree of overtriage is necessary to avoid the preventable morbidity and mortality of trauma patients being transported to non-trauma center hospitals that are ill prepared to manage these victims comprehensively. The American College of Surgeons Committee on Trauma (ACS COT) concedes that a 5–10% undertriage is unavoidable and is associated with an overtriage rate of up to 30–50%.[1]

The ACS COT has established the Field Triage Decision Scheme as an algorithm for prehospital providers to use as a guide for the optimal care of trauma patients (see algorithm).[1] This document is based on the consensus of experts. Much of the trauma triage literature has focused on attempts to validate this and other trauma triage systems.[2–7] Despite this body of literature, the Holy Grail of prehospital trauma triage – a system with 100% sensitivity and 100% specificity for identifying patients with major trauma – remains elusive. Indeed, it is evident that human judgment plays an important role in enhancing triage accuracy, a variable that cannot be readily quantified.[4–5,8]

The ACS Field Triage Decision Scheme is the most widely accepted algorithm for field triage decision making. This document is augmented to some extent by the scientific literature and will serve as the primary algorithm for this chapter.

## Vital signs and level of consciousness (Step One)

A systolic blood pressure of less than 90 mmHg has been shown to be a strong predictor of serious injury.[3,4,9]

Interestingly, even a single determination of hypotension by prehospital personnel and subsequent normotension upon trauma center arrival was still predictive of more serious injuries.[9]

A Glasgow Coma Scale score of less than 14 as an indicator of serious trauma has been best supported by alterations in the motor score component of the scale.[3,4,10] In one large retrospective study, Meredith determined that a gross motor score of less than 6 (i.e. does not follow commands) was the single best predictor of subsequent trauma death.[10] In his study, the gross motor score was more predictive than a full GCS, Trauma Score or ISS. In another study, Baxt identified a gross motor score of less than 5 as a sensitive and specific predictor of identifying the major trauma patient.[3]

The inclusion of an abnormal respiratory rate as a vital sign criterion for trauma alert criteria is clinically intuitive but anecdotal. Because both systolic hypotension and the gross motor score of the Glasgow Coma Scale are components of the Revised Trauma Score, it perhaps can be extrapolated that the RTS has some validity as determined by the literature. However, the full RTS as a primary discriminator of major trauma has been shown in retrospect to be a predictor of mortality but not an accurate discriminator of serious injury.[2]

## Anatomy of injury (Step Two)

To a certain degree, common sense will indicate when an anatomic derangement, which is the result of trauma, defines a patient who should be transported to a trauma center and warrants activation of the trauma team. It would be unlikely that any investigator would conduct a randomized trial to test the hypothesis that "open and depressed skull fractures" should be treated anywhere other than at a trauma center and that this injury by its nature defines serious trauma. It is for this reason that most of the injuries listed in Step Two are based on common sense, yet anecdotal grounds.

The true prehospital utility of these anatomic findings for trauma triage may be further questioned because the ability of prehospital providers to identify accurately some of these injuries that ultimately require radiographic confirmation (e.g. flail chest or pelvic fractures) has not been tested in the literature. It is perhaps for this reason that these broad anatomic injuries have only been shown to have an "intermediate yield" when used as a single criterion for identifying major trauma patients in prehospital trauma triage.[5]

Penetrating trauma to the head, neck or torso has been demonstrated to be an accurate predictor of major trauma.[3,4] Not only do these patients tend to have a high ISS score but the definition of "major trauma" in much of the trauma triage literature is usually based on the need for operative intervention, which is frequently the case in penetrating trauma victims.[2–4]

## Mechanism of injury (Step Three)

In general, mechanism of injury (MOI) must be linked with anatomic and physiologic criteria to have value as a trauma triage predictor of serious injury.[6,7] In one study, however, Esposito identified prolonged prehospital time, death of another occupant in the same vehicle and a pedestrian being struck at greater than 20 mph (32 km/hour) as "high yield" for identifying major trauma victims, even when used as a single criterion.[5] The remainder of the MOIs listed are anecdotal but based on the sound premise that the greater the energy involved in a trauma, the greater propensity for serious injury.

The algorithm for Step Three recommends that if there is a significant MOI encountered, then medical direction should be contacted. This step introduces the human judgment factor into trauma triage. Champion has described that the real-time input of physician judgment on trauma triage decisions enhances the identification of serious injuries.[8]

Similarly, it is at this point in the algorithm that prehospital provider judgment may come into play in the "consider transport to a trauma center" based on the MOI. Both Esposito and Fries have independently reported that paramedic judgment enhances the accuracy of established trauma triage schemes.[4,5] Importantly, both studies demonstrated that paramedic judgment alone, in the absence of other trauma triage criteria, was not a reliable single indicator of serious injury.

If the decision is made to transport the trauma victims to a trauma center based on MOI or comorbidity, there is an option to consider a "trauma team alert". Presumably, if the patient is transported to a trauma center and the team is not "alerted" prior to arrival, then it is likely that the patient will be initially evaluated by the on-duty emergency medicine physician.

There is a growing body of literature suggesting that hemodynamically stable trauma patients transported to a trauma center can be appropriately evaluated and managed without a full-scale trauma team alert.[6,11–13] The utilization of emergency medicine physicians in a "two-specialty, two-tiered" triage not only saves money and resources, but also accelerates the emergency department throughput time of these patients whether to discharge, the ICU or the operating room.[12,13]

## Comorbidity (Step Four)

The patient categories listed in Step Four represent comorbidities that are likely to result in complications of trauma management. This portion of the scheme is supported by clinical logic, expert opinion, and anecdotal experience that trauma victims with complex medical conditions are best managed in tertiary centers with more extensive resources. Although there are no controlled trials that randomize these patients to a trauma center one day and a community hospital the next day, there is support in the literature for the impact that tertiary care resources can make in the care of trauma patients. For example, Scalea reported decreased mortality of geriatric trauma patients who underwent early invasive monitoring as part of comprehensive trauma care.[14]

## Traumatic cardiac arrest in the field

### Blunt trauma

Blunt trauma victims who succumb to cardiac arrest in the field have a uniformly dismal prognosis.[15–17] Given the high cost of the futile management of traumatic cardiac arrests and the low yield for tissue harvesting of these patients, Rosemurgy concluded that attempts at resuscitation of these patients are unwarranted.[15] Durham *et al.* supported this conclusion when evaluating the survival of blunt trauma patients who underwent emergency thoracotomy and found there to be no survivors.[16]

### Penetrating trauma

Penetrating trauma victims who suffer cardiac arrest in the field appear to have a higher survival rate than those who arrest in the setting of blunt trauma.[16,17] The sur-vival of these patients is, however, highly dependent on their physiologic status, duration of cardiac arrest, and level of prehospital care at the time of presenta-tion to the trauma center.[16,17] Lorenz found that no patients who were in cardiac arrest upon EMS arrival survived emergency thoracotomy.[17] A study conducted in Houston showed that survival of cardiac arrest patients undergoing thoracotomy correlated with duration of CPR by EMS, with survivors having an average of 5.1 minutes of CPR prior to ED arrival as compared to 9.1 minutes for non-survivors.[16] Interestingly, in that same study, endotracheal intubation by paramedics lengthened the viability window of cardiac arrest survivors from 4.1 minutes for unintubated patients to 9.4 minutes for those who were intubated in the field.

## Class II references

2. Baxt WG, Berry CC, Epperson MD *et al*. The failure of prehospital trauma prediction rules to classify trauma patients accurately. *Ann Emerg Med* 1989; **18**:1–8.

    This is a retrospective review of 2434 patients entered in the trauma registry of the San Diego Regional Trauma System. The researchers abstracted data to calculate predicted ISS score and mortality based upon the CRAMS Scale, Trauma Score, Revised Trauma Score, and Prehospital Index for this large sample of patients. Although all these various rules for injury prediction were generally accurate in identifying patients who subsequently died, none of these prehospital scales consistently predicted accurate ISS scores of trauma patients.

3. Baxt WG, Jones G, Fortlage D. The trauma triage rule: a new, resource-based approach to the prehospital identification of major trauma victims. *Ann Emerg Med* 1990;**19**:1401–6.

    This prospective study of 1004 trauma patients is an attempt to identify more accurate prehospital criteria that will accurately predict major trauma patients in light of the limitations of existing systems as previously identified by the same principal investigator. The paper defines a new "Trauma Triage Rule (TTR)" that states that patients with any of the following prehospital findings are at high risk for major trauma: systolic blood pressure of less than 85 mmHg, motor component of the Glasgow Coma Scale less than 5 or those who have sustained penetrating trauma to the head, neck or torso. The authors report that application of this TTR resulted in a 97% sensitivity and specificity in identifying major trauma patients. Of the 17 major trauma patients that the TSS failed to identify in the study, all were the victims of blunt trauma and the majority of these had intraabdominal injuries.

4. Fries GR, McCalla G, Levitt MA *et al*. A prospective comparison of paramedic judgment and the trauma triage rule in the prehospital setting. *Ann Emerg Med* 1994;**24**:885–9.

    This prospective study of 653 patients enhanced the Trauma Triage Rule described by Baxt with the augmentation of paramedic judgment when TTR criteria for major trauma identification were not present. This enhancement of paramedic "gut feeling" raised sensitivity to 100% while resulting in an decrease in the specificity to 75%.

5. Esposito TJ, Offner PJ, Jurkovich, GJ *et al*. Do prehospital trauma center triage criteria identify major trauma victims? *Arch Surg* 1995;**130**:171–6.

    The study retrospectively evaluated objective anatomic, physiologic, and mechanism of injury criteria as well as the subjective "gut feeling" of prehospital providers as single criteria to identify major trauma patients. These investigators identified prolonged scene times, pedestrians struck by cars at greater than 20 mph, and physiologic criteria as the most reliable indicators of major trauma patients. Prehospital provider "gut feeling" was not a reliable indicator as a single criterion, but enhanced mechanism of injury findings when the two criteria were applied together.

6. Simon BJ, Legere P, Emhoff T *et al*. Vehicular trauma triage by mechanism: avoidance of unproductive evaluation. *J Trauma* 1994;**37**(4):645–9.

    A retrospective study of 1235 consecutive patients presenting to a trauma center as "trauma activations" identified 349 patients with significant mechanisms in vehicular crashes upon which the study was based. The authors found that major trauma patients most often presented with a combination of both mechanisms and abnormal physiologic and/or anatomic findings. They conclude that patients transported to a trauma center by EMS solely for mechanism of injury reasons can safely be subjected to secondary triage upon ED arrival prior to activation of the trauma team.

7. Shatney CH, Sensaki K. Trauma team activation for "mechanism of injury" blunt trauma victims: time for a change? *J Trauma* 1994;**37**(2):275–82.

    Another retrospective study of blunt trauma victims presenting to a trauma center based solely on the prehospital triage criteria of mechanism of injury. The authors conclude that if such patients are hemodynamically stable, can be safely and more cost-effectively evaluated by the emergency medicine physician than by the automatic activation of the trauma team based on the mechanism.

10. Meredith W, Rutlage R, Hansen AR *et al*. Field triage of trauma patients based upon the ability to follow commands: a study in 29 573 injured patients. *J Trauma* 1995;**38**(1):129–35.

Utilizing a state trauma registry, the authors identified that the Glasgow Coma Scale's motor score (GMS) was the most accurate discriminator as compared to full GCS, Trauma Score, and ISS using both discriminating analysis and logistic regression methods. Simply stated, the inability to follow simple commands (GMS 1–5) was the single best predictor of subsequent trauma death in this study.

11. Ochsner MG, Schmidt JA, Rozycki GS *et al*. The evaluation of a two-tiered trauma response system at a major trauma center: is it cost effective and safe? *J Trauma* 1995;**39**(5):971–7.

The authors utilized a protocol based on prehospital criteria that modified the number of personnel responding to evaluate trauma victims (both blunt and penetrating). The authors concluded that such a system was both safe and resulted in a cost saving of $250 per patient.

12. Tinkoff GH, O'Connor RE, Fulda GJ. Impact of a two-tiered trauma response in the emergency department: promoting efficient resource utilization. *J Trauma* 1996;**41**(4):735–40.

A prospective observational study with historical controls evaluated the effectiveness of a two-tiered trauma response based on mechanism of injury, anatomic, and physiologic criteria, as well as logistical considerations. This study found that the utilization of such a system decreased the length of ED stay of trauma patients – whether reducing the length of ED stay prior to discharge with minor injuries or facilitating the movement of more critical patients through the ED either to the operating room or the ICU.

## Class III references

1. Committee on Trauma, American College of Surgeons. *Resources for optimal care of the injured patient.* Chicago: ACS, 1999.

The most complex Field Triage Decision Scheme currently available is based upon expert and consensus opinion with some referenced input from the trauma triage literature.

8. Champion HR, Sacco WJ, Gainer PS *et al*. The effect of medical direction on trauma triage. *J Trauma* 1988;**28**:235–9.

The study of patients flown to a trauma center by helicopter demonstrated that real-time physician input in field or emergency department trauma triage decisions identified patients with higher ISS scores than those flown to the trauma center without physician input.

9. Chan L, Bartfield J, Reilly K. The significance of out-of-hospital hypotension in blunt trauma patients. *Acad Emerg Med* 1997;**4**:785-8.

In this small (54 patient) retrospective case control study it was found that patients who had documented hypotension (systolic BP <90 mmHg) by EMS personnel but were normotensive in the emergency department had higher ISS scores, higher incidence of mortality, ICU admissions, pelvic and femur fractures than controls.

13. Plaisier BR, Meldon SW, Super DM *et al*. Effectiveness of a 2-specialty, 2-tiered triage and trauma team activation protocol. *Ann Emerg Med* 1998;**32**:436–41.

A retrospective study which found that a cooperative two-tiered response system of emergency medicine and trauma surgery based on prehospital information was safe and effective. In addition, the authors estimated that the use of such a system saved 578 trauma team physician hours over the six-month study period by avoidance of unnecessary trauma team activations.

14. Scalea TM, Simon HM, Duncan AO *et al*. Geriatric blunt multiple trauma: improved survival with early invasive monitoring. *J Trauma* 1990;**30**(2):129–36.

A prospective study of selected geriatric blunt trauma patients who underwent early central invasive monitoring found they had increased survival compared with historical controls.

15. Rosemurgy AS, Norris PA, Olson SM *et al*. Prehospital traumatic cardiac arrest: the cost of futility. *J Trauma* 1993;**35**(3):468–74.

The authors retrospectively reviewed the 138 trauma arrest victims who were treated by advanced life support prehospital providers over an 18-month period. This study group (made up of 70% blunt and 30% penetrating trauma) included those patients who underwent CPR either at the scene or while in transport to the hospital. The authors report that there were no survivors despite an aggregate care cost of $871 000 dollars. In addition, only 11 of these patients were harvested for organ procurement (corneas only). The authors conclude that allocating significant resources (including the use of aeromedical services) for these patients is a costly and futile endeavor.

16. Durham LA, Richardson RJ, Wall MJ *et al*. Emergency center thoracotomy: impact of prehospital resuscitation. *J Trauma* 1992;**32**(6):775–9.

The authors reviewed their urban trauma center's five-year, 389 patient experience of emergency thoracotomies. They reported an overall survival rate of 8.3% (no victims of blunt trauma survived). The authors then examined prehospital data and noted that survivors had prehospital CPR for an average of 5.1 minutes as compared to 9.1 minutes of CPR in non-survivors. Of the survivors, it was found that endotracheal intubation by paramedics prolonged "successful toleration of CPR" to 9.1 minutes as compared to an average of 4.1 minutes of CPR tolerance in survivors who were not intubated. The study suggests that prehospital intubation may further extend the window of opportunity for the successful resuscitation of patients with penetrating trauma.

17. Lorenz HP, Steinmetz B, Lieberman J *et al*. Emergency thoracotomy: survival correlates with physiologic status. *J Trauma* 1992;**32**(6):780–8.

A retrospective review of a decade of patients who underwent emergency thoracotomy either in the ED (n = 424) or in the OR (n = 39). The authors found that no patients found to be in traumatic cardiac arrest by paramedics survived.

**Field triage**

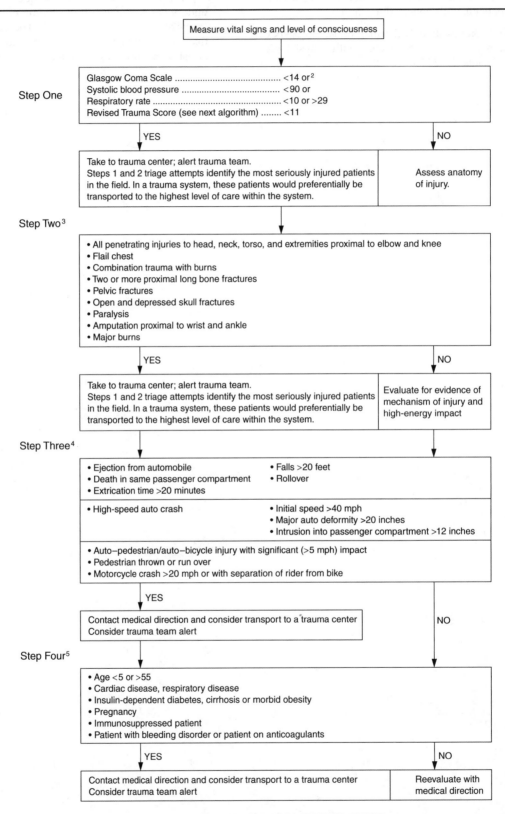

Measure vital signs and level of consciousness

**Step One**

Glasgow Coma Scale ......................................... <14 or [2]
Systolic blood pressure ..................................... <90 or
Respiratory rate ............................................... <10 or >29
Revised Trauma Score (see next algorithm) ........ <11

YES — NO

Take to trauma center; alert trauma team.
Steps 1 and 2 triage attempts identify the most seriously injured patients in the field. In a trauma system, these patients would preferentially be transported to the highest level of care within the system.

Assess anatomy of injury.

**Step Two[3]**

• All penetrating injuries to head, neck, torso, and extremities proximal to elbow and knee
• Flail chest
• Combination trauma with burns
• Two or more proximal long bone fractures
• Pelvic fractures
• Open and depressed skull fractures
• Paralysis
• Amputation proximal to wrist and ankle
• Major burns

YES — NO

Take to trauma center; alert trauma team.
Steps 1 and 2 triage attempts identify the most seriously injured patients in the field. In a trauma system, these patients would preferentially be transported to the highest level of care within the system.

Evaluate for evidence of mechanism of injury and high-energy impact

**Step Three[4]**

• Ejection from automobile
• Death in same passenger compartment
• Extrication time >20 minutes

• Falls >20 feet
• Rollover

• High-speed auto crash

• Initial speed >40 mph
• Major auto deformity >20 inches
• Intrusion into passenger compartment >12 inches

• Auto–pedestrian/auto–bicycle injury with significant (>5 mph) impact
• Pedestrian thrown or run over
• Motorcycle crash >20 mph or with separation of rider from bike

YES

Contact medical direction and consider transport to a trauma center
Consider trauma team alert

NO

**Step Four[5]**

• Age <5 or >55
• Cardiac disease, respiratory disease
• Insulin-dependent diabetes, cirrhosis or morbid obesity
• Pregnancy
• Immunosuppressed patient
• Patient with bleeding disorder or patient on anticoagulants

YES — NO

Contact medical direction and consider transport to a trauma center
Consider trauma team alert

Reevaluate with medical direction

**WHEN IN DOUBT, TAKE TO A TRAUMA CENTER**

**Traumatic arrest in the field**

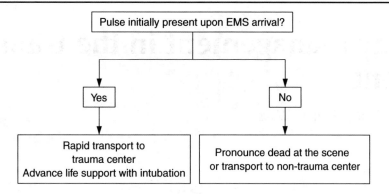

# 2 Airway management in the trauma patient

*Michael A Gibbs, Ron M Walls*

## Introduction

Airway management is the most critical intervention in acute trauma care. Early intubation has been shown to improve outcome in the severely injured patient. Conversely, failure to manage the airway adequately is the number one cause of preventable mortality in trauma.[1]

Airway management in the trauma patient poses several unique challenges. Success requires excellent assessment skills, an understanding of the physiology of injury, a thorough knowledge of airway pharmacology, and strong leadership.

## Airway management algorithm

### Rapid airway assessment

By definition, the trauma patient should be considered at least a *potentially difficult* airway. During the initial assessment, the treating physician should immediately assess the patient for:

- injury to the face, mouth or neck that may make intubation difficult or impossible
- the potential for cervical spine injury and the need for in-line cervical stabilization
- chest injury that may limit respiratory reserve
- the presence of traumatic brain injury (TBI) that may alter airway management decision making and drug selection[2]
- signs of obvious or occult hemodynamic instability that can be worsened or unmasked by the pharmacologic agents used for rapid sequence intubation (RSI).

This information will be forthcoming during the primary and secondary survey. Some of the essentials can be rapidly determined at the bedside in 10–20 seconds. As soon as the patient is moved to the stretcher in the trauma room, ask the following four questions:

- What is your name?
- Are you having trouble breathing?
- Can you move your toes?
- Where do you hurt?

Answers to these questions will immediately help you establish the patient's level of consciousness and Glasgow Coma Score, elicit signs of upper airway obstruction or labored breathing, assess the integrity of the spinal cord, and focus in on the predominant injury(ies).

Next, examine the mouth and posterior pharynx carefully for edema, intraoral bleeding or foreign body. The airway should be cleared of all blood and debris with a suction catheter and/or MacGill forceps. While it is important to determine the patient's ability to handle secretions, testing the gag reflex is not recommended, as this maneuver may precipitate vomiting and worsen intracranial hypertension. Instead, test the patient's ability to swallow. Intact swallowing is a reasonable reflection of retained airway protection. An assessment of the patient's cardiopulmonary status will give additional information crucial to the airway management plan.

Remember to document a brief neurologic examination (GCS, pupillary response and symmetry, and the presence or absence of lateralizing motor findings) *before* neuromuscular blocking agents are given. This information will assist with subsequent management of the patient with traumatic brain injury.

### Is intubation required?

The decision to intubate requires experience and judgment. "Standard" indications for endotracheal intubation in the trauma patient include:

- inadequate ventilation and oxygenation despite high-flow oxygen
- airway injury with impending obstruction
- profound hemodynamic instability
- traumatic brain injury (TBI) with a GCS ≤ 8.

These criteria are by no means absolute and the threshold for early intubation should be lowered in patients with severe multisystem injuries, in the elderly, and in situations where constant medical oversight cannot be provided.

Another part of the decision-making paradigm should be a prediction of the patient's anticipated course. For example, early intubation of the patient with significant blunt chest injury, the patient with blunt or penetrating anterior neck trauma, or the patient with early signs of smoke inhalation may avert disaster when the clinical situation progresses to respiratory failure or airway obstruction. Measures must also be taken to ensure definitive airway control when patients are expected to be out of a critical care area for prolonged periods of time (e.g. radiology suite), and certainly before interfacility transport.

## Supplemental oxygen, monitor and reassess

All patients suffering significant trauma should receive supplemental oxygen. High-flow oxygen via non-rebreather mask is essential for patients with altered mentation, respiratory distress, hemodynamic instability, and blunt or penetrating chest trauma and in trauma victims with preexisting pulmonary pathology or coexistent pregnancy.

Careful patient monitoring is fundamental during acute trauma resuscitations. All patients should be placed on a cardiac monitor, pulse oximeter, and automated blood pressure cuff. In addition, serial examinations during the first few hours postinjury are important to detect early signs of clinical deterioration that may ultimately require endotracheal intubation. This is especially important in patients with traumatic brain injury, hemodynamic instability, injuries that may progress to upper airway obstruction (e.g. inhalation injury, blunt or penetrating maxillofacial or neck trauma), and in those with significant chest trauma.

## Can patient be oxygenated?

In the spontaneously breathing patient, oxygenation and ventilation should be assessed clinically at the bedside. Clinical signs of inadequate oxygenation include altered mental status, respiratory distress, tachycardia, and dysrhythmias. A pulse oximetry reading of <90% despite high-flow oxygen should be considered a sign of inadequate oxygenation. In the apneic patient the adequacy of oxygenation and ventilation is determined by assessing the ease of breath delivery with a bag-valve-mask, chest wall rise, and pulse oximetry measurements.

When oxygenation remains inadequate, measures must be taken immediately to improve ventilation and, if possible, increase the concentration of delivered oxygen. Clear the posterior pharynx of blood, debris or foreign body and open the airway with a jaw thrust. If there are no concerns about cervical injury, place the patient in the "sniffing position". Insert an oral or nasal airway if tolerated, keeping in mind that this may precipitate coughing and vomiting. When these simple measures fail to improve the patient's clinical status and oxygen saturation, the airway should be secured, preferably using endotracheal intubation.

## Is laryngoscopy possible?

In the patient who cannot be oxygenated (SaO$_2$ <90%) with either high-flow oxygen and/or a bag-valve-mask, one rapid attempt at laryngoscopy is reasonable. The clinician should quickly determine the likelihood that this attempt will be successful. It must be recognized that if laryngoscopy fails, the patient may deteriorate rapidly. Multiple intubation attempts in the hypoxic patient are strongly discouraged. The use of neuromuscular blockade in this situation should be individualized. The authors believe that RSI will provide the most ideal intubating conditions and should be used, provided a plan and the equipment for airway rescue is immediately available. Should this attempt at laryngoscopy be unsuccessful, the airway must then be immediately secured using a surgical airway or alternative technique.

## Difficult airway anticipated?

The difficult airway must be identified during the rapid airway assessment. A difficult airway may be the result of intrinsic airway anatomy, extrinsic airway injury or both. The patient with distorted airway anatomy presents a significant challenge. The very condition that may mandate intubation will also render it much more difficult and prone to failure.

Direct airway injury may be the result of:

- maxillofacial trauma
- blunt or penetrating anterior neck trauma
- smoke inhalation
- caustic ingestion.

In cases of distorted anatomy, the approach to airway management must be one that minimizes the potential for catastrophic deterioration. A careful approach must be planned, taking into account the expertise of the physician(s) in the department and in the hospital, the equipment at hand, the need for transfer, the urgency of the need for surgery, the need for diagnostic studies, and many other factors. If there is a theme that unifies the approach to this type of airway problem, it is "plan ahead". The optimal approach for airway management will vary, depending on the clinical scenario. In patients with signs of significant airway compromise (e.g. stridor, drooling, respiratory distress, expanding neck hematoma) the risk of using neuromuscular blockade is high and it may be most appropriate to attempt awake intubation with sedation or proceed directly to a surgi-cal airway. When symptoms are modest but elective intubation is still indicated (e.g. before interfacility transport), a combined approach may be used, in which an awake technique is used to assure visibility of the glottis, then RSI is used for the actual intubation. This can be accomplished by gentle laryngoscopy or nasopharyngoscopy.

### Cricothyrotomy

When laryngoscopy is not possible (e.g. massive facial trauma) or when intubation fails, an immediate cricothyrotomy may be required. While this procedure is usually not technically difficult to perform, the tenuous clinical scenario in which it is most often required will challenge the fortitude of even the most experienced physician. A few seconds of preparation early on can mean the difference between success and failure.

First, *anticipate* the situation in which a surgical airway may be needed before laryngoscopy is attempted and certainly before the patient is paralyzed. Second, *assess* the anatomic landmarks of the neck and identify the cricothyroid membrane. Lastly, *assemble* the necessary equipment at the bedside.

### Consider TTJV, LMA or Combitube

Traditionally, the failed airway in the trauma patient has been managed using surgical cricothyrotomy. While this technique does provide a definitive airway, it is invasive and associated with significant complications. Several alternative techniques are available that may provide a temporary "bridge" to intubation by restoring oxygenation and ventilation, often obviating the need for cricothyrotomy. These include transtracheal jet ventilation (TTJV), the laryngeal mask airway (LMA), and the Combitube airway (CT). The decision to use one of these techniques rather than a surgical airway clearly must be individualized and based on the clinical situation at hand and the experience of the clinician.

### Postintubation care

After intubation is accomplished and ETT position is verified:

- perform a repeat neurologic examination
- complete any remaining components of the secondary survey
- be sure the patient is adequately sedated
- take measures to prevent inadvertent self-extubation (e.g. restraints)
- consider giving a dose of a long-acting neuromuscular blocking agent.

### RSI

Rapid sequence intubation is considered the standard for emergency airway management in the trauma patient.[2-5] See the RSI algorithm for a complete description of the procedure.

### Alternative technique

Several airway adjuncts are available for the management of the difficult or failed airway.[6,7] *Supraglottic* techniques (e.g. digital intubation, laryngeal mask airway, Combitube airway, fiberoptic intubation) use devices introduced through the mouth either blindly or under direct visualization. *Infraglottic* techniques (transtracheal jet ventilation, retrograde intubation, percutaneous or surgical cricothyrotomy) rely on invasive access to the airway below the vocal cords.

In general, supraglottic techniques are preferred in patients with normal airway anatomy and are discouraged in patients with abnormal upper airway anatomy or obstruction. Infraglottic techniques are usually required when obvious upper airway injury or obstruction exists. While infraglottic techniques usually provide a definitive airway, they require considerable surgical skill and are relatively contraindicated in patients with anterior neck injury. Obviously, technique selection will depend on both the clinical situation at hand and the experience of the operator.

### Cuffed endotracheal tube placed in trachea?

If an airway adjunct with a cuffed tube is inserted (e.g. I-LMA, surgical cricothyrotomy) this can be replaced electively once the patient is stabilized. Devices without a cuffed tube protecting the trachea from aspiration (e.g. TTJV, conventional LMA, Combitube) should be replaced with a conventional endotracheal tube or tracheostomy as soon as possible by the clinician best qualified to perform this procedure.

## Definitive airway

When an airway adjunct without a cuffed endotracheal tube (e.g. conventional LMA, Combitube, TTJV) is used as a temporary device this must be replaced with a cuffed ETT that provides adequate ventilation and protects the patient from aspiration. When, where, and by whom this is done will depend on the clinical situation, the device used, and local resources.

## Rapid sequence intubation algorithm

Rapid sequence intubation (RSI) is the standard for emergency airway management. This technique involves the rapid administration of short-acting sedatives and rapidly acting neuromuscular blocking agents to facilitate immediate endotracheal intubation in the unstable patient. The goals of RSI are to:

- provide immediate muscle relaxation
- minimize the risk of aspiration
- provide adequate sedation, analgesia, and amnesia
- protect the patient from the acute rise in intracranial pressure associated with laryngoscopy.

Several different mnemonics for the RSI sequence have been proposed. We recommend the 7 Ps:

Preparation
Preoxygenation
Pretreatment
Paralysis and sedation
Position and protection
Pass the tube
Post-RSI patient care

## Preparation

In tandem with the primary and secondary survey, preparation for airway management should be ongoing.

- Be sure the patient is adequately monitored (BP, HR, SAO$_2$).
- Secure at least two large-bore intravenous catheters.
- Assemble and test all necessary equipment.
- Draw up and label the drugs selected for RSI.
- Formulate a back-up plan, should RSI not succeed.
- Assign specific tasks to all team members.
- Begin preoxygenation.

## Preoxygenation

RSI is predicated on the fact that patients requiring emergent intubation have full stomachs and are therefore at risk for aspiration of gastric contents. Because positive pressure ventilation causes gastric distension

and increases this risk, every effort should be made to complete the RSI sequence *without interposed assisted ventilation*. For this to be possible, an oxygen reservoir must be established within the lungs and body tissues, allowing the apneic patient to remain well saturated for several minutes. The principal reservoir is the functional residual capacity (FRC) in the lungs. Administration of 100% oxygen for five minutes will replace the predominantly nitrogenous mixture of the FRC with oxygen and should provide 3–5 minutes of "apnea protection". A bag-valve-mask placed over the patient's mouth provides the highest concentration of oxygen available in most emergency departments. Pulse oximetry monitoring throughout the procedure allows the physician to monitor the oxygen saturation and eliminate guesswork.

If the clinical situation at hand does not allow for five minutes of preoxygenation, the patient should be instructed to take 3–5 vital capacity breaths in rapid succession. If the patient is hypoventilating or apneic, assisted ventilation will be the only means of preoxygenation. Gently delivered breaths should continue until the oxygen saturation rises above 95%.

## Pretreatment

Pretreatment is the administration of drugs to mitigate the adverse effects associated with endotracheal intubation. This is especially vital in the trauma patient with TBI and impaired cerebral autoregulation, where physical stimulation of airway structures during laryngoscopy may cause or worsen intracranial hypertension.[8] This is mediated by a direct neural response and an indirect sympathetically driven response consisting of hypertension and tachycardia. Several pharmacologic agents may blunt this response.

*Lidocaine* has been shown to suppress the direct response to laryngoscopy and blunt the cough reflex. In the recommended dose (1.0–1.5 mg/kg IV) it has essentially no side effects or contraindications.[9] For best results it should be administered 2–3 minutes prior to intubation.

*Fentanyl* can be used to suppress the indirect response to laryngoscopy by preventing hypertension and tachycardia. The recommended dose is 3–5 μg/kg IV. Because fentanyl is a vasodilator and myocardial depressant, it must be used with caution in patients who are volume depleted and in those with impaired left ventricular function.

*Defasciculation* is thought to abate the rise in ICP associated with succinylcholine-induced fasciculations.[10] The recommended dose is one-tenth of the standard intubating dose (e.g. vecuronium 0.01 mg/kg IV). It must be remembered that defasciculation may occasionally cause complete paralysis and apnea and the clinician must be ready to intervene immediately after this process is initiated.

## Paralysis and sedation

The rapid administration of a neuromuscular blocking agent and sedative should provide immediate muscle relaxation and the most ideal intubating conditions possible. In general, succinylcholine is the preferred muscle relaxant because of its rapid onset and short duration. While there are several contraindications to the use of succinylcholine, these are usually not a factor in the acutely injured patient.

A number of sedatives are available for use during RSI. These include the benzodiazepines (e.g. midazolam, lorazepam, diazepam), the ultra short-acting barbiturates (e.g. thiopental, methohexital), ketamine, and etomidate.[11,12] A detailed discussion of these agents is beyond the scope of this chapter. Recommended doses for the sedative agents are provided in Table 2.1.

It should be recalled that patients suffering significant multisystem trauma may have obvious or occult hypotension from many different sources.[13,14] Remember

that patients on the verge of cardiovascular collapse often maintain a "normal" blood pressure, especially if they are young. Several of the sedative agents used for RSI may cause significant myocardial depression and vasodilatation that will worsen shock in the hypovolemic patient. This is especially true for the barbiturates (e.g. thiopental) and the benzodiazepines (e.g. midazolam). Both drugs are contraindicated in the hemodynamically unstable patient and should be used with caution in "normotensive" patients at risk. Although fentanyl has an excellent hemodynamic profile, it can significantly worsen shock in patients who are dependent on sympathetic drive because of its sympatholytic effect. If RSI is planned, etomidate, which possesses a favorable hemodynamic profile, is the preferred induction agent. Ketamine is also an excellent choice, provided there is no evidence of intracranial hypertension. Patients with cardiac dysfunction are equally vulnerable. When intubation is required in the patient with cardiogenic shock, induction agents should be used with care.

## Position and protection

All severely injured blunt trauma patients have cervical injury until proven otherwise. If urgent airway management is needed, DO NOT waste time getting a cross-table lateral cervical spine X-ray prior to intubation. This single view is inadequate to exclude injury, with a sensitivity of 85% at best. Waiting for the X-ray will waste precious time, and give the operator a false sense of security when the film is interpreted as "normal". Instead, assume all patients have cervical injury and maintain in-line stabilization at all times.[15–19]

The application of cricoid pressure (Sellick's maneuver) is a fundamental component of the RSI algorithm. This maneuver should be initiated during the preoxygenation phase in the unresponsive patient and immediately following the administration of paralytics and sedatives in the awake patient. Cricoid pressure should never be removed until proper tube placement has been confirmed and the ETT cuff has been inflated.

## Pass the tube

The endotracheal tube should be passed gently and atraumatically. Overzealous advancement of the ETT may result in airway injury and/or right main stem intubation. Verify correct endotracheal tube position immediately following intubation.[20] This can be done with a disposable qualitative end-tidal $PCO_2$ detector, or by continuous quantitative measurement of end-tidal $PCO_2$.

**Table 2.1** Rapid sequence intubation pharmacology

| Drug | Dose/kg | Dose (70 kg adult) |
| --- | --- | --- |
| *Pretreatment drugs* | | |
| Lidocaine | 1.5 mg | 100 mg |
| Fentanyl | 3.0 µg | 200 µg |
| Atropine | 0.02 mg | N/A |
| Defasciculation (vecuronium/pancuronium) | 0.01 mg | 1 mg |
| *Induction agents* | | |
| Etomidate | 0.3 mg | 20 mg |
| Midazolam | 0.2 mg | 14 mg |
| Ketamine | 1–2 mg | 100 mg |
| Thiopental | 3.0 mg | 250 mg |
| *Neuromuscular blocking agents* | | |
| Succinylcholine | 1.5–2.0 mg | 100 mg |
| Rocuronium | 1.0 mg | 70 mg |
| Vecuronium/pancuronium | 0.15 mg | 10 mg |
| Rapacuronium | 1.5 mg | 100 mg |
| *Maintenance drugs* | | |
| Lorazepam | 0.05 mg | 3.0 mg |
| Vecuronium/pancuronium | 0.1 mg | 7.0 mg |

Adapted with permission from Advanced Airway Management Card, The Airway Course, Airway Management Education Center, 2000

## Post-intubation care

After intubation is accomplished and ETT position is verified:

- perform a repeat neurologic examination
- complete any remaining components of the secondary survey
- be sure the patient is adequately sedated (e.g. midazolam + morphine)
- consider a dose of a long-acting neuromuscular blocking agent.

## Three unsuccessful attempts — can patient be oxygenated?

If laryngoscopy is unsuccessful after three attempts by an experienced clinician, the likelihood that subsequent attempts will succeed is remote. The physician should immediately call for assistance (e.g. a colleague, anesthesiologist or nurse anesthetist).

At this juncture oxygenation and ventilation must be immediately assessed. In the paralyzed patient the adequacy of oxygenation and ventilation is determined by assessing the ease of breath delivery with a bag-valve-mask (BVM), chest wall rise, and pulse oximetry measurements. When oxygenation remains inadequate, measures must be taken immediately to improve ventilation and, if possible, increase the concentration of delivered oxygen. Clear the posterior pharynx of blood, debris or foreign body and open the airway with a jaw thrust. If there are no concerns about cervical injury, place the patient in the "sniffing position". Insert an oral or nasal airway at once.

## Consider TTJV, LMA or Combitube

Traditionally, the failed airway in the trauma patient has been managed using surgical cricothyrotomy. While this technique does provide a definitive airway, it is invasive and associated with significant complications. Several alternative techniques are available that may provide a temporary "bridge" to intubation by restoring oxygenation and ventilation, often obviating the need for cricothyrotomy. These include transtracheal jet ventilation (TTJV), the laryngeal mask airway (LMA), and the Combitube airway (CT). The decision to use one of these techniques rather than a surgical airway clearly must be individualized and based on the clinical situation at hand and the experience of the clinician.

## Cricothyrotomy

When intubation fails, an immediate cricothyrotomy may be required. While this procedure is usually not technically difficult to perform, the tenuous clinical scenario in which it is most often required will challenge the fortitude of even the most experienced physician. A few seconds of preparation early on can mean the difference between success and failure.

First, *anticipate* the situation in which a surgical airway may be needed before laryngoscopy is attempted and certainly before the patient is paralyzed. Second, *assess* the anatomic landmarks of the neck and identify the cricothyroid membrane. Lastly, *assemble* the necessary equipment at the bedside.

## Continue BVM, use alternative technique

Ventilation with a BVM should be continued. It is reasonable to attempt placement of an alternative airway provided oxygenation is maintained.

## Cuffed endotracheal tube placed in trachea?

If an airway adjunct with a cuffed tube is inserted (e.g. I-LMA, surgical cricothyrotomy) this can be replaced electively once the patient is stabilized. Devices without a cuffed tube protecting the trachea from aspiration (e.g. TTJV, conventional LMA, Combitube) should be replaced with a conventional endotracheal tube or tracheostomy as soon as possible by the clinician best qualified to perform this procedure.

## Definitive airway

When an airway adjunct without a cuffed endotracheal tube (e.g. conventional LMA, Combitube, TTJV) is used as a temporary device this must be replaced with a cuffed ETT that provides adequate ventilation and protects the patient from aspiration. When, where, and by whom this is done will depend on the clinical situation, the device used, and local resources.

## Clinical pearls

- A rapid bedside assessment should help you anticipate the difficult airway.
- Essentials of the physical examination should elicit clinical evidence of spinal injury, traumatic brain injury, occult hypovolemia, direct airway trauma, and pulmonary dysfunction.
- All blunt trauma patients have injury to the cervical spine until proven otherwise. In-line stabilization should be performed and documented.
- The priority in the initial management of the patient with traumatic brain injury is to maintain adequate CNS perfusion and oxygenation at all costs.

- In the patient with direct injury to the airway, the clinician must always have an immediate plan (and the equipment) for airway rescue should RSI fail.
- Remember that many of the drugs used for RSI (the opiates and barbiturates, in particular) may precipitate hypotension in the hypovolemic patient.

## Conclusion

Oral endotracheal intubation using RSI is the airway maneuver of choice in the majority of trauma patients. A well thought-out management plan, taking into account the patient's known or suspected injuries and hemodynamic status, will help the clinician rapidly orchestrate an individualized airway management plan. During the often chaotic environment of a trauma resuscitation, effective reasoning, communication, and leadership are the ingredients for success.

## Class I references

8. Ebert JP, Pearson JD, Gelman S *et al*. Circulatory response to laryngoscopy: the comparative effects of placebo, fentanyl, and esmolol. *Can J Anaesth* 1989;**36**:301–6.

    The circulatory response of 30-second laryngoscopy and orotracheal intubation was assessed in 60 patients undergoing a variety of non-cardiac surgical procedures. Patients were randomized to receive either placebo, esmolol (500 μg/kg/min for six minutes, followed by 300 μg/kg/min for nine minutes) or fentanyl (0.8 μg/kg/min for 10 minutes). Observers were blinded to the infusion. Fentanyl decreased and maintained heart rate, systolic and diastolic blood pressures, and mean arterial blood pressures below baseline despite laryngoscopy. Esmolol blunted the HR response but BP (SBP, DBP, MAP) were all slightly elevated in this group.

9. Hamill JF, Bedford RF, Weaver DC, Colohan AR. Lidocaine before endotracheal intubation: intravenous or laryngotracheal? *Anesthesiology* 1981;**55**:578–91.

    Lidocaine given topically to the larynx and trachea or intravenously has been shown to blunt the increases in heart rate and blood pressure associated with laryngoscopy and intubation. The purpose of this study was to determine the preferred route of lidocaine administration in patients at risk for intracranial hypertension. Twenty-two patients with brain tumors were studied. ICP, arterial and central venous pressure were continuously monitored. Following induction with thiopental and succinylcholine, 11 patients received laryngotracheal lidocaine (4 cc of 4%) under direct vision and 11 patients received intravenous lidocaine (1.5 mg/kg). In the group given intravenous lidocaine, ICP decreased after administration and did not increase after intubation. In contrast, the group given laryngotracheal lidocaine developed a significant increase in ICP after intubation, with three of these patients sustaining ICPs in excess of 40 torr.

10. Koenig KL. Rapid-sequence intubation of head trauma patients: prevention of fasciculations with pancuronium versus minidose succinylcholine. *Ann Emerg Med* 1992;**21**:929–32.

    Forty-six head trauma patients requiring RSI received lidocaine (1 mg/kg) and were randomized to receive either minidose succinylcholine (0.1 mg/kg) or pancuronium (0.03 mg/kg) one minute prior to the full paralytic dose of succinylcholine (1.5 mg/kg). Fasciculations were noted using a graded visual scale. Eight of 19 (42%) in the pancuronium group and six of 27 (22%) in the minidose succinylcholine group experienced fasciculations (P = NS).

11. Sivilotti ML, Ducharme J. Randomized double-blind study on sedatives and hemodynamics during rapid-sequence intubation in the emergency department: the SHRED Study. *Ann Emerg Med* 1998;**31**:313–24.

    The hemodynamic effects of three different agents used for RSI were compared. This double-blind study randomized 86 ED patients with standard indications for intubation to induction with thiopental (5 mg/kg), fentanyl (5 μg/kg) or midazolam (0.1 mg/kg). All patients were paralyzed with succinylcholine, or vecuronium if succinylcholine was judged to be contraindicated. Ease and speed of intubation, changes in pulse and blood pressure, and frequency of complications were compared. Of the patients who received thiopental, 93% were intubated within two minutes of paralysis (P = 0.037), but systolic blood pressure fell an average of 38 mmHg in this group (P = 0.045). The midazolam group had a greater number of delayed intubations (31%) and an average heart rate increase of 17 bpm (P = 0.008). Fentanyl provided the most neutral hemodynamic profile during RSI. Mortality was not affected by drug assignment.

13. Chesnut RM, Marshall LF, Klauber MR *et al*. The role of secondary brain injury in determining outcome from severe head injury. *J Trauma* 1993;**34**:216–22.

    The outcome of 717 patients with severe brain injury (GCS <8) was prospectively studied. The impact on outcome of hypotension (SBP <90 mmHg) and hypoxemia ($PaO_2$ <60 mmHg or apnea or cyanosis in the field) as secondary brain insults was studied. Both variables were independently associated with significant increases in morbidity and mortality. Hypotension was profoundly detrimental, occurring in 35% of patients and associated with a 150% increase in mortality.

20. Knapp S, Kofler J, Stoiser B. The assessment of four different methods to verify tracheal tube placement in the critical care setting. *Anesth Analg* 1999;**88**:766–70.

Prospective trial comparing the efficacy of end-tidal $PCO_2$ detector ($ETCO_2$), esophageal detector device (EDD), transillumination using a Trachlight™ lighted stylet (TL), and auscultation. Investigators placed a second endotracheal tube in the esophagus of each of 38 consecutive tracheally intubated patients, and then asked inexperienced senior medical students and experienced critical care physicians to assess tube placement. The tube and the method to be tested were selected at random. Of the tubes tested, 74 were in the trachea and 78 were in the esophagus. The accuracy of the four methods as used by the inexperienced and experienced clinicians, respectively, was 100% and 100% for $ETCO_2$, 98% and 97% for EDD, 66% and 100% for auscultation, and 87% and 84% for TL. All cases of esophageal intubation were detected by both $ETCO_2$ and EDD and by both experienced and inexperienced clinicians.

## Class II references

1. Esposito TJ, Sanddal ND, Hansen JD, Reynolds S. Analysis of preventable trauma deaths and inappropriate trauma care in a rural state. *J Trauma* 1995;**39**:955–62.

Trauma deaths in the state of Montana were reviewed to determine the rate and cause of preventable mortality and inappropriate care. Trauma deaths occurring between October 1990 and September 1991 were identified using ICD-9 E-CODES. A panel of physicians and prehospital care providers judged cases as either preventable, possibly preventable or non-preventable. Six hundred and twenty-nine deaths related to trauma were identified. The overall preventable death rate was 13%. The most common cause of inappropriate care was inadequate management of the airway in either the prehospital setting (6.8% of cases) or emergency department (5.4% of cases).

3. Li J, Murphy-Lavoie H, Bugas C, Martinez J, Preston C. Complications of emergency intubation with and without paralysis. *Am J Emerg Med* 1999;**17**:141–4.

Retrospective study comparing the complication rate in patients intubated with neuromuscular blockade (RSI) and without neuromuscular blockade. All patients received a sedative during intubation. There were 166 patients in the RSI group and 67 patients in the sedation-alone group. Complications (multiple intubation attempts (>4), inability to intubate, esophageal intubation, airway trauma, aspiration, and death) were compared between groups. RSI was associated with a marked decrease in all measured complications. Multiple attempts

at intubation were required in 2% of patients in this group and recognized esophageal intubation occurred in 3%. No cases of airway trauma, aspiration or death occurred in the RSI group. In the patients intubated without neuromuscular blockade, multiple intubation attempts were required in 24% of cases, esophageal intubation occurred in 18% of cases, and intubation was not accomplished in 18% of cases. Airway trauma, aspiration and death occurred in 28%, 15%, and 2% of patients respectively.

14. Stocchetti N, Furlan A, Volta F. Hypoxemia and arterial hypotension at the accident scene in head injury. *J Trauma* 1996;**40**:764–9.

This study was conducted to quantify the incidence of hypotension and hypoxemia in a series of head-injured patients rescued by helicopter. Arterial saturation and blood pressure were measured immediately prior to intubation at the accident scene in 49 patients with severe traumatic brain injury (mean GCS 6, SD 2). Mean arterial saturation was 81% (SD 24.24) and mean systolic blood pressure was 112 (SD 37.25). Airway obstruction was detected in 22 cases. Twenty-seven patients showed a saturation of less than 90% on scene and 12 had an arterial blood pressure of less than 100 mmHg.

19. Shatney CH, Brunner RD, Nguyen TQ. The safety of orotracheal intubation in patients with unstable cervical spine fracture or high spinal cord injury. *Am J Surg* 1995;**170**:676–9.

Prospective study of airway management practice and associated neurologic outcome in 150 patients subsequently diagnosed with cervical spine injury. A standardized neurologic examination was performed before intubation and in-line stabilization was maintained in all patients during the procedure. Endotracheal intubation was required in 26 (32%) of 81 patients without a neurologic deficit on presentation. No patient manifested a subsequent neurologic deficit. Sixty-nine additional patients had high cervical injury and intubation was required in 29 (42%) of these. No patient experienced further neurologic deficit following intubation.

## Class III references

2. Silber S. Rapid sequence intubation in adults with elevated intracranial pressure: a survey of emergency medicine residency programs. *Am J Emerg Med* 1997;**15**:263–7.

A survey assessing RSI protocols in patients with elevated ICP was distributed to directors of 100 emergency medicine residency programs in February 1995. Sixty-seven programs responded. Five programs performed 0–10 RSIs annually; six performed 10–30; 19 performed 30–50; 17 performed 50–100; 18 performed more than 10. Succinylcholine was the most frequently used neuromuscular blocker and was used exclusively by 23% of programs. Vecuronium was ranked second. Midazolam was the most frequently used sedative (87%), followed by thiopental (69%), etomidate (34%), diazepam (25%), and methohexital (6.2%). Lorazepam, fentanyl, and haloperidol were each used 1.5% of the time. Defasciculation was performed prior to succinylcholine administration by 81% of respondents. Intravenous lidocaine was administered as a pretreatment medication 88% of the time. Other pretreatment drugs used in the RSI protocol included fentanyl (49%), midazolam (34%), morphine (22%), and diazepam (12%).

4.  Vijayakumar E, Bosschner H, Renzi FP, Baker S, Heard SO. The use of neuromuscular blocking agents in the emergency department to facilitate tracheal intubation in the trauma patient: help or hindrance? *J Crit Care* 1998;**13**(1):1–6.

    Retrospective trauma registry analysis of 160 patients requiring emergent endotracheal intubation or establishment of a surgical airway over a 3.5-year period. Risk factors for difficult intubations were identified and analyzed using multivariate logistic regression analysis. Neuromuscular blockade was used in 75% of patients requiring intubation. Fifteen per cent of the intubations were considered difficult. No association was found between the presence of airway injuries and difficult intubations; however, the use of succinylcholine was associated with a lower risk of difficult intubations compared with intubations where a paralytic was not used.

5.  Sing RF, Rotondo MF, Zonies DH *et al.* Rapid sequence induction for intubation by an aeromedical transport team: a critical analysis. *Am J Emerg Med* 1998;**16**:598-602.

    Records of a consecutive series of injured patients undergoing RSI by a university-based aeromedical transport team were reviewed for demographics, intubation mishaps, and pulmonary complications. Eighty-four patients with a mean age of 30 years were studied. The mean RTS was $11.3 \pm 2.4$ and the mean ISS was $19.6 \pm 11.5$. RSI was successful in 96% of patients, 87% on the first attempt. Intubation "mishaps" occurred in 15 patients (18%), the most common being multiple intubation attempts. Pulmonary complications occurred in 22 patients (29%), the most common being pulmonary aspiration and pneumonia. Pulmonary complications were *not* related to intubation mishaps.

6.  Levitan RM, Kush S, Hollander JE. Devices for difficult airway management in academic emergency departments: results of a national survey. *Ann Emerg Med* 1999;**33**:694-8.

    A national survey of emergency medicine residency programs was conducted to determine which alternative devices were available in the emergency department for airway management. Respondents were asked if they had alternative *intubation* devices (fiberoptic bronchoscope, rigid Bullard laryngoscope, lighted stylet, retrograde intubation kit) and alternative *ventilation* devices (transtracheal jet ventilation (TTJV) system, Combitube, laryngeal mask airway). Information was obtained from 95 of 118 programs (81%). Concerning intubation devices: 64% had a fiberoptic bronchoscope, 45% a retrograde intubation kit, 35% a lighted stylet, and 0.06% a rigid Bullard laryngoscope. Forty-nine percent of programs had two or more devices and 21% had none. Concerning ventilation devices: 67% had a TTJV system, 26% had a Combitube, 26% had a laryngeal mask airway. Thirty-one percent of programs had two or more devices and 21% had none.

7.  Mercer MH, Gabbott DA. Insertion of the Combitube airway with the cervical spine immobilized in a rigid cervical collar. *Anaesthesia* 1998;**53**:971–4.

    The Combitube (CT) airway has been marketed as a device for airway rescue when RSI fails. Placement of the CT was attempted in 15 ASA class 1 or 2 patients (mean age, 32 years). Patients were paralyzed under general anesthesia for elective surgery after each had a semi-rigid collar (Philadelphia or Nec-Loc) applied. When blind CT placement failed, standard laryngoscopy was performed. Blind insertion of the CT was possible in only five patients; in the remaining 10 the investigators were unable to advance the device through the mouth into the hypopharynx. Once placed, the CT functioned effectively. These results cast doubt on the use of the Combitube in the immobilized trauma patient.

12. Moss E, Powell D, Gibson RM, McDowell DG. Effect of etomidate on intracranial pressure and cerebral perfusion pressure. *Br J Anaesth* 1979;**51**:347–51.

    Ten patients with intracranial mass lesions anesthetized with thiopentone and nitrous oxide received etomidate 0.2 mg/kg IV. Intracranial pressure (ICP) and cerebral perfusion pressure (CPP) were recorded. ICP decreased significantly in all patients (P < 0.001). The changes in cerebral perfusion pressure and heart rate were not clinically or statistically significant.

15. Criswell JC, Parr MJ, Nolan JP. Emergency airway management in patients with cervical spine injuries. *Anaesthesia* 1994;**49**:900–3.

    Retrospective study of 393 patients with traumatic cervical spine injuries. On admission 278 patients (71%) had no neurologic deficit and 115 (29%) had some neurologic deficit. All 36 patients intubated urgently and 37 of the 68 patients intubated between 30 minutes and 24 hours were intubated orally using RSI with cervical in-line stabilization. There were no neurologic sequelae in these 73 patients.

16. Suderman VS, Crosby ET, Lui A. Elective oral tracheal intubation in cervical spine-injured adults. *Can J Anaesth* 1991;**38**(6):785–9.

Retrospective review of 150 patients with known cervical spine injuries electively intubated. Preoperative neurologic deficit was present in 33% of patients. Intubation occurred after induction of general anesthesia in 83 patients (55%) and in 67 patients (45%) the tracheas were intubated with the patient awake. Cervical immobilization with in-line stabilization was documented in 86 patients (57%). After surgery two patients (1.3%) had new neurologic deficits. There were no differences in neurologic outcome whether intubation was performed while the patient was awake or under general anesthesia. Oral tracheal intubation with in-line stabilization, performed either after induction of general anesthesia or with the patient awake, remains an excellent option for elective airway management in patients with cervical spine injuries.

17. McCrory C, Blunnie WP, Moriarty DC. Elective tracheal intubation in cervical spine injuries. *Irish Med J* 1997;**90**(6):234–5.

Patients presenting for surgical stabilization of an unstable cervical spine are at risk of sustaining a further iatrogenic spinal cord injury during intubation of the trachea. Controversy exists regarding the optimal anesthetic technique for securing the airway. Techniques employed for intubating the trachea over a five-year period are reviewed. Tracheal intubation was achieved using two different techniques: awake fiberoptic intubation with local anesthesia and general anesthesia via the intravenous or inhalational route with neuromuscular blockade. Forty-five patients were included; 16 patients demonstrated a preoperative neurological deficit. Awake fiberoptic intubation was used in 27 cases, general anesthesia was employed via the intravenous route in 17 cases and the inhalational route in one case. Weighted traction was employed in all cases to immobilize the cervical spine during intubation. There were no new neurological sequelae with any of these techniques. The study suggests that there is no optimal anesthetic technique for intubating the trachea in patients with cervical spine injuries and it is noteworthy that in-line traction was used in every case.

18. Holley J, Jorden R. Airway management in patients with unstable cervical spine fractures. *Ann Emerg Med* 1988;**18**:1237–9.

Retrospective review of airway management techniques in 113 patients with cervical spine fractures requiring operative repair. Eighty (70%) had no neurologic deficit and 33 (30%) had a partial neurologic deficit. Nasal intubation with stabilization of the head was performed in 86 (76%) patients, while oral intubation with in-line cervical stabilization was performed in 27 (24%). No neurologic complication occurred in any patient.

**Airway management**

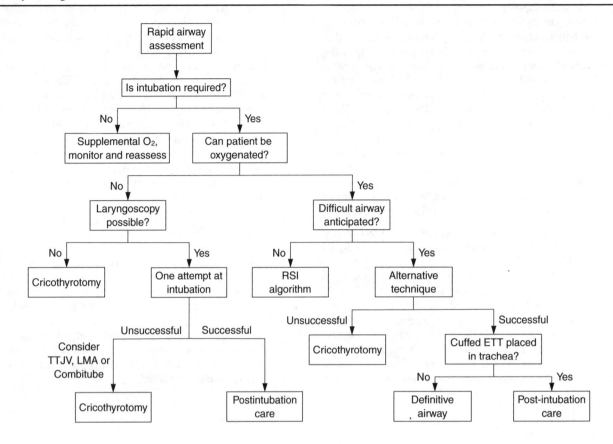

**Rapid sequence intubation**

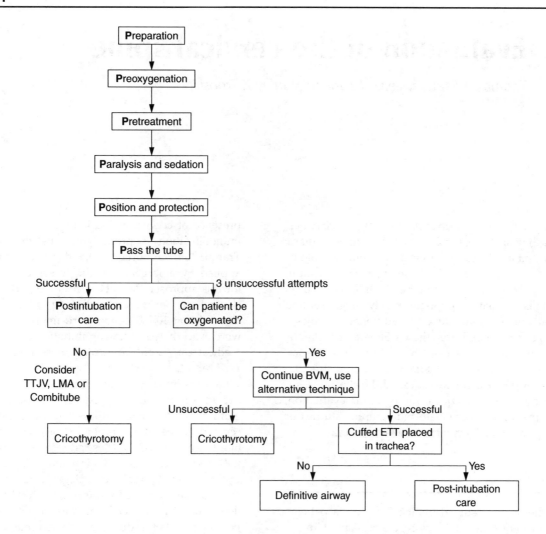

# 3 Evaluation of the cervical spine

*Thomas A Santora, Lewis J Kaplan, Stanley Z Trooskin*

Spinal cord injury occurs in approximately 10 000 Americans each year. It is estimated that four times as many cervical spine injuries (CSI) occur without neurologic sequelae.[1] The incidence of CSI in most series of blunt injuries is between 0.9% and 5%.[2-7] It is clear from these statistics that appropriate, timely diagnosis and management are imperative if additional neurologic injury is to be avoided from these CSI. Potential pitfalls in the management of patients with CSI can result from: lack of appreciation for the potential of CSI, distracting factors/injuries which may confound the clinical manifestations of CSI, inadequate radiographic evaluation, misinterpretation of adequate radiographic studies or inappropriate management of known injuries.

## Blunt trauma

A CSI should be assumed in all blunt trauma patients until proven otherwise; therefore, cervical spine immobilization should be maintained until a CSI is reliably excluded.

- Nearly every blunt mechanism of injury has been associated with cervical spine injury. The most common mechanisms cited in clinical series were motor vehicle crashes, motorcycle crashes, pedestrians struck by motor vehicles, assaults, sporting accidents, and falls.[2,4,8] Anecdotally, Jacobs and coworkers[8] found that individuals who fell from a level surface had a greater incidence of cervical spine injury than those who fell from a height. This counterintuitive finding may be explained by the patient population studied.
- In the presence of a hemodynamically unstable patient, the cervical immobilization should be maintained and diagnostic efforts to "clear the cervical spine" should be foregone until the life-threatening injuries are addressed.[9-11]
- The mere presence of a rigid cervical immobilization device and long backboard does not indicate the presence of cervical spine injury. This type of field immobilization is promulgated by the Advanced Trauma Life Support course and is nearly universally applied by emergency medicine services. Rationale for this approach dates back to the report by Rogers (*Journal of Bone and Joint Surgery*, 1957) which showed that 10% of spinal cord injuries occurred or were exacerbated following initiation of professional medical care; Reid confirmed these findings in his 1987 report.[12]
- What constitutes a "reliable" method of evaluation to exclude CSI has been extensively addressed in the literature.[1,6,13-17] Some authors[18] recommend routine cervical spine radiographic (CSR) assessment in blunt trauma patients. These advocates cite the potential of significant neurological morbidity of missed CSI as well as the medicolegal consequences as appropriate rationale for this approach. The low incidence of CSI, reduced radiation exposure to the patient and staff, reduced evaluation time which can be utilized to perform other emergent procedures, and decreased costs have been reported as the imputes for a more selective CSR assessment.

## Critical diagnostic elements

In the hemodynamically stable patient, the diagnostic evaluation to "clear the cervical spine" begins with assessment of critical diagnostic elements (CDE).[19] The presence of even *one* of the following CDEs has been correlated with CSI.[3,5]

(1) The initial assessment of the injured patient, though systematic and thorough, should be directed by subjective complaints. One of the many clinical challenges imposed by the acutely injured patient is the assessment of the reliability of the subjective information obtained. An altered mental status, as a result of a closed head injury (loss of consciousness),

presence of intoxicants, dementia or mental illness/ retardation can compromise the communication between patient and examining physician.[15] This compromised communication may prevent the patient expressing pain or the examiner from detecting a subtle neurologic deficit or tenderness over the cervical spine, either of which might indicate spinal column injury. Insight into the presence of these important diagnostic elements is gained by obtaining a thorough history. This same limitation to patient–physician communication can occur in patients without altered mental status who are intubated for mechanical ventilation or present with a language barrier.

(2) Neck pain is a common complaint following blunt CSI. Reports show the sensitivity is greater than 90% but specificity is poor, usually in the 40% range.[14] In a prospective study of 1000 patients, Hoffman[5] showed that neck pain was not statistically correlated to the presence of CSI and that when the complaint of neck pain was the only CDE, CSI was not found in this population. He suggested that if neck pain in isolation was eliminated as a CDE, no CSI would have been missed and 37% of the radiographic evaluations of the neck could have been foregone. This suggestion would require a much larger study population to validate.[13] This extreme position, even if validated, may never be adopted by some physicians for fear of the medicolegal ramifications of an undiagnosed CSI.[18,20]

(3) Once the historical evaluation has assessed the absence of any of the above subjective CDEs (neck pain, altered mental status, communication barrier), the secondary survey of the physical examination should assess the objective CDEs.

- A complete neurologic examination should be performed. Any motor or sensory neurologic deficit with or without associated head injury should raise concerns of spinal cord injury (SCI).
- When a SCI is suspected, radiographic evaluation of the neck is indicated. These patients should be considered to have an unstable spinal column until radiographically proven otherwise. Neurologic deficits, which are more profound in the upper extremities, should raise concern for central cord syndrome that frequently arises from hyperextension of the cervical spine. The presence of a neurologic deficit indicative of a SCI outside the cervical region should prompt radiographic evaluation for a concomitant CSI. Clinical reports[12] suggest that multilevel spinal column injuries occur in approximately 10% of patients and may involve different vertebrae within the same region or different spinal

column regions. Suspected SCI is best delineated by MRI.

- The presence of a distracting (painful) injury may mask the patient's ability to appreciate subtle pain symptoms in the neck or to cooperate during examination of the neck. A cooperative patient, capable of concentrating on the directions of the examining physician, is necessary to detect subtle sensory neurologic deficits. What constitutes a distracting injury is somewhat subjective. In a methodological descriptive paper, the authors of the multiinstitutional NEXUS study suggest criteria that make distracting injuries more objective.[21]
- The neck is evaluated for tenderness to palpation by removal of the cervical immobilization device while an assistant maintains in-line skeletal immobilization/stabilization. Palpation of all structures of the neck should be undertaken. Midline posterior neck tenderness occurs due to manipulation of fractured posterior elements. Since the anterior elements of the spinal column are more deeply placed within the soft tissues of the neck, direct manipulation of fractured anterior elements is more difficult, hence less likely to produce tenderness. Tenderness in the lateral or muscular structures of the neck is more commonly seen with strain or whiplash.[15,22]

(4) Numerous reports have suggested the safety of the clinical examination alone (no radiographs) in the "asymptomatic" neurologically intact evaluable patient.[3–6,20] There have been anecdotal case reports that describe CSI in "asymptomatic" patients.[23] In all of these reports, the "asymptomatic" patient was either intoxicated, head injured, or neurologically impaired or there was no mention of associated injuries. The National Emergency X-Radiography Utilization Study (NEXUS) is a multiinstitutional study that seeks to prove that absence of any of the CDEs defines a "no-risk" patient population. To make this bold statement, at least one of the CDEs must exist in a patient with CSI (100% sensitivity) and a CSI could never occur in a patient who lacked any of the CDEs (100% negative predictive value). The power analysis done in the planning of this study showed that, to approach this level of confidence, approximately 850 CSI patients would be needed. Using the lowest prevalence rate for CSI (2%), approximately 43 000 patients will be enrolled to encounter the needed CSIs. This prospective study is being undertaken at 21 medical centers throughout the US. Until a study like NEXUS validates that absence of any of the CDEs defines a no-risk population of injured patients,

many clinicians will continue to rely on cervical radiographs to confirm their clinical examinations and avoid potential allegations of clinical negligence.

## Dynamic neck exam

If there is absence of all CDEs, a clinical evaluation alone without the need for radiographic study appears justifiable.[5] Once the neurologic examination is proven normal and palpation of the neck reveals no tenderness, a dynamic (range of motion) evaluation of the neck should be undertaken to assess the mobility of the cervical spine. Pathologic mobility can occur as a result of fracture of the vertebral elements or ligamentous disruption. This evaluation not only looks for cervical tenderness with motion but also the development of sensory or motor neurologic deficits. If this dynamic evaluation produces no tenderness or neurologic deficits, the stabilization device (collar) can be removed and the cervical spine considered clinically cleared of potential injury. If motion produces tenderness or neurologic deficits, even if transient, the cervical stabilization should be maintained and a radiographic evaluation pursued.

## Radiographic screen

If any of the CDEs are present, a radiographic evaluation is warranted.

Radiographic screening tools include the cross-table lateral view (CTLV), an anteroposterior (AP) view, and an open mouth view to evaluate the odontoid process.

- The three-view cervical spine series begins with a cross-table lateral view with the X-ray beam and X-ray plate on opposite sides of the patient. An assistant should apply steady and continuous caudal traction on the patient's shoulders by grasping the patient's hands or wrists. The technique may be modified for patients with upper extremity injuries by looping a sheet over the top of each shoulder and pulling on the sheet. Of course, the person performing this maneuver should be dressed in a protective lead apron and vest with an additional thyroid shield. All seven cervical vertebrae need to be visualized as well as the junction of C7–T1 (see below). The bony integrity is evaluated as well as the alignment of the anterior and posterior borders of the vertebral bodies with the bodies above and below. The spinous processes are similarly evaluated. The position of the

dens may be evaluated, as well as any associated bony abnormalities of the skull base visualized on the film. The soft tissues of the neck are inspected for foreign bodies, pathologic gas shadows, and increases in the prevertebral soft tissue spaces (see below) on the CTLV as well.

- The AP view also evaluates the integrity and alignment of the cervical vertebrae. This view is the least problematic in terms of adequacy of visualized bony structures and needs no special maneuvers to obtain other than the alignment of the X-ray beam at a right angle to the patient's long axis. Review of this film undergoes a process similar to the one outlined previously. This view has been used primarily to assess the potential of a unilateral facet dislocation ("jumped facet"); the Penn State group has questioned the need for this view, stating the low incidence of this injury and the likelihood of visualizing its existence on either the CTLV or the odontoid view.[24]

- The open mouth (odontoid) view is technically challenging. An adequate odontoid view requires that the entirety of the odontoid, including the tip, is visualized as well as the alignment to the lateral masses of C1 with the articulating surfaces of the base of the skull and the lateral masses of C2. To prevent overlying shadows from the teeth requires a cooperative patient who can open widely his/her mouth (without extension of the neck) or the use of retracting devices in the uncooperative or unresponsive patient. Padded tongue blades placed with the wide-side dimension between the maxillary and mandibular molars can be used for this purpose. The standard AP odontoid view aligns the X-ray beam with a line drawn between the caudal surface of the upper incisors and the tip of the mastoid process perpendicular to the plate. When the tip of the odontoid is obscured with this technique, the X-ray beam can be aligned with the tip of the C1 transverse process on a line that is equidistant between the upper and lower incisors ("foramen magna view"). This method may not be appropriate for trauma patients who are rigidly immobilized in a collar as it may require extension at the atlantooccipital joint.[25]

Potential pitfalls in the radiographic evaluation of the cervical spine involve inadequacy of the radiographs, due either to poor penetration, presence of overlying shadows that obscure the cervical spine structures or insufficient visualization of the necessary vertebral levels. The two most problematic areas for adequate visualization on the initial radiographic screen are the cervicothoracic junction (C7-T1)[9] and the C1-C2 interface.[26]

- Enhanced evaluability of the C1–C2 relationship is obtained by modifying the method of obtaining the open mouth view as outlined above. When this technique fails to improve visualization, computed tomography (CT) or conventional tomography is frequently utilized. Since CT images are usually obtained in an axial plane, one is cautioned about the potential difficulty of detecting a type II odontoid fracture because the axial orientation of the fracture line may reside completely between the axial images obtained through the base of the dens.

- Imaging of the C7–T1 interface may be enhanced by the use of a lead-lined acrylic filter attached to the portable X-ray device beam collimator.[27] The use of supine oblique views of the incompletely visualized cervical spine to image C7–T1 is equally efficacious in evaluating alignment when compared to the standard swimmer's view and results in less radiation delivery.[28] Cervicothoracic junction injury has been estimated to occur in 9% of patients.[29] In this study, 24% of patients had neither pain nor neurologic deficit upon presentation with a radiographically apparent injury; 59% of these patients with a cervicothoracic junction injury were discharged with a neurologic deficit.

- The width of the prevertebral space may indirectly suggest CSI, especially fractures of the anterior vertebral bodies and/or disruption of the anterior longitudinal ligament, where bleeding is contained in these soft tissues. The value of the prevertebral soft tissue measurements (>5 mm at C3) in identifying cervical spinal injury is somewhat limited if the width of the prevertebral tissue at C3 is ≤7 mm as there is significant overlap with normals. The prevertebral space will vary in width physiologically; deep inspiration results in narrowing and crying or coughing leads to widening. Templeton *et al.* showed that significant likelihood of injury was predicted by a width >9 mm.[30]

- Misinterpretation of the radiographs is not an infrequent occurrence;[31] the exact incidence is difficult to quantify. Misinterpretation has been attributed to inexperienced personnel performing the interpretations or experienced interpreters doing the interpretation in less than ideal situations or with suboptimal X-rays.

## Abnormal radiograph

An abnormal radiograph indicating fracture, dislocation or subluxation leads to consultation with a spine injury specialist. In addition, the spine injury specialist should evaluate any patient with neurologic deficits, regardless of the results of the CSR. To plan the definitive treatment of the CSI, the spine specialist frequently

requires further delineation of the injury which can be obtained by CT, magnetic resonance imaging (MRI) or a combination of both imaging modalities.[21,31,32]

## Suspicious or inadequate radiograph

Any suspicious or inadequate radiographic screen requires further study.[1,12,25,31–33] Inadequate views can be repeated or different plain film techniques can be applied in an attempt to visualize the necessary structures. If repeat attempts fail or a suspicious area is discovered, a CT is frequently used to image the cervical spine. CT provides good bone detail in cooperative patients and is capable of detecting most cervical spine fractures. Since the standard CT protocols use 3 mm slices, imaging the cervical spine is time consuming. In addition, CT has difficulty imaging axially oriented fractures such as the type II odontoid, facet fractures or laminar fractures.[32] Three-view radiographic screens complemented by directed CT scanning have resulted in a sensitivity of 100% for CSI detection.[33]

## Evaluability of the patient

An adequate radiographic evaluation of all the cervical vertebrae, including the junction of C7 with T1, leads into a decision point with regard to the evaluability of the patient to report adequately pain or other manifestation of cervical spine injury such as paresthesias.

Unevaluable patients are maintained in a rigid cervical immobilization device. Pain, an altered level of consciousness, alcohol intoxication, and a painful injury elsewhere (distracting) are all associated with an increased likelihood of cervical spinal fracture in the setting of an appropriate mechanism of injury.[5]

- In obtunded patients, with a normal three-view radiographic screen, Davis *et al.*[34] has used fluoroscopically imaged flexion-extension studies to evaluate the ligamentous stability of the patients' cervical spines. This intervention was done to facilitate removal of the cervical collar to avoid the morbidity of collar-induced decubiti. At this point, this practice cannot be recommended as a standard of care based on study limitations.

- If dynamic fluoroscopy is not utilized, cervical immobilization is maintained until the patient is deemed to be evaluable or for a period of six weeks. If the patient is still unevaluable at six weeks, the CSR should be repeated. If no fractures or dislocations are seen, especially when compared to the initial CSR, the collar can be removed. Most feel that any injury that may be missed on these studies would be adequately treated with six weeks of immobilization. Bone SPECT may have a role in the diagnostic approach to patients with persistent neck pain.[35]

Evaluable patients are thought to be reliable and cooperative. Clinical clearance is begun by the assessment of the objective CDEs as outlined above. This evaluation starts with palpation of the cervical spine. The absence of pain, crepitus, and malalignment on initial examination allows progression to a passive range-of-motion examination (PROM). If the PROM does not produce pain or other neurologic sequelae, then active ROM is performed. If the AROM examination is normal, then the patient's cervical immobilization device may be removed.[12]

An abnormal PROM or AROM leads to a dynamic study of the integrity of the ligamentous structures of the neck with flexion-extension views. An abnormal dynamic study results in consultation with a spine specialist. A negative study in a patient who still complains of pain is managed by maintenance of cervical immobilization for 2–3 weeks followed by a repeat physical examination and another dynamic evaluation. Functional radiographic evaluation of the cervical spine is best performed using dynamic motion analysis and the Penning method of measurement.[36]

## Class II references

1. Gerrelts BD, Petersen EU, Mabry J, Petersen SR. Delayed diagnosis of cervical spine injuries. *J Trauma* 1991;**31**(12):1622–6.

   This is a retrospective review of 1331 patients that occurred over a 32-month period. CSI occurred in 61 (4.6%) patients. Neurologic deficit occurred in 24 (39%); nine died as a result of an atlantooccipital dislocation. A delay in diagnosis occurred in five (10% of the surviving patients); the delay resulted from incomplete CSR in all cases. The sensitivity of CSR was 85.2% whereas CT sensitivity was 97.2%. These authors recommend the early use of CT when conventional CSRs result in inadequate visualization of the cervical spine.

2. Cadoux CG, White JD, Hedberg MC. High-yield roentgenographic criteria for cervical spine injuries. *Ann Emerg Med* 1987;**16**(7):738–42.

   Retrospective study of 749 patients who underwent CSR at an urban referral teaching hospital in 1985. The authors attempted to correlate an abnormality seen on five-view CSR with clinical findings. Straightening and/or arthritic changes were seen in 102 patients whereas a fracture and/or dislocation was seen in 18 (2.4%). When all abnormal CSRs were considered, the presence of direct cervical trauma, loss of consciousness, cervical tenderness or involvement in a motor vehicle crash correlated positively with an abnormal CSR and use of seatbelts correlated negatively with an abnormal CSR. When only the CSRs that showed fracture or dislocation were used for this comparison, no statistical correlation was found.

3. Lindsey RW, Diliberti TC, Doherty BJ, Watson AB. Efficacy of radiographic evaluation of the cervical spine in emergency situations. *Radiograph Eval Cervical Spine* 1993;**86**(11):1253–5.

   A study of 2283 patients which illustrated the low incidence of CSI. In a retrospective review of 1686 consecutive patients studied with CSR (views not specified), CSI was detected in 32 (1.9%). In a prospective population of 597 patients, clinical presentation was correlated with documented CSI. In the 17 (2.8%) patients with suspected CSI, all had at least one of Fischer's criteria (neck pain, neurologic deficit or altered mental status). The authors recognize that a larger study is required to validate these findings before selective radiographic evaluation can be safely undertaken.

4. Stiell IG, Wells GA, Vandemheen K *et al*. Variation in emergency department use of cervical spine radiography for alert, stable trauma patients. *Can Med Assoc J* 1997;**156**:1537–44.

   A large retrospective, multiinstitutional Canadian study conducted at eight centers that enrolled 6855 alert and stable patients. Eligible patients had obvious trauma to the head or neck as a result of high-risk mechanisms of injury such as motor vehicle crashes, motorcycle crashes, pedestrians struck, falls from heights greater than or equal to 1 meter, diving accidents or other contact sports. These authors documented that CSR was used in the evaluation of possible neck injury in 3979 patients (58%). Use of CSR varied greatly between emergency centers and there was significant variation in use of CSR by attending emergency center physicians at seven of the eight centers. CSI was found in 60 patients (0.9%); no CSIs were missed in this study. This study illustrates that clinical evaluation alone is being performed at a variable rate at many centers despite the establishment of scientifically studied evaluation protocols. Though no CSI was missed, the authors acknowledge the possibility that a patient may have presented to another nonparticipating center where the CSI was discovered.

5. Hoffman JR, Schriger DL, Mower W *et al*. Low-risk criteria for cervical-spine radiography in blunt trauma: a prospective study. *Ann Emerg Med* 1992;**21**(12):1454–60.

   This prospective study of 974 patients, completed over the 19-month period ending December 1989, sought to correlate clinical evaluation with the findings of at least a three-view CSR evaluation. A questionnaire was completed prior to the CSR examination with specific documentation of critical diagnostic elements (CDE) such as neck pain, neck tenderness, neurologic deficits, evidence of intoxication or other alterations of mental status and the presence of a "distracting" injury. CSI occurred in 27 (2.8%) patients, all of whom had at least one of the CDEs. There were 353 (37%) patients lacking any of the CDEs; none of these patients sustained a CSI. The authors suggest that if the results of this study can be scientifically validated, more than one third of the CSRs could be eliminated. This well thought-out study was the foundation for the multicenter NEXUS project which, if completed with the above results, will have the statistical power to conclude that the clinical evaluation of the cervical spine in select patients is scientifically proven as safe and reliable.

6. Kreipke DL, Gillespie KR, McCarthy MC *et al*. Reliability of indications for cervical spine films in trauma patients. *J Trauma* 1989;**29**:1438–9.

   This one-year study of 860 patients sought prospectively to correlate radiographically documented CSI with clinical findings upon presentation. CSI occurred in 24 (2.8%) patients. No CSI occurred in the 324 (38%) alert, asymptomatic patients, defined by lack of neck pain or tenderness and a normal neurologic examination. Significant correlation was found between CSI and respiratory distress upon presentation, motor and/or sensory deficits, and communication barrier. This study further elongates the list of clinical elements that may indicate an increased risk for CSI but the small numbers do not allow the authors' conclusion that CSR can be eliminated in the alert asymptomatic patient.

8. Jacobs LM, Schwartz R. Prospective analysis of acute cervical spine injury: a methodology to predict injury. *Ann Emerg Med* 1986;**15**(1):44–9.

   Prospective study of 233 patients over a four-month period ending July 1984. All patients underwent a two-view CSR (CTLV and AP). This study addressed the question of whether the clinician (general surgery residents), based on a study-controlled standard history and physical examination, can predict which patients need CSR and whether CSI will be present. The CSR was abnormal in 24 (10.3%); however, eight of these abnormalities were straightening. The clinicians predicted CSI with a sensitivity of 50% and a specificity of 92%. Interestingly, the only historical variable which statistically correlated with a CSI was a fall of less than 10 feet. This latter finding seems counterintuitive but may be explained by the population studied, which is not provided in the manuscript.

9. Cohn SM, Lyle WG, Linden CH, Lancey RA. Exclusion of cervical spine injury: a prospective study. *J Trauma* 1991;**31**(4):570–4.

   Cross-table lateral (CTL) cervical spine X-ray was studied prospectively in 60 consecutive trauma patients as a screen for CSI. CSI occurred in seven patients (12%); three CSI were missed. All missed injuries occurred in CTL X-rays that failed to visualize all vertebral levels. Only 54% of the CTL X-rays in this study adequately visualized all vertebral levels. The authors recommend emergent procedures should not be delayed to perform CTL to evaluate for possible CSI; rather, all patients should be treated with spinal immobilization until full cervical spine radiologic evaluation is completed.

11. Davis JW, Phreaner DL, Hoyt DB, Mackerskie RC. The etiology of missed cervical spine injuries. *J Trauma* 1993;**34**(3):342–6.

    A large retrospective trauma registry study from the San Diego Trauma System reporting on patients in the 7.5-year period ending February 1991. Of the 32 117 patients entered into the registry from the six trauma centers, CSI occurred in 740 (2.3%). A delay or missed CSI occurred in 34 (4.6%). The delay in diagnosis was attributed to inadequate CSR in 23 (67%) and/or misinterpretation in 16 (47%). An adequate three-view CSR would have allowed a timely diagnosis in 94% of these missed injuries. The missed injuries, which consisted of 29 fractures and 10 subluxations, occurred at all cervical spine levels; 71% of these missed injuries were unstable. A neurological deficit or death resulted as a consequence of the missed CSI in 29% of these patients. This paper places into perspective the incidence of CSI that can be expected in an urban trauma environment as well as the consequences of the missed CSI. One is left to ponder the medicolegal and monetary consequences of these "overlooked" injuries. A follow-up study from these authors on this aspect of the missed CSI would undoubtedly provide additional imputes to adequately evaluate the cervical spine.

12. Reid DC, Henderson R, Saboe L, Miller JDR. Etiology and clinical course of missed spine fractures. *J Trauma* 1987;**27**(9):980–6.

    This is a prospectively designed cohort study of 253 patients with spinal injuries, 153 of which occurred in the cervical region of the spinal column. Injury occurred at two levels in 20 (8%) and one patient had injury at three levels. CSI occurred at or cephalad to C3 in 49 patients (Group I) and between C4 and C7 in 104 patients (Group II). A delay in diagnosis of CSI occurred in 14 (28.6%) of Group I and 21 (20.2%) of Group II. Neurologic deficit occurred or progressed after initial presentation in 10.5% of the patients with delayed diagnosis of spine injury compared with 1.4% in those who had prompt diagnosis. The cause for the delay in diagnosis was misinterpretation of the radiographs in 20 patients, 20% of which occurred due to acceptance of technically suboptimal studies, and lack of initial radiographic evaluation in 17 patients. This study illustrates the consequences of missed injury and suggests means by which missed injury can be avoided.

13. Velmahos GC, Theodorou D, Tatevossian R *et al.* Radiographic cervical spine evaluation in the alert asymptomatic blunt trauma victim: much ado about nothing? *J Trauma* 1996;**40**(5):768–74.

    Prospective study of 549 alert, neurologically intact, non-intoxicated patients done to evaluate the incidence of CSI in this population, the work-up needed to perform this evaluation, and its cost. Adequate visualization of the entire cervical spine was achieved using a three-view series in 41.3% of these patients; 51% required additional studies to visualize the lower cervical spine. Visualization of the cervical spine required 4.1 radiographs per patient; in addition, 78 CTs and one MRI were needed to complete the imaging. Total cost of this radiologic evaluation without professional fees or room/board was $190 000 or $346 per patient. No CSIs were found in this population. Due to the expected low incidence of CSI in this population, the authors recognized that a multicenter trial with enrollment of approximately 30 000 patients is needed to validate these findings.

14. Roberge RJ, Wears RC, Kelly M *et al.* Selective application of cervical spine radiography in alert victims of blunt trauma: a prospective study. *J Trauma* 1988;**28**(6):784–8.

    This prospective study of 476 patients correlated clinical evaluation with five-view CSR documentation of CSI. CSI occurred in eight (1.7%). No alert patient had a CSI without either neck pain (specificity 45%) or neck tenderness to palpation (specificity 57%). Though suggestive that clinical examination in appropriately selected alert patients can be used to diagnose CSI, the small number of CSIs in this study may overestimate the sensitivity of the clinical evaluation.

15. Neifeld GL, Keene JG, Hevesy G *et al.* Cervical injury in head trauma. *J Emerg Med* 1988;**6**:203–7.

    This is a prospective study of 886 patients enrolled at four Chicago hospitals over a nine-month period ending January 1985. The authors correlated abnormalities on a five-view CSR with the clinical evaluation upon presentation. The clinical evaluation resulted in four groups: Group I – alert, no complaints of neck pain and neurologically intact; Group II – alert, complaints of lateral neck pain/tenderness, neurologically intact; Group III – alert, complaints of central neck pain/tenderness, neurologically intact; Group IV – all others (depressed consciousness, intoxication, neurologic injury, painful "distracting" injuries). CSI occurred in 28 (3.2%) patients. There were no CSIs in Groups I or II, seven in 237 Group III patients, and 21 in 387 Group IV patients. The authors emphasize the potential confounding effects of intoxication, mental status changes, and communication barriers on the sensitivity of the clinical evaluation of subtle manifestations of CSI. If scientifically collaborated, the CSR in the 236 (29%) alert patients in Groups I and II can be eliminated.

20. McNamara RM, O'Brien MC, Davidheiser S. Post-traumatic neck pain: a prospective and follow-up study. *Ann Emerg Med* 1988;**17**(9):906–11.

    This study, which occurred over a 15-month period ending November 1986, involved alert trauma patients who complained of neck pain. These authors sought to address what subsequent evaluation patients pursue relative to neck injury following the initial ED evaluation. Follow-up information was available on 263 patients (75%) enrolled. Additional physician evaluation for neck pain was sought in 63% and 88% were treated with physical therapy. Of the 140 patients who did not have CSR at the time of the initial ED evaluation, 52% obtained a CSR upon subsequent evaluation. Involvement in litigation was found in 66% of the 109 patients questioned. This paper documents the high incidence of ongoing evaluation of the neck following the initial ED evaluation as well as the frequent occurrence of legal action that may involve the physician performing the initial evaluation.

22. Borchgrevink GE, Smevik O, Nordby A *et al.* MR imaging and radiography of patients with cervical hyperextension-flexion injuries after car accidents. *Acta Radiologica* 1995;**36**:425–8.

    This study sought to define the role of magnetic resonance imaging in patients who suffer hyperextension-flexion injuries or whiplash injuries. Conventional radiography of the cervical spine may give adequate information with no additional benefit from MR imaging when evaluating common whiplash injuries. This represents a common sense approach to managing patients with whiplash injuries who have no localizing findings. It has medicolegal implications for those patients who have preexisting cervical spine disease as they are the ones likely to have long-term symptoms and/or disability related to whiplash mechanism during motor vehicle crashes.

27. Quinn JV, Cwinn A, Carr B, Grahovac S, Stiell I, Pelland P. Visualization of C7–T1 on portable lateral cervical spine radiographs using a lead-lined acrylic filter. *Ann Emerg Med* 1995;**2**(7):610–14.

    A blinded case-controlled comparison of lateral cervical spine radiographs taken for the evaluation of blunt trauma was utilized. Twenty films in consecutive patients were taken using the filter. A case-matched sample of another 20 patients who also had c-spine films were used for comparison. Two blinded reviewers examined the films. The filter group had acceptable visualization of C7–T1 in 65% of cases, while the standard group's junction was visualized in only 30% of cases. While suggestive, this study is marred by the potential for significant bias in that the technicians who were obtaining the films knew that the filter was being used and may have been more aggressive or attentive in obtaining an appropriate film. The use of a filter to allow the use of more energy while filtering out low-level energy (more associated with neoplasia) is an attractive idea and a potentially useful tool to eliminate unnecessary CT scanning to complete the c-spine survey.

28. Ireland AJ, Britton I, Forresteer AW. Do supine oblique views provide better imaging of the cervicothoracic junction than swimmer's views? *J Accid Emerg Med* 1998;**15**:151–4.

This two-phase study compared 60 patients whose cervical spines were imaged with swimmer's views to image the cervicothoracic junction to those of 62 patients whose junctions were imaged with bilateral supine oblique images. Oblique view identified the junction adequately in 38% compared to 37% in the swimmer's group. However, the facet joints and posterior elements were fully evaluable in 70% of those imaged obliquely compared to only 37% in the swimmer's group. Dose calculations demonstrated a significant reduction in radiation with oblique images (1.6 mGy) versus the swimmer's view (7.2 mGy).

31. Woodring JH, Lee C. Limitations of cervical radiography in the evaluation of acute cervical trauma. *J Trauma* 1993;**34**(1):32–9.

Retrospective review of documented CSI at a university hospital over a five-year period ending June 1990. A three-view CSR and a CT were done on all of the 216 patients. This study discussed detection of specific fractures/dislocations. Symptoms of neck pain, tenderness or neurologic deficit were present in 87%. The 28 asymptomatic patients manifested intoxication (10) or a brief loss of consciousness (7); no mention of potential distracting injuries was made in the 11 patients who had the CSR based on mechanism alone. Prospective and retrospective review of the CTLV and the full three-view CSR was done. The CTLV detected abnormalities of the cervical spine in 85%; the addition of the OMO and AP view increased this yield to 94%. Of the individually missed injuries, 50–63% were felt to be unstable or potentially unstable. This study suggests that plain film radiographs underestimate the extent and severity of CSI. The authors recommend CT for further delineation of any demonstrable injury or if plain film radiographs are inadequate.

32. Clark CR, Igram CM, El-Khoury GY, Ehara S. Radiographic evaluation of cervical spine injuries. *Spine* 1988;**13**(7):742–7.

A retrospective review of 236 patients with 319 cervical spine injuries which occurred at a university hospital over the 8.25-year period ending March 1986. The authors describe use of pleuridirectional tomography and computed tomography to assist in delineation of specific CSIs. For each CSI, the authors mention whether the additional study provided additional useful information. Pleuridirectional tomography appears particularly helpful with identification of facet fractures whereas CT is good for clarification of C1 and laminar or other posterior element fractures.

It is impossible to draw any conclusion from this uncontrolled review.

33. Borock EC, Gabram SGA, Jacobs LM *et al.* A prospective analysis of a two-year experience using computed tomography as an adjunct for cervical spine clearance. *J Trauma* 1991;**31**:1001–6.

This is a prospective analysis over a two-year period ending July 1990 of 179 patients who underwent CT scanning for evaluation of suspected cervical spine injury at a major trauma center. The indications for CT were pain, abnormal CSRs or neurologic deficits in the face of normal X-rays. For 123 of the 179, the neck could not be cleared by simple cervical spine radiographs. The CSR resulted in a false-positive rate of 28% and a false-negative rate of 1.5%. Ninety-eight per cent of the patients with injuries were diagnosed with CT scan. When the three-view CSR was complemented with CT, sensitivity increased to 100%. The authors concluded that CT is an accurate and cost-efficient adjunct to help evaluate and clear the cervical spine. They underscored the importance of combining CT scanning with plain cervical spine films as early as possible to reduce the cost of hospitalization. There is no mention of the incidence of ligamentous injuries missed by these two studies. This study does not deal with the management of patients who continue to have pain with negative plain radiographs and a negative CT. We evaluate patients in this latter situation with flexion-extension views; if those dynamic studies are negative, the patient is kept in a hard collar for six weeks after which repeat CSR ($+/-$ dynamic studies) are obtained.

## Class III references

7. McNamara RM, Heine E, Esposito B. Cervical spine injury and radiography in alert, high-risk patients. *J Emerg Med* 1990;**8**:177–82.

Retrospective study of 286 alert patients over a 14-month period ending December 1987. All of the five CSIs (1.7%) occurred in patients who had neck pain or tenderness. The small size of this study and the retrospective nature limit the conclusions that can be drawn. Interestingly, an adequate CSR series (three-view) was obtained in 159 of the 215 (74%) studied with radiographs.

10. Chong CL, Ware DN, Harris JH. Is cervical spine imaging indicated in gunshot wounds to the cranium? *J Trauma* 1998;**44**(3):501–2.

This retrospective study of 53 patients sought to answer the question: Does a gunshot wound to the cranium predispose to a CSI? These 53 patients underwent two-view CSR. Though none of these patients had a CSI, the limited numbers involved in this study prohibit meaningful interpretation. In the discussion, the authors appropriately highlight that life-saving maneuvers such as endotracheal intubation should not be delayed pending radiographic evaluation of the cervical spine.

16. Turetsky DB, Vines FS, Clayman DA, Northup HM. Technique and use of supine oblique views in acute cervical spine trauma. *Ann Emerg Med* 1993; **22**(4):685–9.

   Retrospective review of 83 patients with documented CSI over a 21-month period ending September 1990. A five-view CSR was completed on all patients; CSI was confirmed in all by CT. Three patients had normal three-view CSR with the fracture seen only on the obliques (30° above horizon). These fractures involved the pedicles and/or lamina of the lower cervical vertebrae. The uncontrolled nature of this study does not allow any conclusions to be drawn about the utility of the oblique views other than they represent a different way to visualize the posterior elements of the lower cervical vertebrae which may occasionally be helpful.

17. Weiss LR, Knopp RK, Morishima MS. Recommendations for evaluation of the acutely injured cervical spine: a clinical radiologic algorithm. *Ann Emerg Med* 1980;**9**(8):422–8.

   This is a "concept" article that proposes an unsubstantiated but logical approach to the evaluation of the cervical spine. It highlights some technical aspects of the radiologic evaluation.

18. Shandera R. Ordering radiographs with the law in mind. *Can Med Assoc J* 1997;**15**:1352.

   A letter from a practitioner with 25 years of experience who uses CSR in everyone to address the potential of legal evidence. This testimonial suggests that the cost of the radiographs may "save" money in the long run by avoiding legal action, but provides no substantiation.

19. Cadoux CG, Spring S, White JD. High-yield radiographic considerations for cervical spine injuries. *Ann Emerg Med* 1986;**15**(3):236–9.

   A review article that highlights the citations which propose high-yield clinical criteria that should increase the index of suspicion for CSI.

21. Hoffman JR, Wolfson AB, Todd K, Mower WR. Selective cervical spine radiography in blunt trauma: methodology of the National Emergency X-Radiography Utilization Study (NEXUS). *Ann Emerg Med* 1998;**32**(4):461–9.

   A descriptive paper which outlines the methodology to be used in a multicenter study to test the predictive power of the following critical diagnostic elements: altered mental status, intoxication, neck tenderness or distracting injuries. Operational definitions are provided for each of these categories. A detailed sample size calculation is included. This must-read paper emphasizes that absence of all the above diagnostic elements must have a 100% negative predictive

value if selective radiographic evaluation of the cervical spine is to be validated.

23. Roberge RJ. Unstable occult cervical-spine fracture. *Ann Emerg Med* 1993;**22**(5):144.

   A letter which questions the occult nature of CSI. The author outlines that no time course was defined in the alcoholic patient who reportedly had the occult CSI. This author reviews the anecdotal case reports of occult CSI and describes the obvious confounding factors which include head injury, intoxication, as well as the presence of distracting injuries, and the "occult" CSI with neurological symptoms.

24. Holliman CJ, Mayer JS, Cook RT, Smith JS. Is the anteroposterior cervical spine radiograph necessary in initial trauma screening? *Am J Emerg Med* 1991;**9**(5):421–5.

   This is a retrospective review of 60 patients with CSI who had a three-view CSR completed on initial evaluation. The lateral showed definitive fracture or dislocation in 43 and suggested an abnormality in an additional 13. The AP view did not show an abnormality that was not seen on the lateral; however, in 15 patients the AP appeared normal when the lateral showed a major vertebral injury. No case of unilateral "jumped" facet was included in this limited study. Though this retrospective study is consistent with my own anecdotal impression of the utility (or uselessness) of the AP view, abandonment of the radiographic principle of obtaining a perpendicular view of an area of suspicion is not warranted by this study.

25. Wylie J. A comparative study of two methods for obtaining the anteroposterior open mouth cervical view. *J Manipulative Physiol Ther* 1995;**18**(4):219–25.

   This is a small case series of open mouth radiographs obtained in a chiropractor's office using two different methods of beam alignment. Patients were not randomized and each patient contributed to only one method. The junction of the occiput with C1, C1–C2 junction, and lateral masses were more readily visualized with the new method of alignment, but the dens was less readily identified in its entirety. The method is also hampered by the need to obtain extension at the atlantoaxial joint for beam positioning.

26. Nunez DB, Zuluaga A, Fuentes-Bernardo DA *et al*. Cervical spine trauma: how much more do we learn by routinely using helical CT? *RadioGraphics* 1996;**16**:1307–21.

   This study retrospectively reviewed 88 severely traumatized patients, 32 of whom had a spine fracture that was either not seen or not clearly revealed on plain films of the cervical spine. The authors noted that the injuries missed on plain films were either located in C1, C2, C6 or C7. These were mostly transverse process fractures and the posterolateral element injuries. One third of the patients with missed injuries had unstable fractures. These authors suggest that helical CT should be routinely added to the initial screening in polytrauma patients in the following circumstances: plain film CSR suggests or shows a CSI, the CSR inadequately visualizes the cervical spine, or severe pain persists despite apparently negative CSRs. This is the approach that we follow at our trauma center.

29. Nichols CG, Young DH, Schiller WR. Evaluation of cervicothoracic junction injury. *Ann Emerg Med* 1987; **36**(6):640-2.

Cervicothoracic junction injury was identified in 9% (37) of patients in this retrospective review of 397 patients who underwent cervical spine radiography for suspected blunt cervical spine injury. Nineteen per cent had only pain, 22% had only a neurologic deficit, and 35% had both pain and neurologic deficit. Distressingly, 24% of patients had neither pain, nor neurologic deficit with a radiographically apparent injury. Fifty-nine per cent of all patients with a cervicothoracic junction injury were discharged with a neurologic deficit in this same patient population. Interestingly, the radiographs from 17 of these patients were reevaluated along with six normal controls. One of the control films was read as positive for indirect evidence of cervicothoracic junction injury.

30. Templeton PA, Young JWR, Mirvis SE, Buddemeyer EU. The value of retropharyngeal soft tissue measurements in trauma of the adult cervical spine. *Skeletal Radiol* 1987;**16**:98–104.

A series of patients with a complete cervical spine series was evaluated with soft tissue measurements taken from C2–C5 to evaluate the utility of these measurements in identifying patients with cervical spine injury. Significant overlap with normal patients (trauma patients with no c-spine abnormality) was identified up to a prevetebral tissue thickness of 7 mm. Above 9 mm width, the likelihood of cervical spine injury greatly exceeded the likelihood of overlap with normals.

34. Davis JW, Parks SN, Detlefs CL, Williams G, Williams JL, Smith RW. Clearing the cervical spine in obtunded patients: the use of dynamic fluoroscopy. *J Trauma* 1995;**39**(3):435–8.

The authors undertook a logically sound and provocative study to clear the cervical spine of obtunded patients (GCS ≤13 for >48 hours after admission). These patients underwent a standard three-view cervical spine series and/or CT scans to exclude cervical spinal fracture. Patients who required anesthesia for an operative procedure (i.e. endotracheal intubation) then underwent dynamic fluoroscopic evaluation (n = 116). Examination technique was excellent and total examination time under fluoro was less than 20 minutes. There was only one positive examination

and there was no neurologic compromise from the examination. Cervical collars had been in place for an average of 5.9 ± 4.2 days prior to fluoroscopic examination; pressure ulceration was present in 44%. Editorial comments identify that the study is sound, but lacks an adequate "n" to be convincing. Also, one must question the values used to define "normal" vertebral body motion identified on dynamic analysis, as the method of measurement is not provided.

35. Seitz JP, Unguez CE, Corbus HF *et al.* SPECT of the cervical spine in the evaluation of neck pain after trauma. *Clin Nucl Med* 1995;**20**:667–73.

This is a retrospective study that examined 35 patients with persistent neck pain posttrauma. Nineteen patients had normal bone SPECT studies and 16 had abnormal studies. SPECT proved to be quite useful in identifying fractures with a sensitivity of 100% and a specificity of 78% and excluded recent fractures in six of nine. It therefore appears to be useful in diagnosing occult fractures in those patients with normal X-rays and for differentiating recent versus remote fractures. It may also have a role in diagnosing patients with persisted pain after injury in spite of negative films. It is not clear from this study how SPECT compares to CT scan and MR. Should SPECT studies have a role before proceeding with CT or MR or vice versa? There are no cost data presented to make economic sense of this dilemma. Therefore, the role for SPECT scanning in relationship to CT and MR remains unclear. For practical purposes, patients with persistent pain and negative plain radiographs of the cervical spine routinely have a CT of the cervical spine or MRI. What remains to be demonstrated is whether SPECT scanning has a role with patients with a negative MR and CT scan.

36. Dvorak J, Froehlich D, Penning L, Baumgartner H, Panjabi MM. Functional radiographic diagnosis of the cervical spine: flexion/extension. *Spine* 1988;**13** (7):748–55.

This interesting study calls into question the techniques utilized in dynamic evaluation of the integrity of the cervical spine ligamentous supports. Patients without any injury served as controls. Additional patients with soft tissue injuries of the cervical spine served as the study group. Active range of motion was imaged and then the patients were put through a passive range of motion by one of the authors and repeat imaging was performed. The passive studies more frequently demonstrated segmental hypermobility, but more infrequently demonstrated hypomobility. The technique of Penning (one of the authors) was found to be a more reliable measurement method than the comparison method of Buetti-Baumi.

**Evaluation of the cervical spine**

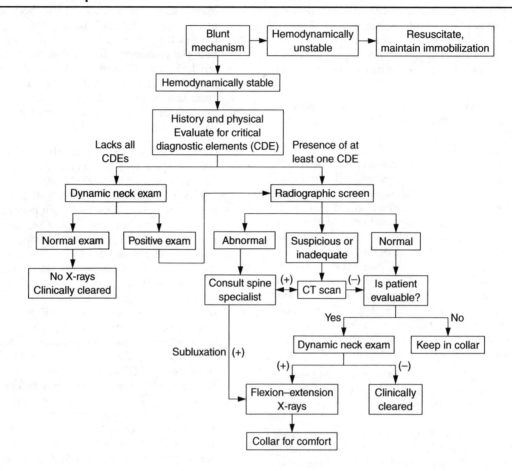

# 4 Evaluation of thoracolumbar vertebral column injury

*Glen H Tinkoff*

## Introduction

The reported incidence of thoracolumbar (TL) fractures in victims of blunt trauma is 2–5%.[1,2] Seventy-five percent of these patients have associated injuries and as many as 30% have neurologic deficits.[3]

Evaluation for specific injury should be initiated in the secondary survey after management of life-threatening injuries.[4,5] Spine precautions (see below) should be maintained throughout the primary survey; the trauma team should note the patient's complaints relating to back pain, neurologic deficits, and/or signs of direct injury to the back.

Patients at risk for injury to their thoracic and lumbar spine include those who have sustained falls, high-velocity motor vehicle crashes (as an occupant or pedestrian), and direct trauma to the back.[1,2,6] Specific high-risk mechanisms include falls from a significant height (greater than 10 feet),[1,2,6,7] use of a lap belt in a motor vehicle crash,[8] and ejection from a vehicle.[1] If in doubt, treat as if the patient is at risk.

## Spine precautions[5]

These precautions include application and maintenance of a rigid cervical collar and strict bedrest. Patients requiring transfer should maintain the body in neutral alignment, thereby minimizing any untoward movement of the spine. Four people are required to perform a safe logroll procedure.

## Mental status

Patients with Glasgow Coma Scale score of 15, non-intoxicated, and cooperative to physical examination are considered alert. Patients with decreased mental status or altered sensorium for any reason should be considered unreliable for examination.[1,2,4,6–10] Spinal precautions should be maintained and radiologic assessment considered.

## Multiple injuries

The presence of multiple injuries that distract the patient from the physical examination renders the clinical examination of the TL spine unreliable.[1,2,4,6–11] In addition, the presence of a vertebral fracture is associated with a 10–15% incidence of another non-contiguous vertebral fracture.[3] Radiologic assessment of the TL spine should be considered in patients with these findings.

## Physical examination

All patients at risk for TL spine injuries should undergo a thorough physical examination, including an indepth neurologic assessment. If the patient reports back pain and/or tenderness and/or has neurologic symptoms, spine precautions should be maintained and radiologic assessment obtained.[1,2,4–11] The presence of neurologic deficits calls for prompt consultation with the appropriate service or specialist who addresses spinal cord injuries (see Chapter 5).

## Radiologic assessment

AP and lateral views of the TL spine must include all 12 thoracic and five lumbar vertebral bodies and disc spaces. Suspicious areas, obvious fractures of the vertebrae or areas obscured or indistinct on plain film radiography should be evaluated with computed tomography, including the vertebrae above and below the area of concern.[5,12–14] In the presence of neurologic deficits, including paraplegia, paresis, and/or radiculopathy, magnetic resonance imaging of the area of concern should be obtained[12,13] (see Chapter 5).

## Abnormalities

The transition zone of the thoracolumbar junction is particularly prone to injury; 60% of the TL fractures occur between T11 and L2 and 90% occur between T11 and L4.[13] Major TL fractures are categorized by the applied force causing the injury: axial compression, axial distraction or translational forces in a transverse plane. These forces cause four distinct fracture patterns: wedge compression fractures, burst fractures, flexion-distraction injuries, and fracture dislocation. All major fracture patterns should be considered potentially unstable and spine precautions maintained. Minor TL fractures include those involving the transverse processes, spinous processes or pars interarticularis. Isolated minor fractures devoid of accompanying neurologic deficits can be considered stable injuries.[12]

## Consultation

Major TL fractures require prompt consultation with the appropriate service or specialist who addresses injuries to the vertebral column. Spine precautions should be maintained until consultation is completed and recommendations are made.

If neurologic deficits persist despite absence of radiologic or MRI abnormality, consider conversion disorder.[14,15] Neurology, psychiatry or physiatry consultation may be beneficial. Patients can be mobilized with assistance under direct observation.

## Class II references

1. Frankel H, Rozycki G, Oschsner MG *et al*. Indication for obtaining surveillance thoracic and lumbar spine radiographs. *J Trauma* 1994;**37**:673–6.

   This is a four-month prospective cohort study with 167 BTVs entered by admission criteria, defined by a preceding 12-month retrospective observational study using risk ratios. Fifteen (9%) of the patients in the prospective group had TL fractures. When the data of both groups are coupled, 26 patients with TL fractures presented without back pain or tenderness. However, this cohort of asymptomatic patients had

a mean of four associated injuries, a mean ISS of 16, and a mean ETOH of 122. The authors conclude that the absence of back pain does not exclude significant TL trauma. This study is limited by its small injury cohort in the prospective group and the combining of data from unmatched cohorts.

2. Cooper C, Dunham CM, Rodriguez A. Falls and major injuries are risk factors for thoracolumbar fractures: cognitive impairment and multiple injuries impede the detection of back pain and tenderness. *J Trauma* 1995;**38**:692–6.

   Three-year retrospective registry analysis of 4142 BTVs to assess risk factors for TL fractures and the occurrence of back pain/tenderness. TL fractures were identified in 183 (4.4%) patients. Falls and major associated injuries were significant risk factors for TL fractures. Of the 110 patients with TL fractures and a GCS of 13–15, 34 (31%) did not have back pain or tenderness. The majority of these patients had GCS of 13 or 14 and/or associated major injuries. The authors conclude that TL films should be considered in all BTVs with altered mentation or major injury. Clinical care algorithm is provided.

9. Terregino CA, Ross SE, Lipinski MF *et al*. Selective indications for thoracic and lumbar radiography in blunt trauma. *Ann Emerg Med* 1995;**26**:126–9.

   Prospective case control study comparing two groups of blunt trauma victims (BTV) to determine clinical indications for TL spine X-rays. Group 1 consisted of 136 BTVs with seven TL fractures who could not be clinically evaluated (GCS <13, intubated or neuro deficit); Group 2 had 183 BTVs with 17 TL fractures who could be clinically evaluated. Negative predictive value of pain and tenderness was 95%. Authors conclude that routine radiography may be unnecessary in asymptomatic patients without distracting injuries.

## Class III references

3. Saboe LA, Reid DC, Davis LA *et al*. Spine trauma and associated injuries. *J Trauma* 1991;**31**:43–8.

   Review of 508 consecutive patients with spine fractures admitted to a tertiary referral center to assess the number and type of associated injuries. The 21% incidence of thoracolumbar junction (T11–L2) fractures in this study was far greater than incidences of thoracic or lumbar fractures alone. Patients with TL fractures were more likely to have associated injury than those with cervical spine fractures (82% thoracic; 72% lumbar). Fifteen per cent of patients in this series had multiple non-contiguous vertebral fractures. Associated neural deficits occurred in 50% of thoracic fractures, 43% of thoracolumbar junction fractures, and 27% of lumbar fractures.

4. Stanislas MJC, Latham JM, Alpar EK *et al*. A high risk group for thoracolumbar fractures. *Injury* 1998;**29**:15–18.

   Retrospective analysis of 110 BTVs with radiologic evidence of TL fractures. Ninety-four had GCS ≥ 11 and 16 had GCS ≤ 10. Four patients in the latter group had a delay in radiologic diagnosis. Common characteristics in these patients were high-velocity injury, decreased loss of consciousness on admission, head injury, and pelvis or lower extremity injury. Limitations include lack of statistical analysis and small study cohort.

5. American College of Surgeons Committee on Trauma. Spine and spinal cord trauma. In *Advanced trauma life support for doctors*. Chicago: American College of Surgeons, 1997.

   This expert consensus opinion of the American College of Surgeons Committee on Trauma on current research and clinical practice in trauma care outlines one safe method of initial care for the injured patient. The chapter includes suggestions for the initial evaluation and management of TL injuries, including recommendations for radiologic assessment and principles of spine immobilization and logrolling.

6. Samuels L, Kerstein M. Routine radiologic evaluation of the thoracolumbar spine in blunt trauma patients: a reappraisal. *J Trauma* 1993;**34**:85–9.

   Seven-month retrospective analysis of registry data on 756 BTVs to assess the value of routine radiologic evaluation of the TL spine. Ninety-nine of 106 (13%) TL spine X-ray examinations were available to review, with 15 (2%) TL fractures identified. The authors concluded that in the absence of clinical evidence of TL injury, TL spine films are unnecessary (based on the 55 patients in their series that did not have clinical evidence of injury and had negative radiologic evaluations.) This study is limited by its small injury cohort, selection bias, and lack of statistical analysis.

7. Scalea T, Goldstein A, Phillips T *et al*. An analysis of 161 falls from a height: the 'jumper syndrome'. *J Trauma* 1986;**31**:706–12.

   A two-year retrospective analysis of 171 adult patients who fell one to seven stories; 21% (35) suffered TL fractures with nearly three-fourths of these fractures being of major type.

8. Anderson PA, Frederick PR, Maier RV *et al*. The epidemiology of seatbelt-associated injuries. *J Trauma* 1991;**31**:60–7.

   Five-year retrospective observational cohort study examining the association of spine and abdominal injury with seatbelt use. Statistical analysis of the group with lumbar fractures, especially those with chance-type fractures, was associated with rear seat passenger position and the use of the lap belt.

10. Meldon S, Maltus L. Thoracolumbar spine fractures: clinical presentation and the effect of altered sensorium and major injury. *J Trauma* 1995;**39**:1110–14.

    Retrospective observational study comprising 145 patients with TL fractures; 81% had back pain or tenderness on presentation. The remainder had altered sensorium, concomitant major injury, and neurologic deficit. Authors conclude that routine TL X-rays are not needed in asymptomatic, neurologically intact patients with clear sensorium and no concomitant major injuries. Limitations include selection bias and assessments from chart review only.

11. Anderson S, Biros MH, Reardon RF. Delayed diagnosis of thoracolumbar fractures in multiple trauma patients. *Acad Emerg Med* 1996;**3**:832–9.

    Retrospective observational study of 181 patients with 310 TL fractures to determine frequency of delayed diagnosis and characteristics of patients whose diagnosis is delayed. Twenty-four per cent had TL fractures diagnosed after ED disposition with the majority (88%) suffering severe multiple trauma requiring immediate resuscitation and high-priority diagnostic or management procedures for stabilization. Most (97%) fractures were found within 36 hours of admission. Limitations include selection basis and data assessment by chart review only.

12. Savitsky E, Votey S. Emergency department approach to acute thoracolumbar spine injury. *J Emerg Med* 1997;**15**:49–60.

    Excellent review article with 72 references.

13. (a) Meyer S. Thoracic spine trauma. *Semin Roentgenol* 1992;**27**:254–61.

    (b) Kricun ME, Kricun R. Fractures of the lumbar spine. *Semin Roentgenol* 1992;**27**:262–70.

    Reviews of radiologic assessment and classification of thoracic and lumbar vertebral injuries.

14. Vollmer DG, Gegg C. Classification and acute management of thoracolumbar fractures. *Neurosurg Clin North Am* 1997;**8**(4):499–507.

    A recent review of the mechanical and anatomic aspects of TL fractures as they relate to classification systems and stability.

15. (a) Silver FW. Management of conversion disorder. *Am J Phys Med Rehabil* 1996;**75**:134–40.

    (b) Watanabe TK, O'Dell MW, Togliatti TJ. Diagnosis and rehabilitation strategies for patients with hysterical hemiparesis: a report of four cases. *Arch Phys Med Rehabil* 1998;**79**:709–14.

    Up-to-date literature reviews and specific case reports on the diagnosis and management of conversion disorder, a psychologically produced alteration or loss of physical functioning suggestive of a physical disorder.

**Evaluation of thoracolumbar vertebral column injury**

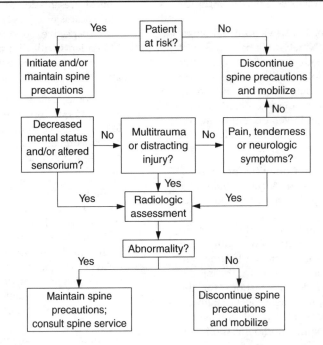

# 5 Evaluation and management of blunt spinal cord injury

*William S Hoff*

## Introduction

In the United States, approximately 10 000 patients sustain injuries to the spinal cord annually. The age distribution for spinal cord injuries is bimodal, with the vast majority occurring in patients less than 30 years old. The second peak incidence occurs in the sixth and seventh decades. In this age group, various degenerative processes (e.g. cervical stenosis) place the spinal cord at risk from minor trauma. Over half of spinal cord injuries are localized to the cervical spine. Spinal cord injuries represent a considerable financial burden in terms of acute hospitalization costs, rehabilitation, and the subsequent loss of income.

## Pathophysiology of spinal cord injury

Much like brain injury, injuries to the spinal cord have a primary and secondary component. Primary mechanical injury, in the form of compression, distraction or shearing, results from blunt trauma. In the case of penetrating trauma, the spinal cord sustains a direct laceration. Secondary spinal cord injury consists of a cascade of cellular, vascular, and biochemical insults which are stimulated by the initial injury. Some of these processes include posttraumatic ischemia, free radical synthesis, destruction of cell membrane integrity, and increased intracellular calcium. Most recent advances in the early management of spinal cord trauma are directed at the secondary mechanisms of injury.

A *complete* spinal cord injury is characterized by the loss of all motor and sensory function below the level of the injury. Patients with *incomplete* spinal cord injury have preservation of various degrees of neurologic function depending on which elements of the spinal cord have been injured. The Brown–Sequard syndrome is an incomplete cord lesion which results from hemitransection of the spinal cord. Patients with this syndrome present with ipsilateral loss of motor function and contralateral loss of sensory function. Some degree of functional improvement frequently occurs in incomplete injuries. Therefore, a detailed neurologic assessment becomes important for prognosis.

## Evaluation

### Spinal cord

Protection of the spine has been appropriately advanced as a major theme in instructional courses aimed at providers of early trauma care (e.g. BTLS, ATLS). As a result, the vast majority of patients who have sustained blunt injury arrive at the hospital immobilized to protect the spine. In the early phases of care, manipulation of an improperly immobilized spine may exacerbate a spinal cord injury. Full immobilization is achieved using a spine board along with one of several commercially available cervical collars. Immobilization should be maintained until an injury to the spine has been excluded.

The diagnosis of spinal cord injury is based on a detailed clinical examination. Regardless of history or mechanism of injury, a patient who presents with neurologic signs or symptoms of spinal cord injury requires an aggressive diagnostic evaluation (see Chapter 3). Once a diagnosis of spinal cord injury has been made, a more refined examination is performed to estimate the anatomic level and extent (i.e. complete versus incomplete) of the injury. This examination involves a thorough assessment of motor function specific to spinal cord level graded on a 0–5 scale (Tables 5.1 and 5.2). The Motor Trauma Index Score of the American

**Table 5.1**  Motor examination of spinal cord injury

| Level | Muscles tested |
|---|---|
| C3–C5 | Diaphragm |
| C5 | Biceps, brachialis, brachioradialis (elbow flexion) |
| C6 | Wrist extension |
| C7 | Triceps (elbow extension) |
| C8 | Finger flexion |
| T1 | Intrinsic muscles of the hand (finger abduction) |
| L4 | Ankle dorsiflexion |
| S1 | Ankle plantarflexion |

**Table 5.3**  Sensory examination of spinal cord injury

| Level | Surface landmark |
|---|---|
| C2 | Occipital protuberance |
| C3 | Supraclavicular fossa |
| C6 | Thumb/index finger |
| C7 | Middle finger |
| C8 | Little finger |
| T4 | Nipple line |
| T10 | Umbilicus |
| L1 | Inguinal crease |
| L3 | Medial aspect of knee |
| L5 | Dorsum of foot |
| S1–S3 | Posterior leg |
| S4–S5 | Perianal area |

Spinal Injury Association (ASIA) provides a more detailed system for scoring motor function. Both light touch and pinprick sensation are evaluated over 28 dermatomes from C2 to S5. Detailed diagrams of the dermatomes are available to assist in the precise localization of a patient's sensory level. However, for the purposes of initial evaluation a more abbreviated set of landmarks may be helpful (Table 5.3). Position sense (proprioception) provides information regarding the dorsal columns.

Following a complete spinal cord injury, all neurologic activity below the level of the lesion is interrupted and patients may present with paralysis, flaccidity, and loss of reflex activity. This period of "spinal shock" results from the mechanical injury to the spinal cord and physiologic changes which impede normal impulse propagation. Resolution of spinal shock, marked by the return of reflex activity, typically occurs over a period ranging from several days up to eight weeks. Any motor and sensory deficits which persist beyond this period will be permanent. Thus, a complete evaluation of deep tendon reflexes has both diagnostic and prognostic implications. The reflex exam corresponds with

spinal cord level as follows: biceps (C5–C6); triceps (C6–C7); patellar (L4); achilles (S1).

The etiology of the spinal cord injury (i.e. cervical spine fracture, ligamentous injury) is best determined using an organized combination of clinical examination and radiographic modalities. While spinal cord injury without radiographic abnormality (i.e. SCIWORA) has been described, the initial diagnostic step is complete radiographic evaluation to exclude a fracture of the cervical spine.

**Associated injuries**

The blunt trauma "strategy" involves the simultaneous resuscitation of normal hemodynamics with comprehensive diagnostic evaluation. In patients with spinal cord trauma, the incidence of associated injuries to other organ systems is between 47% and 60%.[1] Once the spine has been stabilized, a full diagnostic regimen must be applied. Evaluation includes a detailed physical examination, laboratory testing, and radiographic evaluation as indicated.

Evaluation of the abdomen is complicated in patients with cervical spine injuries. In the presence of a neurologic deficit, loss of abdominal muscle tone, dermal sensation, and visceral pain perception limit the utility of physical examination of the abdomen. Physical findings which suggest an intraabdominal injury include progressive abdominal distension, bleeding per rectum or bloody aspirate from the nasogastric tube. Patients with detectable extraabdominal injuries on physical examination have a higher likelihood of having sustained an intraabdominal injury. CT scan and ultrasound are notoriously inaccurate for the diagnosis of hollow visceral injury. In this select group of patients in whom the development of peritoneal signs is unreliable, diagnostic peritoneal lavage is particularly useful.[2]

**Table 5.2**  Evaluation of spinal cord injury – motor strength scoring

| Score | Findings on examination |
|---|---|
| 0 | Total paralysis |
| 1 | Palpable or visible muscle contraction |
| 2 | Active movement; full range of motion – gravity eliminated |
| 3 | Active movement; full range of motion – against gravity only |
| 4 | Active movement; full range of motion – moderate resistance |
| 5 | Normal movement; full range of motion – full resistance |

## Management of spinal cord injuries

The comprehensive approach to the management of spinal cord injuries is summarized in the algorithms. The first algorithm presents the important management principles relative to the primary survey. The second summarizes the major diagnostic and therapeutic approach from secondary survey to the early definitive management phase of resuscitation.

## Cervical immobilization

The potential morbidity of a missed cervical spine injury cannot be overemphasized and several case reports have documented asymptomatic cervical spine fractures.[3] Thus, the currently accepted practice is to presume that an injury to the spinal cord is present. It is common practice for blunt trauma patients with the appropriate mechanism of injury to be immobilized by prehospital providers. In the rare event that such patients arrive in the emergency department with an unprotected cervical spine, immobilization should be performed prior to moving the patient.

Proper immobilization requires a rigid cervical collar. Soft cervical collars are inappropriate for this purpose. A number of rigid cervical collars are commercially available for application in the prehospital phase or the emergency department. The ideal goal is to limit cervical motion in all directions to 11° from the neutral position. Studies have demonstrated that none of the currently available cervical collars achieve this goal.[4,5]

The efficacy of any rigid cervical collar is enhanced by complete spinal immobilization, which is typically provided by a long spinal board. The patient's head is secured to the board using straps, with the head placed between cervical immobilization blocks. If this equipment is not available, towel rolls may be placed on either side of the head and tape placed across the frontal scalp and chin to secure the head to the spine board. On occasion, due to body habitus, placement of a rigid cervical collar may not be possible. In such instances, a towel rolled lengthwise and placed around the neck in the shape of a horseshoe (i.e. open end anteriorly) may be substituted for a cervical collar. The ability of this device to effectively limit cervical motion is severely limited. Therefore, under these circumstances, complete spinal immobilization, as described above, is of the utmost importance.

## Airway management

Evaluation of the airway involves a rapid but critical assessment of the patient's ability to maintain a patent natural airway. In addition to the usual causes of airway obstruction in trauma patients, depending on the level of the injury, spinal-cord injured patients may have difficulty clearing pulmonary secretions. Edema in the prevertebral space is another source of airway obstruction specific to patients with spinal cord injury. In general, endotracheal intubation should be considered in patients in whom there is *any* suspicion of airway problems.[6] This approach avoids the obvious problems associated with emergency intubation in this patient population. To prevent further injury in patients with known spinal cord injury, airway management must be carefully orchestrated.

A well-organized team approach is essential to safe endotracheal intubation. The cervical collar is maintained until the patient has received appropriate induction medications. Ideally, a "three-person" technique is used to ensure proper immobilization during the intubation procedure. With the front portion of the collar removed, one person maintains the cervical spine in the neutral position manually. By virtue of position, the respiratory therapist is ideally suited for this task. A second individual, positioned at the patient's side, maintains cricoid pressure (Sellick maneuver). This person should be prepared to perform a cricothyroidotomy if necessary. The third person is responsible for intubating the trachea. In patients with a difficult airway, the presence of a cervical spine injury should lower the threshold for performing nasotracheal intubation or, perhaps, considering a surgical airway.

## Pulmonary and hemodynamic management

During the early management phase of spinal cord injuries, the major therapeutic modalities are directed at the secondary mechanisms of injury. All intervention efforts are directed toward optimization of oxygen delivery and preservation of cellular integrity. Support of intravascular volume and provision of supplemental oxygen are imperative.[7,8]

In addition to auscultation of the lung fields, the patient with spinal cord injury must have a detailed assessment of respiratory capacity. Normal respiratory drive is largely dependent on the function of the diaphragm which is innervated by the phrenic nerve (C3–C5). However, respiratory depression may also occur following injuries below C5 due to paralysis of the intercostal muscles (T1–T8), particularly in patients with marginal pulmonary reserve. Moreover, following injuries below C4, subsequent ascending spinal cord edema may result in delayed respiratory depression at higher levels. Forceful expiration and coughing are dependent on the abdominal musculature. Traumatic lesions above T12, through paralysis of the abdominal muscles, reduce the ability to clear normal pulmonary secretions.

In these situations, the need for intubation and ventilatory support may not be immediately evident and therefore serial evaluation is imperative.[9]

Evaluation of forced vital capacity ($V_C$) provides the most objective assessment of pulmonary function in patients with cervical spinal cord injuries. Due to ascending spinal cord edema and general deterioration which may occur, serial determination of the $V_C$ should be performed throughout the early phase of management. Intubation and mechanical ventilation should be considered for patients who cannot maintain $V_C \geq 10$ ml/kg. Other criteria suggestive of depressed respiratory function include tachypnea, hypoventilation ($\uparrow PaCO_2$), and hypoxia ($\downarrow PaO_2$).[7] Because the consequences of hypoxia are so disastrous, mechanical ventilation should be considered at the earliest suggestion of impairment.

Following cervical or high thoracic (T1–T5) cord injuries, neurogenic shock may develop. This phenomenon results from complete sympathetic denervation in the presence of intact parasympathetic activity.[10] In addition, due to skeletal muscle paralysis, venous pooling of blood occurs below the level of the injury. Neurogenic shock is characterized by the triad of systemic hypotension, inappropriate bradycardia, and warm peripheral extremities. Despite initial clinical impressions, especially in the blunt trauma population, hypovolemic shock must first be excluded as the source of hypotension. A thorough evaluation for associated injuries must be completed before assigning the diagnosis of neurogenic shock.

The primary goal in the management of neurogenic shock is maintenance of the mean arterial pressure in the normal range.[6,7] This goal can usually be achieved by careful administration of intravenous fluids. Inotropic support (e.g. dobutamine) or vasopressor agents (e.g. dopamine, neosynephrine) may be required if hypotension is refractory to adequate fluid replacement. Atropine may be used for hemodynamically significant bradycardia. In these more difficult cases or in older patients with unknown cardiac reserve, a pulmonary artery catheter should be considered to guide therapy.

## Gastrointestinal management

In most instances, as a manifestation of spinal shock, gastric atony accompanies spinal cord injury. Intestinal peristalsis subsequently ceases within 24 hours.[6] In addition, due to unopposed parasympathetic stimulation, the volume of gastric secretions and hence the risk of stress ulcer formation increases.[7] Subsequent abdominal distension has a deleterious effect on an already marginal respiratory status. In addition, these patients are at increased risk for aspiration with subsequent pulmonary complications. It is imperative that all patients with spinal cord injury, regardless of the level, have effective gastric decompression via the nasogastric or orogastric route. In addition, $H_2$-antagonists should be prescribed, particularly if high-dose steroids are utilized.

## Genitourinary management

Another visceral manifestation of spinal shock is denervation of the urinary bladder, resulting in loss of contractile function of the bladder (i.e. areflexic bladder). Following resolution of spinal shock, reflex bladder activity may return and, with bladder training, some degree of normal bladder function may be realized.[7] However, immediately following spinal cord injury, a urinary catheter should be placed to prevent overdistension of the bladder and aid in fluid management.

## Medical intervention

In 1990, the second National Acute Spinal Cord Injury Study (NASCIS II), a prospective randomized study, established the clinical efficacy of high-dose methylprednisolone therapy in patients with spinal cord injury.[11] As a result, "steroid protocols" have become a routine part of the acute management of cervical spine injuries that present with neurologic deficit. Retrospective research has failed to demonstrate a benefit of steroid protocols in penetrating spinal cord injuries.[12]

The high doses required to achieve this effect exceed the dose necessary to activate corticosteroid receptors. Steroids promote microvascular perfusion and act as free radical scavengers. In addition, it has been proposed that high-dose steroid therapy functions through inhibition of lipid peroxidation. Ultimately, these actions stabilize cell membranes and inhibit edema formation, theoretically limiting further injury to the spinal cord. While demonstrated improvements in motor and sensory function are subtle, the functional result in a quadriplegic is significant.

Based on initial studies, a 30 mg/kg bolus dose of methylprednisolone should be administered within eight hours of injury. The bolus dose is followed by a continuous infusion of 5.4 mg/kg/h for 23 hours. Recent studies (NASCIS III) confirm the efficacy of this 24-hour regimen for patients who receive the bolus within three hours of injury but suggest a role for extended therapy. For patients who receive the initial bolus between three and eight hours following injury, improved motor function has been demonstrated when the infusion is maintained for 48 hours.[13,14] While not statistically significant, a slight improvement in functional independence measurement (FIM score) is also conferred by the extended infusion in this population. It has been presumed that the improved FIM is secondary to the improved motor function.

While the steroid protocol outlined by NASCIS II and NASCIS III is strictly limited, the potential complications of steroids should not be discounted.[15,16] Electrolytes and blood glucose should be monitored closely and the immunosuppressive effects of steroids must be considered. In addition, patients should be placed on a stress ulcer prophylaxis regimen.

## Surgical intervention

A detailed description of the various cervical spine fractures or of the technical aspects of surgical management is beyond the scope of this chapter. In general, the definitive treatment of cervical spine fractures is dependent upon the mechanical stability of the specific injury and the potential threat to the spinal cord. However, issues regarding timing of intervention and the specific approaches (non-surgical and surgical) selected remain controversial. Ultimately, decisions regarding surgical management must be made in consultation with a neurosurgeon or orthopaedic surgeon experienced in management of these patients. If surgical expertise and necessary support staff are not available, early transfer to a tertiary facility or regional spinal cord center should be considered.

The role of decompressive surgery in the management of spinal cord injuries continues to be debated in the literature.[16] Proponents feel that persistent compression of the spinal cord may impede any functional recovery of the injured segment. Opponents indicate that the anatomic injury is defined at the initial event and that decompression, particularly in the presence of a complete injury, will do little to improve neurologic recovery. In general, most studies of complete cervical spinal cord injuries demonstrate no benefit in terms of neurologic outcome from early decompression. Thus, the decision to perform a decompressive procedure in a patient with a complete injury may be governed by the overall hemodynamic stability and the presence of

associated injuries. In the presence of a fixed incomplete injury or a progressive neurologic deficit referable to the spinal cord injury, decompression of the spinal cord should be considered as soon as possible.

Surgical decompression requires that the patient be hemodynamically stable and free of any significant associated injuries. Unstable or multiply injured patients may be effectively decompressed using skeletal traction to reduce the fracture or dislocation and maintain alignment until a more definitive surgical procedure can be safely performed. Contraindications to cervical traction include associated disc herniation, atlantooccipital dislocation, comminuted skull fracture, and anticipated need for craniotomy. A recent study demonstrated the utility of the halo-vest for early reduction and immobilization in patients with multiple injuries.[17] The authors were able to effectively reduce the majority of fractures without the use of cervical traction which facilitates the continued evaluation and treatment of these patients.

Regardless of the severity of the neurologic injury (i.e. incomplete versus complete), some intervention is eventually required to stabilize the osseous or ligamentous component. Mechanical stabilization permits early mobilization, facilitates rehabilitation, reduces complication rates, and reduces length of stay in the acute hospital. Several externally worn orthotic devices are available for definitive stabilization or as a temporary treatment until surgical fixation may be performed. These devices include Philadelphia collar, sternal-occipital-mandibular immobilizer (SOMI), halo-vest, and Minerva jacket. Sufficient stability may be achieved with an external orthotic device in approximately 60% of cervical spine injuries. The need for surgical fusion is determined by the specific type of injury sustained, which predicts the overall mechanical stability.

The major upper cervical fracture types are summarized in Table 5.4. Isolated Jefferson fractures and type I odontoid fractures may be managed non-surgically. A hangman's fracture may require skeletal traction if significant displacement is present, followed by an external

**Table 5.4** Major fractures of the upper cervical spine

| Fracture | Description | Stable |
| --- | --- | --- |
| Jefferson fracture | C1 burst fracture with widening of spinal canal | Yes* |
| Hangman's fracture | C2 bipedical fracture | No |
| Odontoid fracture: | | |
|     Type I | Fracture through tip of odontoid | Yes |
|     Type II | Fracture at base of odontoid | No |
|     Type III | Fracture at base of odontoid into body of C2 | No |

*May be unstable in the presence of an associated odontoid fracture

orthosis. A surgical procedure is required for type III odontoid fractures and, depending on the degrees of displacement of the dens, may be necessary for type II fractures.

Fractures of the lower cervical spine are frequently associated with dislocation and ligamentous injury. As a result, reduction is often required prior to either surgical stabilization or external fixation (i.e. halo-vest). The extent of angular deformity may be considered in the management plan. Patients who are neurologically intact with a minor degree of angulation (i.e. less than 11°) may be managed in a rigid cervical collar or a halo-vest. Surgical fusion is indicated in the presence of a neurologic deficit or an angular deformity greater than 11°. Due to the potential risk to the spinal cord, surgical repair is also required for burst fractures with retropulsed bone fragments and traumatic disc herniation.

## Class I references

4.  Cline JR, Scheidel E, Bigsby EF *et al*. A comparison of methods of cervical immobilization used in patient extrication and transport. *J Trauma* 1985;**25**:649.

    Prospective evaluation of seven methods of cervical spine immobilization using combinations of short-board and commercially available cervical collars using radiographic assessment in healthy adult volunteers. Cervical collars reduced flexion/extension by 51% to 69%, lateral bend by 28% to 55%, and axial rotation by 39% to 50%. No consistently superior device among the three cervical collars tested. Addition of short-board decreased range of motion when used with all three collars.

5.  Rosen PB, McSwain NE, Arata M *et al*. Comparison of two new immobilization collars. *Ann Emerg Med* 1992;**21**:1189.

    Prospective comparison of four cervical collars. Range of motion calculated in healthy adults using head goniometer. No device limited cervical motion to ideal (i.e. 11° relative to neutral). Cervical immobilization requires use of additional devices along with commercial immobilization collars.

11. Braken MB, Shepard MH, Collins WF *et al*. A randomized, controlled trial of methylprednisolone or nalaxone in the treatment of acute spinal cord injury. *N Engl J Med* 1990;**322**:1405.

    Multicenter study of patients with SCI randomized to receive methylprednisolone, nalaxone or placebo for 24 hours. Significant improvement in motor function and pinprick/light touch sensation documented at six weeks and six months in patients who received methylprednisolone ≤8 hours following injury.

13. Braken MB, Shepard MJ, Holford TR *et al*. Methylprednisolone or tirilazad mesylate administration

after acute spinal cord injury: 1-year follow up. *J Neurosurg* 1998;**89**:699.

    One-year follow-up to NASCIS III (*JAMA* 1997; **277**:1597). For patients who receive initial therapy between three and eight hours postinjury, motor function recovery improved with 48-hour methylprednisolone protocol compared with 24-hour protocol. Although not statistically significant, improvement was also demonstrated in self-care and sphincter control.

14. Braken MB, Shepard MJ, Holford TR *et al*. Administration of methylprednisolone for 24 or 48 hours or tirilazad mesylate for 48 hours in the treatment of acute spinal cord injury. *JAMA* 1997;**277**:1597.

    A multicenter study of patients with spinal cord injury (SCI) randomized to receive methylprednisolone, tirilazad mesylate or placebo. Improved motor function at six weeks and six months in patients receiving methylprednisolone for 48 hours compared with 24 hours. 48-hour regimen recommended for patients receiving bolus between three and eight hours after injury; 24-hour regimen for patients who receive bolus ≤3 hours from injury.

## Class II references

15. Galandiuk S, Rague G, Appel S *et al*. The two-edged sword of large-dose steroids for spinal cord trauma. *Ann Surg* 1993;**4**:419.

    Retrospective review of immunologic parameters and incidence of clinical invection in 32 patients: 18 neurologically intact; 14 with SCI receiving steroid protocol. No significant difference in clinical infection demonstrated despite serum markers of immunosuppression in steroid group.

17. Heary RF, Hunt CD, Krieger AJ *et al*. Acute stabilization of the cervical spine by halo/vest application facilitates evaluation and treatment of multiple trauma patients. *J Trauma* 1992;**33**:445.

    Review of protocol in which halo-vest is applied in the emergency department in 78 patients with potentially unstable cervical spine injuries. Majority of patients may be safely immobilized in halo-vest without use of cervical traction. Halo-vest facilitates subsequent diagnostic evaluation and therapeutic intervention in multiply injured patients with no deterioration in neurologic status.

## Class III references

1.  Reiss SJ, Rogue GH, Shields CB *et al*. Cervical spine fractures with major associated trauma. *Neurosurgery* 1986;**18**:327.

    Review of 88 patients with radiographically proven CSI. Major associated injuries identified in 60%:

extraneural head injury (64%); intracranial lesions (67%); concomitant spinal fractures (6%); thoracic injuries (46%); abdominal injuries (26%); extremity injuries (23%). Patients with CSI require meticulous evaluation to exclude multisystem injury.

2.  Soderstrom CA, McArdle DQ, Ducker DB *et al*. The diagnosis of intra-abdominal injury in patients with cervical cord trauma. *J Trauma* 1983;**23**:1061.

    Review of 288 patients with SCI over six years. Shock on presentation in 58 patients with neurologic deficit. Eighteen patients had extraabdominal injuries identified by physical examination; three of 18 (5.2%) had occult intraabdominal injuries. In patients with no major injuries identified on physical examination, management priorities should be directed at cervical stabilization followed by complete evaluation for intraabdominal injuries.

3.  Davis JW, Phreaner DL, Hoyt DB *et al*. The etiology of missed cervical spine injuries. *J Trauma* 1993;**34**:342.

    Review of 5.5-year experience with CSI. CSI diagnosed in 740 patients (2.3% incidence). Diagnosis delayed in 34 patients (4.6%); 70% had closed head injury, intoxication or altered mental status. Majority (94%) of errors leading to delayed diagnosis due to failure to obtain adequate CSR or misinterpretation. Recommend that spinal precautions be maintained in patients with altered mental status until reliable assessment can be performed. Presume occult CSI in symptomatic patients with normal CSR until further diagnostic testing is performed.

6.  Mattera CJ. Spinal trauma: new guidelines for assessment and management in the out-of-hospital environment. *J Emerg Nurs* 1998;**24**:523.

    Reviews the biomechanics and pathophysiology of spinal cord trauma. Author presents contemporary management of patients with spinal cord injury in the prehospital and early resuscitative phase.

7.  Luce JM. Medical management of spinal cord injury. *Crit Care Med* 1985;**13**:126.

    Review of pathophysiology of spinal cord injury and resultant organ system complications. Discussion of medical management of patients with spinal cord injuries during the acute phase.

8.  Saul TG. Management of spinal cord injury. *Bull Am Coll Surg* 1995;**80**:27.

    Outline of principles of assessment and initial management developed in conjunction with the Joint Section on Neurotrauma and Critical Care of the American Association of Neurological Surgeons and Congress on Neurological Surgeons.

9.  Claxton AR, Wong DT, Chung F *et al*. Predictors of hospital mortality and mechanical ventilation in patients with cervical spinal cord injury. *Can J Anaesth* 1998;**45**:144.

    Review of 72 cervical spinal cord injury patients with neurologic deficits. Forty-one (57%) patients required mechanical ventilation; in 29 (70%), ventilation was required for respiratory failure. The following were predictors of the need for mechanical ventilation: neurologic level at C5 and above, complete spinal cord injuries, copious sputum, pneumonia, and atelectasis.

10. Zipnick RT, Scalea TM, Trooskin SZ *et al*. Hemodynamic responses to penetrating spinal cord injuries. *J Trauma* 1993;**35**:578.

    Review of 75 patients with penetrating injuries to the spinal column: cervical (24%); thoracic (56%); lumbar (20%). Twenty-three patients (31%) presented with hypotension; 18 (78%) with hemorrhagic shock. The true incidence of neurogenic shock (22%) was lower than reported in blunt SCI (70%).

12. Prendergast MR, Saxe JM, Ledgerwood AM *et al*. Massive steroids do not reduce the zone of injury after penetrating spinal cord injury. *J Trauma* 1994;**37**:576.

    Retrospective review of 54 patients with SCI; 25 managed without high-dose methylprednisolone (MP) and 29 received MP. No significant difference in neurologic function demonstrated in blunt SCI in patients who received MP. Impaired neurologic improvement demonstrated in penetrating SCI in patients receiving MP. MP therapy discouraged in patients with penetrating SCI.

16. Amar AP, Levy ML. Surgical controversies in the management of spinal cord injury. *J Am Coll Surg* 1999;**188**:550.

    Review of evaluation strategies and contemporary management of spinal cord injuries. Includes discussion of controversies regarding surgical approach to spinal cord injury along with recent advances in pharmacologic treatment.

**Management of spinal cord injury (primary survey)**

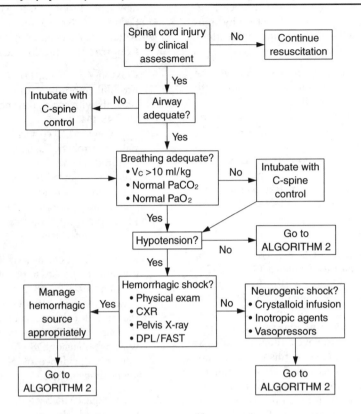

**Management of spinal cord injury (secondary survey, resuscitation, definitive care)**

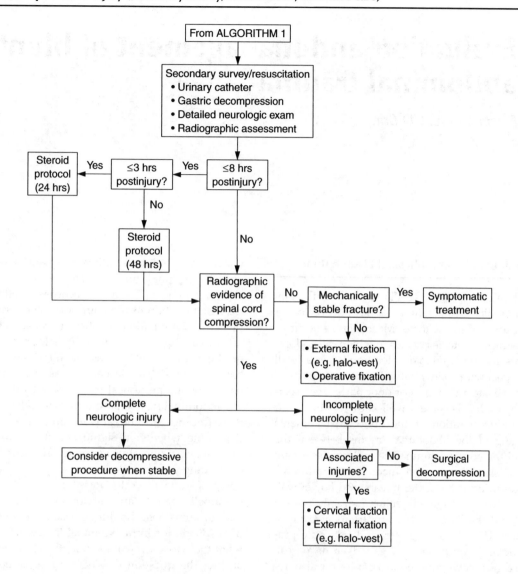

# 6 Evaluation and management of blunt abdominal trauma

*Frederic Cole, L D Britt*

## Background, history, and physical examination

Blunt abdominal trauma (BAT) occurs with any mechanism which results in a significant vector of force being applied to the torso. Most injuries occur as the result of motor vehicle crashes in which the abdominal contents are subjected to deceleration forces as well as direct impact with solid, relatively immobile parts of the vehicle, e.g. steering wheel or door parts. The "seatbelt syndrome" has become a well-known entity.[1-3] It results from deceleration of the abdominal contents with crushing of the abdominal organs between the seatbelt and the spinal column. The hollow viscera are subjected to shear forces and increased intraluminal pressure, resulting in mesenteric tears and bowel wall rupture. The most commonly injured organs remain the spleen and the liver, which rupture as a result of direct impact. High falls (>12 feet) and falls onto projecting structural components (e.g. ledges or wires), along with direct blows suffered in assaults, are also frequent mechanisms of BAT.

There have been major changes in the evaluation and management of BAT over the last 35 years. These changes involve the evolution of management to avoid non-therapeutic laparotomies with their associated morbidity and recognition that many solid organ injuries can be safely managed non-operatively.[4-10] This evolution began with the advent of diagnostic peritoneal lavage introduced by Dr Root in 1964.

With the subsequent widespread application of computed tomography in the 1980s and the recent addition of focused abdominal ultrasonography as an adjunct diagnostic modality, non-operative management has become the mainstay approach in blunt abdominal trauma in the hemodynamically stable patient.

After completing the primary survey as outlined in the ATLS manual, the first step in evaluating the injured patient for possible BAT is assessment of whether the mechanism puts him/her at risk for a significant abdominal injury. The next concern is whether the physical examination of the injured patient is reliable. The physical examination is often unreliable because of accompanying head injury, alcohol/drug intoxication or the presence of distracting injuries such as long bone fractures.[11] If the patient has abdominal tenderness, obvious peritoneal signs or gross disruptions of the abdominal wall, laparotomy is mandatory. Without these findings, additional work-up will be necessary to determine whether a significant abdominal injury is present and if operative intervention is required. Physical findings, such as lower rib crepitance and tenderness, a linear ecchymosis across the abdomen ("seatbelt sign"), and abdominal wall ecchymosis and/or abrasions, should increase the clinician's index of suspicion for intraabdominal injury. In determining what that work-up will include, the clinician must first answer the question of whether the patient is hemodynamically stable.

## Hemodynamic assessment

This represents a major point in the BAT algorithm because hemodynamically abnormal patients are not candidates for evaluation by computed tomography. The latest generation of CT scanners are capable of rapid data acquisition and image production. Nevertheless, performing a CT will add approximately 30–60 minutes to the evaluation of the injured patient. There is increasing evidence that administration of gastrointestinal contrast is not mandatory but most centers still use contrast agents.[12-14] The contrast substance must be administered prior to performance of the scan and time allowed for it to move through the gastrointestinal tract, further adding to the time required to complete the diagnostic evaluation. The patient must be transported to and from the radiology department, adding to the evaluation time as well as the inherent risk associated with any intrahospital transfer. This is time and risk the hemodynamically abnormal patient cannot afford.[15]

Although seemingly intuitive, the assessment of hemodynamics can be challenging. Obviously, patients who are frankly hypotensive (SBP <90 mmHg) have abnormal hemodynamics. However, significant tachycardia (>120/bpm) is also suggestive of abnormal hemodynamics in the trauma patient. The clinician must take the response to therapy into account, along with adequately assessing the patient's hemodynamic status. For example, there is a clear difference in the patient who is initially hypotensive but in whom the hemodynamic status normalizes after 1500 cc of crystalloid fluid as compared with the patient who remains hypotensive and tachycardic, with a significant base deficit, in spite of infusion of isotonic fluids and blood products.

## Abnormal hemodynamics

The patient with BAT and abnormal hemodynamics must have the source of bleeding rapidly identified and controlled. Time-consuming studies like CT are unnecessary and dangerous for the patient. Diagnostic peritoneal lavage has been the standard for the evaluation of the abdomen for significant injury since its introduction in 1964 by Dr Root. In experienced hands, this relatively simple diagnostic procedure can answer the question of whether there is gross blood within the abdomen in 5–10 minutes. Aspiration of gross blood from the lavage catheter in a hemodynamically labile patient mandates immediate laparotomy. If the aspiration is negative, the peritoneal cavity is lavaged with 1000 cc of saline and the effluent is analyzed by cell count, biochemical testing, and microscopic examination. This information must be obtained to complete the examination and, possibly, rule out the need for a laparotomy. However, the absence of gross blood on aspiration of the lavage catheter is strong evidence that the source of the abnormal hemodynamics is elsewhere.

Over the last decade, surgeons in the United States have been catching up with their European and Asian colleagues with respect to the use of surgeon-performed ultrasound in the management of BAT.[16–22] The surgeon performing the four standard views of the focused assessment for the sonographic examination of the trauma patient (FAST), popularized by Rozycki and others, can determine within 2–5 minutes whether there is free fluid (blood) within the peritoneal cavity. This allows for rapid triage of injured patients to the operating room for laparotomy, if the patient is hemodynamically labile and free intraabdominal fluid is detected.[18,23] Further resuscitation, along with pursuit of other possible sources causing hemodynamic instability, should be done if there is no free intraabdominal or pelvic fluid. The four views necessary in performing FAST are a right subcostal view of Morrison's pouch, a subxiphoid view of the pericardium, a left subcostal view of the perisplenic region, and a suprapubic view of the pelvis. This last view is facilitated by the presence of a fluid-filled bladder, which can be achieved by clamping the Foley catheter and/or instilling sterile saline into the bladder via the catheter. Characteristic sonolucent regions are indicative of hemoperitoneum.

If the DPL or ultrasound examination is negative, the clinician must also consider other sources for a patient's hemodynamic lability. These include long bone fractures, pelvic fractures, massive hemothorax, tension pneumothorax, cardiac tamponade, and myocardial contusion.

## Normal hemodynamics

In the presence of normal hemodynamics and the absence of the obvious indications for laparotomy outlined above, the clinician has several options in evaluating the patient for BAT: DPL, CT or US examination of the abdomen. Which modality the clinician selects will be dictated by hospital resources and the surgeon's experience.[5,19,24–31]

Diagnostic peritoneal lavage remains a highly predictive tool in the detection of significant intraabdominal injury. It is considered to be simple, rapid, and relatively inexpensive. The major objections to this technique are the relatively high (20%) non-therapeutic laparotomy rate, possibility for technical error/injury, and the fact that this diagnostic modality is invasive with all the risks attendant on interventional procedures. DPL is also operator dependent in the sense that there is a learning curve associated with being able to perform this procedure expeditiously. When performed only occasionally, it can become an exercise in futility.

FAST essentially provides the same information as DPL: confirmation (or not) of free intraperitoneal fluid (blood). If there is no such confirmation and no other clear indication for operative intervention (see above), expectant management of the patient could be considered. This may involve repeat US examination after several hours, as well as repeat physical examination.[16–18,32,33] The patient should also undergo further work-up for additional injuries as dictated by the clinical situation.

Free fluid on ultrasonographic examination or gross blood on aspiration of the lavage catheter in the hemodynamically abnormal patient mandates immediate laparotomy. However, free fluid on ultrasound examination, gross blood or positive DPL by RBC criteria in the hemodynamically normal patient may be indicative of a solid organ injury (SOI) amenable to non-operative management. These patients should undergo CT scanning of the abdomen and pelvis to confirm that possibility.

Various criteria for non-operative management of SOI have been proposed since the strategy was first entertained in the mid-1980s. Initial laparotomy for SOI remains a valid management strategy. The central question is whether the patient has normal hemodynamics. Various authors have advocated grade of injury (usually I–III), quantity of hemoperitoneum, and absence of other injuries as additional criteria for non-operative management of SOI. Other considerations are the continuous availability of a dedicated surgical team and operating room so that operative intervention can be expeditiously performed if the patient fails non-operative management. Critical care beds, skilled nurses, and a blood bank should also be available. Non-operative management should only be undertaken in trauma centers by those experienced in this treatment strategy.

The majority of SOI resulting from BAT can be managed non-operatively. Indications for abandoning this approach are continuing solid organ-related bleeding (falling hematocrit, transfusion requirements), development of peritonitis, and clinical deterioration.

If the CT scan obtained following a positive US or DPL is negative for SOI immediate laparotomy must be undertaken. SOI explains the presence of free fluid on US examination and the positive findings on DPL. In the absence of SOI, there is a real possibility that the free fluid/blood is the result of hollow visceral injury with spillage of intestinal content.[2,3,34–39] DPL may pick up hollow visceral injury through microscopic examination of the lavage fluid looking for food particles, biochemical analysis for alkaline phosphatase or by WBC criteria.[39,40] These results should also lead to immediate laparotomy. The finding of free fluid/blood in the absence of SOI may be the result of mesenteric tears with the risk of secondary bowel ischemia.

The algorithm, with the supporting literature citations and commentary, provides the framework for evidence-based management in blunt abdominal trauma. With the advent of newer technology and more advanced diagnostic modalities, this particular management paradigm should be considered as "work in progress". Also, irrespective of the evidence based documentation, all management paradigms and clinical pathways are institution and operator dependent. Some flexibility should always be allowed for individualized patient management in a given setting.

## Class II references

1. Blow O, Bassam D, Butler K *et al*. Speed and efficiency in the resuscitation of blunt trauma patients with multiple injuries: the advantage of diagnostic peritoneal lavage over abdominal computerized tomography. *J Trauma* 1998;**44**(2):287–90.

   This study compared a group of patients with BAT evaluated using a prospective protocol in which DPL was the primary diagnostic modality in all patients with time-sensitive injuries (e.g. open fractures, severe head injury, hemodynamic lability) and a historic cohort of patients who were preferentially evaluated with CT unless their hemodynamics were grossly abnormal. The protocol patients spent less time in the emergency department and in radiology. There were no missed injuries, non-therapeutic laparotomy rates were similar, and cost was significantly less in the DPL group.

2. Boulanger BR, Brenneman FD, Kirkpatrick AW *et al*. The indeterminate abdominal sonogram in multisystem blunt trauma. *J Trauma* 1998;**45**(1):52–6.

   This prospective study examined the outcome of patients undergoing sonography for the evaluation of BAT who had an indeterminate result. Four hundred and seventeen patients underwent emergent abdominal sonography (EAS) for the evaluation of BAT; 28 (6.7%) had indeterminate findings. They were further evaluated with a combination of repeat sonography, computed tomography, and diagnostic peritoneal lavage (none were managed with repeat sonography alone). The scans were indeterminate because of patient factors such as subcutaneous emphysema or obesity in 20 of 28 patients. Operator factors resulting in equivocal findings included an inability to generate an interpretable image in four patients. All DPLs were negative. Eight of 23 CT scans demonstrated IAI and five of those eight patients underwent therapeutic laparotomy. The authors conclude that indeterminate sonograms are an infrequent result in their institution and mandate further evaluation because those patients have a significant risk for operative injury.

3. Boulanger BR, McLellan BA, Brenneman FD *et al*. Emergent abdominal sonography as a screening test in a new diagnostic algorithm for blunt trauma. *J Trauma* 1996;**40**(6):867–74.

   This prospective evaluation of emergent abdominal sonography (EAS) in the evaluation of BAT supports the use of EAS as a screening test in the diagnostic algorithm for BAT. The authors compared EAS to DPL and CT in a blinded manner. EAS was performed in 400 patients; 293 were further evaluated by CT and 107 with DPL. The accuracy of EAS for detection of free fluid was 94%. Positive and negative predictive values were 82% and 96% respectively. Of 338 patients with a negative EAS, one subsequently underwent a therapeutic laparotomy.

4. Boulanger BR, Brenneman FD, McLellan BA *et al.* A prospective study of emergent abdominal sonography after blunt trauma. *J Trauma* 1995;**39**(2):325–30.

A prospective study of ultrasonography in the evaluation of BAT in 206 adult patients. The US examinations required $2.6 \pm 1.4$ minutes to perform. The positive and negative predictive values of US for intraperitoneal fluid were 90% and 97% respectively. The sensitivity, specificity, and accuracy of US for free fluid were 81%, 98%, and 96%.

5. Branney SW, Moore EE, Cantrill SV *et al.* Ultrasound based key clinical pathway reduces the use of hospital resources for the evaluation of blunt abdominal trauma. *J Trauma* 1997;**42**(6):1086–90.

This interesting prospective study describes and discusses the development of key clinical pathways (KCPs). The authors developed a KCP for patients with BAT and applied it prospectively to patients with BAT admitted to their institution. They demonstrated a reduction in use of DPL from 17% in the pre-KCP period to 4% and a reduction in CT use from 56% pre-KCP to 26%. This was despite an overall increase in injury severity over the study period. No differences were noted with respect to demographics, number of laparotomies or types of injuries between the two periods. They conclude that an ultrasound-based KCP can result in savings from decreased resource utilization without risk to the patient.

6. Chandler CR, Lane JS, Waxman KS. Seatbelt sign following blunt trauma is associated with increased incidence of abdominal injury. *Am Surg* 1997;**63**(10):885–8.

This study prospectively analyzed 117 consecutive adult victims of MVCs, the use of seatbelts, and the presence or absence of a seatbelt sign was documented on admission. The patients then underwent further evaluation with CT scanning, DPL, serial clinical examination or laparotomy as clinically indicated. The patients with a seatbelt sign (14 of 117; 12%) were compared to the remaining patients in terms of abdominal injury. Nine of the 14 patients with a seatbelt sign (64%) harbored abdominal injuries, five (36%) of whom required operative intervention, and three (21%) had small bowel perforation. This compared to the group without seatbelt sign which had nine patients (8.7%) with abdominal injuries, four (3.8%) required laparotomy, and two (1.9%) experienced small bowel perforation. The authors conclude that the presence of a seatbelt sign is associated with

an increased risk for abdominal and intestinal injuries and thus requires a heightened index of suspicion.

7. Chiu WC, Cushing BM, Rodriguez A *et al.* Abdominal injuries without hemoperitoneum: a potential limitation of focused abdominal sonography for trauma (FAST). *J Trauma* 1997;**42**(4):617–25.

This prospective evaluation of 772 BAT patients undergoing FAST examination raises a cautionary note regarding FAST as the sole diagnostic modality in evaluating BAT. Fifty-two patients (7%) had IAI. Fifteen of the 52 (29%) had no detectable hemoperitoneum on FAST. These included 10 patients with splenic injury, four of whom required laparotomy, and five patients with hepatic injuries, who were managed non-operatively. The authors recommend that the result of FAST examination be considered in light of the overall clinical picture including associated injuries and physical examination findings.

8. Ferrera PC, Verdile VP, Bartfield JM *et al.* Injuries distracting from intraabdominal injuries after blunt trauma. *Am J Emerg Med* 1998;**16**(2):145–9.

This study prospectively analyzed patients who had sustained BAT and had evaluable abdomens (GCS 15, no previous diagnostic study, no spinal cord injury, and no immediate indication for laparotomy). The patients were interviewed specifically about abdominal pain and assessed for tenderness. The presence of distracting injuries and subsequent demonstration of IAI was documented. IAI was demonstrated in 7% of patients presenting with neither abdominal pain nor tenderness. All of these patients had extraabdominal injuries, primarily rib and long bone fractures. One patient with IAI and no pain/tenderness had only concomitant pulmonary contusion. The authors conclude that the absence of pain and tenderness does not preclude IAI.

9. Förster R, Pillasch J, Zielke A *et al.* Ultrasonography in blunt abdominal trauma: influence of the investigators' experience. *J Trauma* 1992;**34**(2):264–9.

This prospective study of surgeons using ultrasonography in the evaluation of BAT demonstrates the learning curve associated with the technique. Surgeons with a learning period of less than one year had a positive predictive value of 60%, surgeons with a learning period of greater than one but less than three years had a positive predictive value of 76%, and surgeons with a learning period of greater than three years had a positive predictive value of 92%.

10. Healey MA, Simons RK, Winchell RJ *et al.* A prospective evaluation of abdominal ultrasound in blunt trauma: is it useful? *J Trauma* 1996;**40**(6):875–85.

A large prospective evaluation of US examination in the evaluation of BAT. Eight hundred US examinations were performed in selected BAT patients. The authors examined the time required to perform the examination (including the time required to get the machine), the ease with which US examination could be integrated into the resuscitation, and the US results compared to DPL/CT findings and clinical course. There were four examinations which were technically inadequate. A sensitivity of 88.2%, a specificity of 97.7%, a positive predictive index of 72.3%, and negative predictive index of 99.2% with an overall accuracy of 97.1% were demonstrated in the other 796 US examinations. Although it took on average 17.3 minutes to get the US machine into the resuscitation area, another 7.0 minutes to prepare to do the examination, and an additional 10.6 minutes to perform the examination, the authors felt that the study could be obtained rapidly, integrated into the resuscitation, and completed quickly.

11. Liu M, Lee C, P'eng F. Prospective comparison of diagnostic peritoneal lavage, computed tomographic scanning, and ultrasonography for the diagnosis of blunt abdominal trauma. *J Trauma* 1993;**35**(2):267–70.

These authors performed a prospective comparison of CT, DPL, and ultrasound examinations in 55 stable multiple trauma patients. They demonstrated sensitivity, specificity, and accuracy of 100%, 84.2%, and 94.5% for DPL, 97.2%, 94.7%, and 96.4% for CT, and 91.7%, 94.7%, and 92.7% for ultrasound. They caution against overstating the capabilities of ultrasound and note difficulties in identifying isolated small bowel injuries. The complementary nature of serial clinical assessment and the various diagnostic studies is highlighted.

12. Livingston DH, Lavery RF, Passannante MR *et al.* Admission or observation is not necessary after a negative abdominal computed tomographic scan in patients with suspected blunt abdominal trauma: results of a prospective, multiinstitutional trial. *J Trauma* 1998;**44**(2):273–82.

This study represents a large, prospective, multiinstitutional effort to determine what additional care is needed for patients with BAT who have negative CT scans. Three thousand eight hundred and twenty-two consecutive patients presented to the four participating institutions during the study period. Two thousand seven hundred and seventy-four met the study eligibility criteria and were enrolled. Two thousand two hundred and ninety-nine fulfilled the study protocol. One thousand eight hundred and nine patients had negative CT scans. The negative predictive value of an abdominal CT was 99.63% and there was no apparent benefit from hospital admission and prolonged observation.

13. McElveen TS, Collin GR. The role of ultrasonography in blunt abdominal trauma: a prospective study. *Am Surg* 1997;**63**(2):184–8.

This study describes the initiation of a trauma ultrasound program at a rural level I trauma center. One trauma attending and one surgical chief resident underwent theoretical and practical training in trauma ultrasound. Data regarding results of US examinations were gathered prospectively and compared to other diagnostic modalities. A sensitivity of 88%, a specificity of 98%, and accuracy of 96% were demonstrated for US examination.

14. McKenney MG, McKenney KL, Compton RP *et al.* Can surgeons evaluate emergency ultrasound scans for blunt abdominal trauma? *J Trauma* 1998;**44**(4):649–53.

This study represents a prospective collection of ultrasound evaluation of BAT by surgeons and surgical housestaff compared to interpretation by attending radiologists. The study period was seven months. There was a wide variability in surgeon experience with ultrasound preceding the study. Minimal training was provided prior to institution of the protocol. Sonogram results were confirmed by computed tomography, diagnostic peritoneal lavage or operation. The surgical team accuracy in interpretation of the sonograms was 99%, which was equivalent to the accuracy of the attending radiologists.

15. Otomo Y, Henmi H, Mashiko K *et al.* New diagnostic peritoneal lavage criteria for diagnosis of intestinal injury. *J Trauma* 1998;**44**(6):991–9.

This prospective study examines the accuracy in detection of intestinal injury of a new criterion for laparotomy using DPL: WBC $\geq$RBC/150 in addition to the traditional criteria of aspiration of gross blood, RBC $\geq$100 000/mm$^3$, WBC $\geq$500/mm$^3$. DPL was performed in 250 BAT patients during the seven-year study period. The new criteria yielded a sensitivity of 96.6% and a specificity of 99.4% after exclusion of 57 patients who underwent DPL within three hours or after 18 hours postinjury. One hundred and thirty-three patients had hemoperitoneum. DPL was negative by WBC:RBC/150 criteria in 85 of those patients. This cohort of patients had no adverse sequelae to non-operative management of these 85 patients.

16. Richards JR, Derlet RW. Computed tomography for blunt abdominal trauma in the ED: a prospective study. *Am J Emerg Med* 1998;**16**(4):338–41.

This study prospectively evaluated indications of obtaining CT evaluation of the abdomen in trauma patients and followed their course to hospital discharge. A total of 196 patients were evaluated. Forty admissions were averted by negative CT. The combination of an abnormal abdomen examination and presence of hematuria had sensitivity of 64%, specificity of 94%, positive predictive value of 56%, and negative predictive value of 95%. A decrease of 5% or more in hematocrit did not correlate with IAI.

17. Rozycki GS, Ballard RB, Feliciano DV *et al.* Surgeon-performed ultrasound for the assessment of truncal injuries. Lessons learned from 1540 patients. *Ann Surg* 1998;**228**(4):557–67.

This report consists of the results of the prospective evaluation of 1540 patients with truncal injuries using the Focused Assessment for the Sonographic examination of the Trauma patient (FAST). One thousand two hundred and twenty-seven of these patients had a blunt mechanism of injury. Sensitivity was 78.3% and specificity was 99.8%. The article reviews the authors' technique for performing FAST and their protocols. The authors conclude that ultrasound should be the initial diagnostic modality for the evaluation of patients with blunt truncal injuries and that immediate surgical intervention is justified in hypotensive victims of blunt torso trauma based on a positive FAST.

18. Shih, HC, Wen Y, Ko T *et al*. Noninvasive evaluation of blunt abdominal trauma: prospective study using diagnostic algorithms to minimize nontherapeutic laparotomy. *World J Surg* 1999;**23**:265–70.

    This prospective study compares a group of 170 patients with blunt abdominal trauma evaluated using a non-invasive assessment algorithm with a cohort of historical controls. The non-invasive algorithm used ultrasonography as an initial screen. Unstable patients with free fluid on ultrasound examination underwent laparotomy. Stable patients with free fluid underwent further evaluation. Computed tomography served as the principal complementary evaluation method. The non-therapeutic laparotomy rate was markedly reduced in the study group versus the historical control group (9.1% versus 32.2%, $P = 0.025$). The authors conclude that non-invasive evaluation of BAT can be performed safely, with a minimal non-therapeutic laparotomy rate using well-designed algorithms.

19. Stanley AC, Vittemberger F, Napolitano L. The use of delayed computerized tomography in the evaluation of blunt abdominal trauma: a preliminary report. *Am Surg* 1999;**65**:369–74.

    These authors instituted a protocol of serial physical examinations and hematocrit determinations in order to decrease the number of routine CT scans obtained to evaluate BAT in their institution. They first reviewed all patients with BAT evaluated over a one-year period. They discovered that 379 of the 813 (46.6%) patients seen during that time period were hemodynamically stable, had a GCS >13, and Hct ≥35. CT scans were obtained because of distracting injuries, possible traumatic brain injury or substance abuse. Only 47 (12.4%) of these scans were positive for intraabdominal injury. Fifty-two patients were then prospectively entered into a treatment protocol of serial physical examination and Hct determinations every six hours. Inclusion criteria were a mechanism for BAT, hemodynamic stability, a normal admission abdominal examination, GCS >13, and admission Hct ≥35. CT scans were obtained in patients whose abdominal examinations became abnormal or who sustained a drop in Hct. Using this protocol, they performed CT scans in only seven (13.5%) of the study patients. The authors conclude that a protocol of serial abdominal examinations and Hct determinations may be useful in decreasing the number of negative routine abdominal CT scans obtained in the evaluation of BAT.

20. Thomas B, Falcone RE, Vasquez D *et al*. Ultrasound evaluation of blunt abdominal trauma: program implementation, initial experience, and learning curve. *J Trauma* 1997;**42**(3):384–90.

    This study describes the initiation of a trauma ultrasound program credentialled through the Department of Surgery under the auspices of Continuous Quality Improvement. The authors describe the didactic and hands-on training in preparation for initiation of the program. The results of US examinations were prospectively obtained and compared to results from CT, DPL diagnostic studies or the clinical course. Three hundred patients were studied over four months. There were 277 true negative examinations, 17 true positives, two false positives, and four false negatives. Sensitivity of US examination was 81%, specificity was 99.3%, and accuracy was 98.0%. The authors estimated that the use of US evaluation versus standard diagnostic evaluation would amount to over $100 000 in cost savings per year.

21. Williams RA, Black JJ, Sinow RM, Wilson SE. Computed tomography-assisted management of splenic trauma. *Am J Surg* 1997;**174**(3):276–9.

    The authors retrospectively evaluated 50 CT scans for BAT and graded splenic injuries with respect to subcapsular hematoma, parenchymal disruption or hilar involvement. The clinical courses of the patients were documented. They then instituted a prospective protocol in which hemodynamically stable patients underwent CT scanning. Patients identified as having splenic injuries without hilar involvement were managed non-operatively. Splenic injuries with hilar injury were operated. Non-operative patients were found to have shorter hospital stays and required fewer blood products. Institution of the protocol resulted in fewer laparotomies compared to the control period.

## Class III references

22. Bain IM, Kirby RM, Tiwari P. Survey of abdominal ultrasound and diagnostic peritoneal lavage for suspected intra-abdominal injury following blunt trauma. *Injury* 1998;**29**(1):65–71.

    A retrospective review of the use of abdominal ultrasound (AUS) in the evaluation of 220 patients with BAT, this study demonstrates comparable sensitivity and specificity for AUS and DPL. The authors note more frequent non-therapeutic laparotomies following DPL than AUS (nine of 25 or 36% compared to three of 23 or 13%). The authors state that AUS is now the first line investigation for BAT in their institution.

23. Baron BJ, Scalea TM, Sclafani SJA *et al*. Nonoperative management of blunt abdominal trauma: the role of sequential diagnostic peritoneal lavage, computed tomography, and angiography. *Ann Emerg Med* 1993;**22**(10):1556–62.

These authors retrospectively analyzed the results of treating 52 BAT patients using an algorithm of sequential DPL, CT scan, and angiography. Patients were initially evaluated by DPL. Those who had positive results were then subjected to CT. If a surgically significant lesion was identified, e.g. small bowel perforation or pancreatic transection, it was subjected to laparotomy. If there were only insignificant visceral injuries identified (e.g. superficial liver laceration), the patients were observed. Patients with significant visceral injuries which did not mandate immediate operation (e.g. splenic injuries, perinephric hematomas, retroperitoneal hematomas, parenchymal liver injuries) underwent angiography with an attempt at embolization of any actively bleeding lesion. Fifteen patients had negative CT scans and were successfully observed. The remaining 37 patients had 17 liver, 16 splenic, and eight kidney injuries, eight extraperitoneal bleeds, and one mesenteric hematoma. Six of the 37 were observed, 30 underwent angiography. Twelve angiograms demonstrated no active bleeding, 17 had successful embolization of the identified bleeding site. An additional patient's injuries could not be embolized successfully and required laparotomy. Six patients underwent delayed laparotomy, but none had bleeding or missed intestinal injury. The authors conclude that DPL and CT are complementary studies in the evaluation of BAT, with DPL providing an effective screening test and CT defining specific organ injury. Angiography may often control bleeding through embolization, limiting the surgery rate.

24. Bloom AI, Rivkind A, Zamir G *et al*. Blunt injury of the small intestine and mesentery – the trauma surgeon's Achilles' heel? *Eur J Emerg Med* 1996;**3**:85–91.

This retrospective study from the Trauma Unit of the Hadassah University Hospital in Jerusalem identified 18 patients over a 34-month period who had sustained small intestinal and/or mesenteric injuries secondary to BAT. Ten of their patients were subjected to early laparotomy, but the other eight had operative intervention delayed from 20 hours to 46 days. The authors attribute the delay to a lack of suspicion for injury in hemodynamically stable patients who have had negative CT scans. They note that late diagnosis was associated with increased morbidity and prolonged hospital stay. They recommend a high index of suspicion particularly when physical examination reveals a "seatbelt sign". They propose a management algorithm, which includes observation following a negative CT or DPL, with repeat study if the results are equivocal.

25. Brasel KJ, Olson CJ, Stafford RE, Johnson TJ. Incidence and significance of free fluid on abdominal computed tomographic scan in blunt trauma. *J Trauma* 1998; **44**(5):889–92.

This retrospective review of 1141 patients with BAT undergoing CT scanning demonstrated free fluid without solid organ injury in 34 (3%) of patients. Thirteen underwent laparotomy, which demonstrated small bowel injury in six, and one diaphragm injury for a therapeutic laparotomy rate of 54%. Ten patients who were deemed to have only trace amounts of free fluid were successfully managed non-operatively. The authors conclude that patients with more than trace amounts of free fluid in the absence of solid organ injury should be explored.

26. Cathey KL, Brady WJ, Butler K *et al*. Blunt splenic trauma: characteristics of patients requiring urgent laparotomy. *Am Surg* 1998;**64**(5):450–4.

In an attempt to delineate characteristics of patients with blunt splenic trauma who require urgent laparotomy, the authors reviewed their cases of blunt splenic injury identified from their trauma registry over a 15-month period. In their 55 patients they determined that hemodynamic instability, multiple injuries, abnormal laboratory parameters, and need for blood transfusion in the emergency department were associated with a need for urgent laparotomy.

27. Clancy TV, Ragozzino MW, Ramshaw D *et al*. Oral contrast is not necessary in the evaluation of blunt abdominal trauma by computed tomography. *Am J Surg* 1993;**166**:680–5.

The authors identified 492 patients who underwent CT scanning of the abdomen for evaluation of BAT. The practice in their institution is to perform these scans without gastrointestinal contrast material. Three hundred and seventy-two (76%) of the scans were negative; 120 (24%) of the scans were positive for intraabdominal injury. Oral contrast was used in eight (1.6%) of the 492 patients. One patient whose initial scan without gastrointestinal contrast was interpreted as negative subsequently required operation. The authors concluded that the omission of gastrointestinal contrast did not represent a disadvantage in evaluating patients for BAT. Such an omission has the advantage of avoiding time delays and hazards associated with the use of gastrointestinal contrast.

28. Cunningham MA, Tyroch AH, Kaups KL, Davis JW. Does free fluid on abdominal computed tomographic scan after blunt trauma require laparotomy? *J Trauma* 1998;**44**(4):599–603.

This retrospective review of patients sustaining BAT and evaluated by CT demonstrated isolated intraperitoneal fluid in 31 patients. All 31 underwent laparotomy, 29 were therapeutic. There were 18 patients with bowel injury, eight with mesenteric injury, and five with intraperitoneal bladder rupture. The authors conclude that isolated intraperitoneal fluid on CT scan after blunt trauma mandates laparotomy.

29. Fang J, Chen R, Lin B. Cell count ratio: new criterion of diagnostic peritoneal lavage for detection of hollow organ perforation. *J Trauma* 1998;**45**(3):540–4.

This retrospective study of 320 patients undergoing DPL over an 18-month period examines the utility of a new criterion for positivity of DPL in detecting hollow visceral perforation. The new criterion, the cell count ratio, is defined as the ratio of WBC to RBC in the lavage fluid divided by the ratio of WBC to RBC in the peripheral blood. A ratio of greater than one is considered a positive lavage result. Forty-four patients had a cell count ratio greater than or equal to one. Thirty-one of these patients were found to have a small bowel perforation at operation, eight had colon perforation, one had a diaphragmatic tear, two each had sustained pancreatic transections and liver lacerations. None of the patients with hollow visceral injury had a cell count ratio less than one. The authors conclude that the cell count ratio appears to be a sensitive and specific indicator of hollow organ perforation and that when greater than one, operation should be undertaken. A criticism of the study is that the average interval from injury to performance of the DPL was five hours and the shortest time to DPL was 1.5 hours. The authors outline in the introduction to their paper that a time lag of approximately three hours is needed to provoke an inflammatory peritoneal reaction. This leaves the question of how discriminating the cell count ratio would be if the DPL had been performed sooner following injury.

30. Federle MP, Courcoulas AP, Powell M *et al*. Blunt splenic injury in adults: clinical and CT criteria for management, with emphasis on active extravasation. *Radiology* 1998;**206**(1):137–42.

This retrospective, blinded review of 270 patients with blunt splenic injury over a five-year period was performed in order to determine the relevance of various clinical and CT criteria for the prediction of outcome in adults with splenic injuries. It concluded that ISS had the best correlation with outcome of the clinical criteria and absence of active extravasation on CT best predicted outcome of the CT criteria.

31. Federle MP, Peitzman A, Krugh J. Use of oral contrast material in abdominal trauma CT scans: is it dangerous? *J Trauma* 1995;**38**(1):51–3.

This review of 506 consecutive patients undergoing CT scanning for the evaluation of BAT utilizing 450 cc of 2.5% diatrizoate meglumine and diatrizoate sodium as the gastrointestinal contrast agent demonstrated no instances of emesis related to the CT scan and no instances of aspiration of contrast material. There was one instance of contrast material being delivered into the tracheobronchial tree by way of a NG tube, which was placed into the airway rather than the GI tract. They reported satisfactory opacification of the stomach and small intestine in all cases.

32. Hulka F, Mullins RJ, Leonardo V *et al*. Significance of peritoneal fluid as an isolated finding on abdominal computed tomographic scans in pediatric trauma patients. *J Trauma* 1998;**44**(6):1069–72.

This study is a retrospective review of abdominal CT scans obtained in the evaluation of BAT and compared to clinical course. The authors identified 24 of 259 patients with free peritoneal fluid as the only finding. They quantified the amount of fluid as small, moderate or large based on the number of anatomic spaces occupied by fluid. Sixteen patients had a small amount of fluid and only two (12%) required operation. Eight had a moderate amount of fluid and four required laparotomy. All six patients had small bowel injuries. The authors concluded that pediatric patients with free fluid in more than one anatomic space have a significant risk for small bowel injury, while patients with only a small amount of intraabdominal fluid may not require operation.

33. Kinnunen J, Kivioja A, Poussa K, Laasonen EM. Emergency CT in blunt abdominal trauma of multiple injury patients. *Acta Radiologica* 1994;**35**:319-22.

The purpose of this review of 110 hemodynamically stable BAT patients undergoing CT scanning of the abdomen was to examine the safety of omitting administration of oral contrast prior to performing the scan. No significant missed injuries were identified.

34. Meredith JW, Young JS, Bowling J, Roboussin D. Non-operative management of blunt hepatic trauma: the exception or the rule? *J Trauma* 1994;**36**(4):529–35.

The authors instituted a protocol of non-operative management of all hemodynamically stable patients with blunt hepatic injury in their institution. They reviewed all cases of blunt hepatic injury over the time course of the protocol to assess efficacy and safety. One hundred and twenty-six patients were identified with blunt hepatic injury. Twenty-four underwent immediate laparotomy without CT scanning because of hemodynamic instability (16), peritoneal signs (2), and positive DPL (2). The remaining 92 patients underwent CT scanning. Twenty of the 92 required operation for hemodynamic instability (7), peritoneal signs (6), non-hepatic injuries (5) or massive hemoperitoneum (2). Seventy-two patients were managed non-operatively (55% of all liver injuries and 78% of liver injuries identified by CT). Seventy of the 72 patients (97%) were successfully managed non-operatively. There were 11 Grade I, 28 Grade II, 16 Grade III, 10 Grade IV, and five Grade V injuries in the non-operative group. There were no instances of hemobilia, intrahepatic bilomas or abdominal abscesses encountered in the non-operative group. The authors conclude that approximately half of all blunt liver injuries, and the majority of liver injuries in patients stable enough to allow CT scanning, can be safely managed non-operatively.

35. Pachter HL, Knudson MM, Esrig B *et al*. Status of non-operative management of blunt hepatic injuries in 1995: a multicenter experience with 404 patients. *J Trauma* 1996;**40**(1):31–8.

This study is a multiinstitutional retrospective analysis of blunt hepatic trauma in the 13 participating level I trauma centers. Four hundred and four patients with blunt hepatic injury were identified at the participating trauma centers. The distribution of Grades was I: 19%, II: 31%, III: 36%, IV: 10%, V: 4%. There were two deaths (0.4%) attributable to the hepatic injury and 21 (5%) complications: hemorrhage 14 patients (only three requiring operation, and four angiographic embolization), two bilomas, three perihepatic abscesses, and two missed enteric injuries. The authors conclude that non-operative management is the treatment modality of choice in hemodynamically stable patients regardless of grade of injury. Complications are infrequent and often amenable to non-operative management. They recommend particular attention to the Grade IV and V injuries since they accounted for 66.6% of those requiring operative intervention but only 14% of the series overall.

36. Talton DS, Craig MH, Hauser CJ, Poole GV. Major gastroenteric injuries from blunt trauma. *Am Surg* 1995;**61**(1):69–73.

This study reviews 50 patients with major gastroenteric injuries sustained as the result of blunt trauma treated at the University of Mississippi from 1982 through 1993. Small bowel perforations and devascularizations were the most frequent problems. These injuries were the result of high-energy torso trauma. Most of the alert patients presented with evidence of peritoneal irritation. The authors found DPL to be more useful than CT in diagnosing these injuries.

37. Sherck J, Shatney C, Sensaki K, Selivanov V. The accuracy of computed tomography in the diagnosis of blunt small-bowel perforation. *Am J Surg* 1994; **168**:670–5.

This retrospective study calls into question the commonly held belief that CT scans are likely to miss isolated small bowel injury. The authors tracked the clinical course of 883 patients undergoing CT evaluation of BAT. Twenty-six (3%) of these patients had small bowel injury. Twenty-four of the 26 had abnormal CT scans. Twelve of the scans were diagnostic (free air, extraluminal contrast) and an additional 12 were suggestive but not diagnostic (free fluid without solid organ injury, small bowel thickening or dilatation). Overall, the authors report a sensitivity of 92%, specificity of 94%, positive predictive value of 30%, negative predictive value of 100%, and accuracy of 94% for CT in the detection of small bowel perforation. The authors conclude that in the rare instances in which intestinal perforation occurs as the result of

BAT, the CT is usually abnormal, although the abnormality may be subtle. They recommend that any unexplained abnormality on the CT signals the possibility of a small bowel perforation and the patient must be attended with vigilance or evaluated with further diagnostic tests.

38. Snyder CJ. Bowel injuries from automobile seat belts. *Am J Surg* 1972;**123**:312–6.

This older reference consists of four case reports of bowel injury resulting from BAT to restrained occupants in motor vehicle crashes. It outlines the mechanism of injury and physical findings of the seatbelt syndrome. It also provides interesting earlier references to this problem in the bibliography.

39. Taylor CR, Degutis L, Lange R *et al*. Computed tomography in the initial evaluation of hemodynamically stable patients with blunt abdominal trauma: impact of severity of injury scale and technical factors on efficacy. *J Trauma* 1998;**44**:893–901.

This retrospective report emphasizes the importance of standardized reporting of injuries and grading of injuries. The authors found a correlation between increasing grade of injury and the likelihood of surgical intervention.

40. Tsang B, Panacek EA, Brant WE, Wisner D. Effect of oral contrast administration for abdominal computed tomography in the evaluation of acute blunt trauma. *Ann Emerg Med* 1997;**30**:7–13.

This retrospective review was undertaken to evaluate the necessity of administration of oral contrast in the assessment of patients with BAT. Blunt trauma victims over a five-year period were identified from the trauma registry. Hospital records and CT scans were reviewed for all patients sustaining intestinal/ mesenteric and pancreatic injuries. Randomly selected cases of splenic, hepatic, and no intraabdominal injury were also reviewed. The oral contrast was not found to be essential in the diagnosis of any of the splenic or hepatic injuries. The oral contrast was deemed essential in the radiographic diagnosis of one pancreatic injury, which was found to be a false positive at operation. The only pancreatic injury requiring operation was missed by CT. There was no oral contrast specific finding found in any of the intestinal/mesenteric injuries. Administration of the contrast material required placement of a NG tube in 21% of patients, 23% of patients vomited the contrast material, and one had a documented aspiration of oral contrast. Administration of contrast added approximately 144 minutes to the time required to obtain the CT. The authors conclude that oral contrast is rarely essential for the CT diagnosis of intraabdominal injury, represents an aspiration risk, and prolongs evaluation time.

**Blunt abdominal trauma**

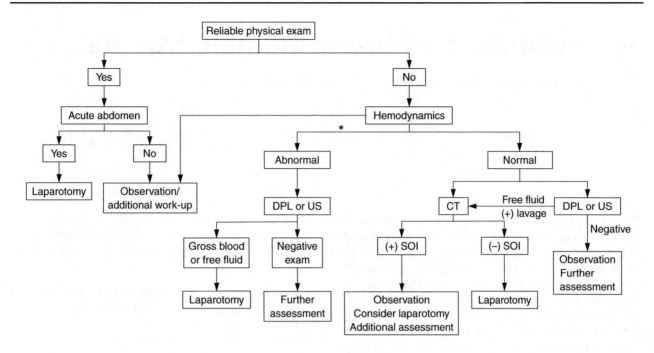

* Immediate laparotomy is indicated for the patient with obvious blunt abdominal trauma along with significant and sustained hemodynamic lability.

# 7 Evaluation of blunt thoracic trauma

*Lena M Napolitano, Thomas Genuit, Aurelio Rodriguez*

Thoracic injuries account for about 30% of admissions in trauma centers and are due to blunt trauma in almost 70% of the cases.[1–5] The in-hospital mortality is 4–8% for isolated thoracic trauma and 35% for multiple trauma. Few patients with blunt thoracic trauma require emergency surgery, most often due to severe intrathoracic blood loss, although delayed surgery may be necessary after more accurate diagnostic investigations. While the overall survival rate of thoracic trauma patients largely depends on the development of posttraumatic complications (partly due to the high incidence of significant associated injuries), the early survival rate depends on the initial resuscitation and the timeliness and correct sequence of diagnostic investigations.

Blunt thoracic trauma is suggested by the history:

- mechanism of injury consistent with rapid deceleration or direct thoracic impact (i.e. high speed motor vehicle crash (majority of patients), ejection from a vehicle, pedestrian struck, fall from a great height, assault)
- patient complaint of chest wall pain, shortness of breath or dyspnea.

Blunt thoracic trauma can be classified into the following:

- chest wall injuries (rib fractures, flail chest, sternal fracture, clavicle fracture, scapular fracture)
- pulmonary injuries (pulmonary contusion or laceration, hemothorax, pneumothorax, tracheobronchial disruption)
- cardiovascular injuries (myocardial contusion, cardiac rupture/tamponade, aortic or other great vessel disruption)
- esophageal injuries (uncommon)
- thoracic spine injuries.

Chest wall and pulmonary injuries are most common, with pulmonary contusion reported in 30–75% of patients, and pneumothorax in 15–50% of patients.

## Physical examination

Blunt thoracic trauma is also suggested by the following:

- external evidence of chest trauma (i.e. steering wheel or seatbelt imprint, chest wall contusion or subcutaneous emphysema)
- chest wall tenderness on examination
- chest wall retractions or decreased chest wall excursion
- palpable rib fractures with or without flail chest segment
- palpable fractures of the sternum, clavicle or scapula
- absent or diminished breath sounds over one or both hemithoraces, coarse rhonci (pulmonary contusion)
- dyspnea or tachypnea
- hemoptysis
- tracheal deviation (signifying tension pneumothorax or hemothorax)
- distended neck veins (from tension pneumothorax or cardiac tamponade)
- hypotension and tachycardia (due to mediastinal shift from tension pneumothorax, blood loss from massive hemothorax, myocardial contusion or cardiac tamponade).

## Hemodynamically unstable patient

Defined as hypotension (SBP <90), tachycardia, base deficit, lactic acidosis, unexplained fall in hemoglobin, and significant fluid requirement to maintain stability.

## Abnormal chest X-ray

(1) Subcutaneous emphysema
(2) Rib fractures

(3) Clavicle fracture
(4) Sternal fracture
(5) Pneumothorax
(6) Hemothorax, pleural effusion
(7) Pulmonary contusion
(8) Mediastinal air
(9) Widened mediastinum:
   - Measured width greater than 8 cm
   - Mediastinal/chest width ratio >0.25
   - Physician impression that mediastinum is widened
(10) Signs suggestive of aortic injury (see Chapter 8)
(11) Abnormal hemidiaphragm (suggesting diaphragmatic rupture):
   - intrathoracic hollow viscus or NG tube
   - elevated hemidiaphragm
   - pleural effusion/hemothorax
   - air–fluid levels or unusual shadows above the diaphragm
   - mediastinal shift away from the injury
   - plate-like atelectasis or "contusion" above an indistinct diaphragm (loss of diaphragmatic contour).

Initial management of the patient with significant thoracic trauma is often guided by the initial trauma AP chest X-ray as a screening tool.[6,7] Sensitivity and specificity for detecting the various potential injuries are far from 100% and depend largely on the quality of the film and experience of the physician providing the radiologic interpretation. Subtle abnormalities in the initial chest film should not be overlooked, but should prompt the consultation of a staff radiologist and/or initiate further investigations.

## Upright or reverse Trendelenburg chest X-ray

When obtaining these X-rays:

(1) place X-ray plate directly between patient and backboard
(2) instruct patient to hold breath or obtain film during maximal inspiration for mechanically ventilated patients
(3) with upright film, elevate head of bed to >10° forward.

## Abnormal ECG

- Dysrhythmias (atrial or ventricular)
- ST-T wave abnormalities
- Conduction disturbances

## Myocardial injury

The initial ECG remains the best screening test for potential cardiac complications from blunt myocardial injury.[8–16] There is controversy as to whether patients should be monitored with telemetry or repeat ECGs, and the optimal duration of monitoring.[13,16] The use of echocardiography (transthoracic or transesophageal)[17–19] can aid in the evaluation of unstable patients to detect cardiac rupture/pericardial tamponade, valvular lesions and wall motion abnormalities due to significant blunt myocardial injury and to reevaluate patients who develop hemodynamic instability after initial ECG or troponin I abnormalities.

Troponin I determination is a more specific indicator than CK-MB of blunt myocardial injury but has little predictive value for the development of complications or need for hospitalization.[20–25] Troponin T measurement has little utility in the diagnosis of blunt myocardial injury.

## Mediastinal abnormality

Air in the mediastinum is not uncommon after trauma to the chest. It can reflect injury to the lung parenchyma, the tracheobronchial tree or thoracic esophagus, but can also dissect caudally from an injury in the head or neck. Findings on chest radiograph can be subtle (sharp outline of the descending aorta, continuous diaphragm sign). Dynamic CT scanning is much more sensitive for the detection of small amounts of air and blood and should be performed whenever there is doubt about the presence of injury in hemodynamically stable patients.[26–35]

## Pulmonary abnormality

Isolated mild pulmonary contusion in healthy patients is not associated with increased mortality but more extensive contusion is a major cause of respiratory failure with blunt chest trauma.[36–47] Factors predicting poor outcome (prolonged hospitalization, mechanical ventilation, infectious and other complications, and death) include the need for chest tube drainage, multiple rib fractures and, most importantly, hypoxia ($PaO_2$ <70, $PaO_2/FiO_2$ <250).[36] Early aggressive pulmonary toilet, supplemental oxygen, and adequate analgesia are important to improve outcome. Quantifying the extent of injury with CT scan and differentiation of contusion from laceration might prove helpful in predicting outcome and need for more aggressive support.[38,39,46] Emergency thoracotomy with lung resection following trauma is associated with high morbidity and mortality rates (10–33%).[40,41,43,44]

## Bony abnormality

Sternal fractures are not associated with an increased incidence of visceral thoracic injury. Sternal fractures occur most often in motor vehicle occupants and are associated more frequently with older age, female gender, and thoracic vertebral fractures (flexion type injury, not associated with an increased incidence of spinal cord injuries).[48,49]

Isolated clavicle, scapula, and upper rib fractures are seldom of clinical importance but in the context of the injury mechanism reflect a significant impact (especially in adult patients). Fractures involving the thoracic outlet may cause injuries to the brachial plexus and adjacent vascular structures in up to 15% of patients. Apical extrapleural hematomas may reflect these fractures or vascular injury.

Flail chest is one of the most serious injuries seen with blunt trauma. The reason for the high associated morbidity is the severe impairment of chest wall function (impaired ventilation, increased work of breathing), the presence of significant parenchymal injury, and the high occurrence rate of other serious injuries. A significant portion of flail chest injuries are not evident during the first several hours and the underlying injury may be underestimated. Multiple rib fractures can be the source of significant blood loss. Pain control is of great importance.

Lower rib fractures should prompt the search for abdominal visceral injury.

## Diaphragmatic abnormality

Diaphragmatic injuries occur in less than 5% of major blunt truncal trauma.[50–57] There is no gold standard for early and reliable diagnosis of traumatic diaphragmatic rupture (TDR).[50] Uniform diagnosis depends on a high index of suspicion, careful interpretation of subtle signs on chest radiographs ($\geq$80% abnormalities, $\leq$50% diagnostic), and utilization of additional diagnostic modalities, including repeat chest X-rays, CT scans, MRI, and thoracoscopy or laparoscopy.[51,54,55] While most TDR occur on the left side, it is especially the right-sided lesions that are difficult to diagnose and positive pressure ventilation can make the diagnosis more difficult. There is a high incidence ($\geq$80%) of significant associated injuries (craniofacial, truncal, and/or extremity injuries) with TDR, which may contribute to the significant mortality of 15–40%. Laparotomy, laparoscopy and thoracoscopy can be used for definitive diagnosis and surgical repair.[52,53,56]

## Class I references

8. Maenza RL, Seaberg D, DiAmico F. A meta-analysis of blunt cardiac trauma: ending myocardial confusion. *Am J Emerg Med* 1996;**14**:237.

   Meta-analysis in 2210 prospective patients and 2471 retrospective patients with possible blunt myocardial injury. Abnormal ECG correlated with complications; odds ratios = 3.2 and 26.0 (prospective and retrospective data); normal ECG correlated with the lack of complications.

## Class II references

3. Dubinsky I, Low A. Non-life-threatening blunt chest trauma: appropriate investigation and treatment. *Am J Emerg Med* 1997;**15**(3):240–3.

   Prospective study of 69 adult patients (after exclusions), seen with non-life threatening blunt chest trauma in a community-based ED and followed up one week after injury. No specific clinical features (chest wall pain, local tenderness, cough, hemoptysis, shortness of breath) had a sufficient positive predictive value to warrant their use as screening tools for further investigations. All abnormalities detected on initial CXR were rib fractures. On follow-up, new findings were detected in five patients (10%); these were all minor (pleural reaction, rib fracture, atelectasis, small consolidation) and required no specific therapy. Routine use of radiologic investigations and follow-up is costly and not warranted in non-life threatening blunt chest trauma.

4. Kalyanaraman R, De Mello WF, Ravishankar M. Management of chest injuries: a 5 year retrospective survey. *Injury* 1998;**29**(6);443–6.

   Five-year retrospective review of 181 patients admitted with blunt (145) and penetrating (36) injuries to the chest. The patients were evaluated and treated according to a standardized protocol. Frequency and distribution for chest and associated injuries, as well as for the use of treatment modalities, are described.

5. Inci I, Ozcelik C, Nizam O, Eren N. Thoracic trauma in the elderly. *Eur J Emerg Med* 1998;**5**(4):445–50.

   Retrospective study of 101 patients over the age of 60 with thoracic trauma, admitted over a six-year period. The epidemiology of thoracic trauma is discussed. Morbidity and mortality rates are related to injury severity scores. Elderly patients with ISS of >25 had a mortality of >70%.

6. Hehir MD, Hollands MJ, Deane SA. The accuracy of the first chest X-ray in the trauma patient. *Aust NZ J Surg* 1990;**60**;529.

   This study documented that 27 of 94 patients had serious injuries missed on the initial CXR. These included pneumothoraces, hemothoraces, injuries to the great vessels, and sternal or thoracic vertebral fractures. The erect AP CXR had a sensitivity of 79% for detecting serious injuries, whereas the supine CXR had a sensitivity of 58%.

9. Fildes JF, Betlej TM, Mangliano R *et al*. Limiting cardiac evaluations in patients with suspected myocardial contusion. *Am Surg* 1995;**61**:832.

Prospective study in 93 patients. All patients with normal initial ECG did not develop cardiac complications.

10. Cachecho R, Grindlinger GA, Lee VW. The clinical significance of myocardial contusion. *J Trauma* 1992; **33**:68.

Prospective study in 336 patients with suspected myocardial contusion. No cardiac complications in those admitted for abnormal initial ECG or mechanism; all 19 complications occurred in patients >60 years old or with otherwise significant chest injury (i.e. four rib fractures, pulmonary contusion, flail chest, major vascular injury or severe associated injuries).

11. Gunnar WP, Martin M, Smith RF *et al*. The utility of cardiac evaluation in the hemodynamically stable patient with suspected myocardial contusion. *Am Surg* 1991;**57**:373.

Prospective study in 123 patients which documented that ECG did not correlate well with cardiac complications or abnormal myocardial nuclear medicine study.

12. Illig KA, Swierzewski MJ, Feliciano DV *et al*. A rational screening and treatment strategy based on electrocardiogram alone for suspected cardiac contusion. *Am J Surg* 1991;**162**:537.

Retrospective study in 133 patients admitted to two institutions with a clinical suspicion for myocardial contusion. Thirteen patients (9.7%) developed cardiac complications; no patient with a normal ED ECG developed a cardiac complication.

13. Miller FB, Shumate CR, Richardson JD. Myocardial contusion: when can the diagnosis be eliminated? *Arch Surg* 1989;**124**:805.

Only four of 172 patients with suspected blunt myocardial injury had dysrhythmias requiring treatment. All four patients had abnormal initial ED ECGs.

14. Soliman MH, Waxman K. Value of a conventional approach to the diagnosis of traumatic cardiac contusion after chest injury. *Crit Care Med* 1987;**15**:218.

Retrospective study in 104 patients documented that ECG did not predict complications that occurred in 23% of patients.

16. Wisner DH, Reed WH, Riddick RS. Suspected myocardial contusion: triage and indications for monitoring. *Ann Surg* 1990;**212**:82.

Retrospective study in 95 patients. Conduction abnormalities on initial ECG predicted serious arrhythmias.

17. Weiss RL, Brier JA, O'Connor W *et al*. The usefulness of transesophageal echocardiography in diagnosing cardiac contusions. *Chest* 1996;**109**(1):73–7.

This is a retrospective review over a 30-month period of 81 transesophageal echocardiographic examinations (TEE) in blunt trauma patients, of which 22 patients were diagnosed as having cardiac contusions. Right ventricular contusions (n = 15) were more common than left ventricular contusions (n = 7), and two patients had both ventricles involved. Corresponding ECGs were non-diagnostic in 73% of these patients with cardiac contusions. There were no complications related to the TEEs. Cardiac contusion patients had an average ISS of 27 and a mortality of 27% compared with the overall trauma group with an average ISS of 33 and a mortality of 9% (P < 0.001). Cardiac contusion diagnosed by TEE in blunt trauma patients carries a high mortality rate.

18. Ognibene A, Mori F, Santoni R *et al*. Cardiac troponin I in myocardial contusion. *Clin Chem* 1998;**44**:889.

Prospective study in 28 patients, five of whom had myocardial contusion diagnosed by TEE, reported 100% sensitivity and specificity of elevated serum troponin I for TEE-documented myocardial contusion.

19. Helling TS, Duke P, Beggs CW *et al*. A prospective evaluation of 68 patients suffering blunt chest trauma for evidence of cardiac injury. *J Trauma* 1989; **29**:61.

Prospective study in 68 patients; 54% of patients with echocardiographic abnormalities after blunt myocardial injury had abnormal ECGs, but the remaining 46% of patients did not. The majority (49%) of the abnormalities were non-specific ST-segment depression and T-wave changes and the rest constituted conduction abnormalities, axis deviation, and dysrhythmias.

20. Adams JE, Davila-Roman VG, Bessey PQ *et al*. Improved detection of cardiac contusion with cardiac troponin I. *Am Heart J* 1996;**131**:308–12.

A prospective study in patients (n = 44) with acute blunt chest wall trauma enrolled within 24 hours of injury and no prior history of cardiac disease. Immediately after admission all patients underwent an ECG and echocardiogram; serial blood samples were obtained for CK, CK-MB, and cTnI every six hours for the first 24 hours, then daily for up to three days. Patients with abnormal echocardiograms underwent serial echocardiograms before discharge. Six patients had evidence of cardiac injury by echo; all had elevations of CK-MB and CTnI. Twenty-six of the 37 patients without contusion had elevations of CK-MB; none had elevations of CTnI. A CK-MB/CK ratio >5% improved specificity at the expense of sensitivity. Measurement of cTnI was a more accurate indicator of cardiac injury in patients with blunt chest trauma.

21. Biffl WL, Moore FA, Moore EE *et al*. Cardiac enzymes are irrelevant in the patient with suspected myocardial contusion. *Am J Surg* 1994;**168**:523.

Retrospective study in 359 patients with possible blunt cardiac injury. Seventeen of 107 patients with contusion developed complications requiring treatment. Only two of 17 patients had an initial ECG that was abnormal; three had sinus tachycardia.

22. Ferjani M, Droc G, Dreus S *et al*. Circulating cardiac troponin T in myocardial contusion. *Chest* 1997; **111**(2):427–33.

Prospective study in 128 patients with blunt trauma to investigate the validity of cardiac troponin T measurement in the diagnosis of myocardial contusion. Patients also had echocardiography and continuous Holter monitoring performed. Myocardial contusion was diagnosed in patients who fulfilled one of the following criteria: (1) an abnormal echocardiograph compatible with myocardial contusion; (2) severe cardiac rhythm abnormalities; (3) severe cardiac conduction abnormalities; and (4) hemopericardium. Myocardial contusion was diagnosed in 29 patients. An elevated cardiac troponin T concentration $(0.5 \mu g/l)$ was more accurate than MB fraction of creatine kinase (CK-MB) and CK-MB/CK ratio in the diagnosis of myocardial contusion but this improvement was not clinically acceptable (sensitivity 0.31; specificity 0.91).

23. Fulda GJ, Gilberson F, Hailstone D *et al*. An evaluation of serum troponin T and signal-averaged electrocardiography in predicting electrocardiographic abnormalities after blunt chest trauma. *J Trauma* 1997; **43**:304.

Another prospective study of troponin T in 71 patients determined 27% sensitivity and 92% specificity of elevated troponin T for predicting clinically significant ECG abnormalities. Only 20 patients in this study had or developed a clinically significant ECG abnormality.

24. Swaaneburg JC, Klaase JM, DeJongste MJL *et al*. Troponin I, troponin T, CKMB activity and CKMB mass as markers for the detection of myocardial contusion in patients who experienced blunt trauma. *Clin Chim Acta* 1998;**272**:171–81.

Prospective study in 89 patients with blunt trauma (38 patients with thoracic injuries and 51 patients without thoracic injuries – normal ECG, normal CXR, no obvious external chest injury, and no complaints of chest pain). All parameters were measured on admission and 24 hours later. CK-MB activity, mass, and ratio were not useful for the detection of myocardial contusion, whereas troponin I and T were equally accurate and more reliable than the other biochemical markers.

26. Blostein PA, Hodgman CG. Computed tomography of the chest in blunt thoracic trauma: results of a prospective study. *J Trauma* 1997;**43**(1):13–18.

Prospective study which evaluated 40 patients (pediatric and adult) with a clinical history of blunt trauma to the chest by thoracic CT when one or more of the following nine criteria were present:

(1) age >1 with more than three rib fractures (falls from heights of less than 10 feet excluded)
(2) age ≥60 with more than two rib fractures (falls from heights of less than 10 feet excluded)
(3) multiple rib fractures with a flail chest
(4) first or second rib fractures with a major deceleration mechanism of injury
(5) plain CXR evidence of pulmonary contusion with abnormal ABG $(PaO_2/FiO_2 <300)$
(6) abnormal mediastinum on CXR with a normal aortogram or unlikely mechanism of injury for aortic rupture
(7) persistence of gross blood via endotracheal tube after adequate suctioning
(8) extensive subcutaneous emphysema without visible pneumothorax on plain CXR
(9) COPD, asthma, obesity (>50% above ideal body weight) or >30 pack per year smoking history with a forced vital capacity on hand-held spirometry <10 cc/kg of ideal body weight.

Thoracic CT detected 76 injuries not found on plain CXR, yet only six patients had therapy changes based on these findings. Routine thoracic CT in blunt trauma is not recommended.

27. Nelson JB, Bresticker MA, Nahrwold CL. Computed tomography in the initial evaluation of patients with blunt trauma. *J Trauma* 1992;**33**(5):722–7.

Retrospective study of 266 of 374 consecutive blunt trauma patients who underwent emergency CT evaluation. Thoracic CT was performed in 26 patients and 10 (38%) were interpreted as abnormal. Thoracic CT provided information about extent of injury but did not alter the initial management of any patient. Therefore thoracic CT is rarely indicated in the acute evaluation of trauma patients.

28. Poole GV, Morgan DB, Cranston PE *et al*. Computed tomography in the management of blunt thoracic trauma. *J Trauma* 1993;**35**(2):296–302.

Prospective study in 67 patients with blunt thoracic trauma, hemodynamically stable, age 18 years, with an estimated AIS thorax score of 2 who underwent a contrast-enhanced thoracic CT. CXR was superior to thoracic CT in identifying rib fractures, but CT was more sensitive than CXR for pneumothorax, fluid collections, and infiltrates $(P < 0.001)$. However, most of these abnormalities had no clinical significance and infrequently led to a change in management.

29. Trupka A, Waydhas C, Hallfeldt KKJ *et al*. Value of thoracic computed tomography in the first assessment of severely injured patients with blunt chest trauma: results of a prospective study. *J Trauma* 1997; **43**(3):405–12.

Prospective study to evaluate whether early thoracic CT is superior to CXR in the diagnostic work-up of blunt thoracic trauma. This study included 103 patients with clinical or radiologic signs of chest trauma (94 multiple injured patients with chest trauma, nine patients with isolated chest trauma) with an average ISS of 30. In 67 patients (65%) thoracic CT detected major chest trauma complications that were missed on CXR (lung contusion, n = 33; pneumothorax, n = 27; residual pneumothorax after chest tube placement, n = 7; hemothorax, n = 21; displaced chest tube, n = 5; diaphragmatic rupture, n = 2; myocardial rupture, n = 1). Thoracic CT was significantly more effective than CXR in detection of lung contusions (P < 0.001), pneumothorax (P < 0.005), and hemothorax (P < 0.05). In 42 patients (41%) the additional thoracic CT findings resulted in a change of therapy. Compared with a historical group of trauma patients that did not undergo thoracic CT, the incidence of respiratory failure and the mortality rate were significantly reduced. The authors conclude that thoracic CT is highly sensitive in the early diagnosis of blunt chest trauma and superior to CXR, and the additional information is useful in the management of major multiple trauma with an ISS >20.

35. Demetriades D, Gomez H, Velmaho GC *et al.* Routine helical computed tomographic evaluation of the mediastinum in high-risk blunt trauma patients. *Arch Surg* 1998;**133**:1084–8.

Prospective one-year study in 112 patients with high-speed deceleration injuries who required CT evaluation of the head or abdomen and underwent helical evaluation of the mediastinum irrespective of the chest radiographic findings. CT scan was diagnostic for aortic injury in eight of nine patients and was suggestive of injury but not diagnostic in one patient with brachiocephalic artery injury. CXR revealed a widened mediastinum in 42 patients (37.5%) and aortic rupture was diagnosed in only five of these patients (11.9%). CT scan is far superior to CXR in evaluation of the mediastinum for blunt aortic injury and angiography should be reserved for patients whose CT scan is indeterminate.

36. Hoff SJ, Shotts SD, Eddy VA, Morris JA Jr. Outcome of isolated pulmonary contusion in blunt trauma patients. *Am Surg* 1994;**60**:138–42.

Retrospective study in 94 adult patients, age 16–49, ISS < 25, with isolated pulmonary contusion by CXR. Variables of poor outcome are examined. Isolated pulmonary contusion is not associated with increased mortality (no deaths in this series). Although contusion on admission CXR (64%), >3 rib fractures (27%), and need for tube thoracostomy (44%) are predictors of poor outcome in univariant analysis, only hypoxia ($PO_2$ <70, $PaO_2/FiO_2$ <250) on admission (21%) remains significant on multivariant analysis. Although 16% needed initial intubation, most patients were extubated after 48 hours. Infectious complications are frequent and necessitate early aggressive pulmonary toilet.

37. Sariego J, Brown JL, Matsumoto T, Kerstein MD. Predictors of pulmonary complications in blunt chest trauma. *Int Surg* 1993;**78**:320–3.

Retrospective one-year study of 98 patients admitted to a level I trauma center with the principal diagnosis of blunt chest trauma; 49% developed pulmonary complications. Of these, 39.6% had immediate complications alone (hemothorax, pneumothorax, ruptured diaphragm present on admission), 20.8% had delayed complications alone (pulmonary contusion, pneumonia, pulmonary embolus developed after 24 hours), and 39.4% had both. TS and ISS predicted mortality but not the occurrence of these complications, gender did not predict mortality or the development of complications, and age >50 years was associated with higher mortality but not higher pulmonary complication rate.

38. Eun-Young Kang, Muller N. CT in blunt chest trauma: pulmonary, tracheobronchial and diaphragmatic injuries. *Semin Ultrasound CT MRI* 1996;**17**(2):114–18.

Review of CT findings in pulmonary contusion, laceration, tracheobronchial and diaphragmatic injury. CT is superior in the diagnosis of these injuries.

39. Wolfman NT, Myers WS, Glauser SJ *et al.* Validity of CT classification on management of occult pneumothorax: a prospective study. *Am J Roentgenol* 1998;**171**:1317–20.

Prospective study in 44 patients with occult pneumothorax (visualized on abdominal CT images of the lower thorax, not detected on CXR) who were classified into three groups: minuscule, anterior or anterolateral according to size and location. Of 36 occult pneumothoraces initially managed with observation, 24 did not require further intervention and 12 required tube thoracostomy. All eight patients with anterolateral pneumothoraces underwent tube thoracostomy. Most small occult pneumothoraces can successfully be managed with close observation.

48. Hills MW, Delprado AM, Deane SA. Sternal fractures: associated injuries and management. *J Trauma* 1993;**35**(1):55–60.

Prospective study of 172 consecutive trauma patients with sternal fractures (of 12 618 total trauma admissions) admitted over a six-year period. Overall, 1.36% of the trauma patient population had sternal fractures; 17.6% of the total trauma patient population were motor vehicle occupants, compared to 89% of patients with sternal fractures. Compared to patients without sternal fracture, significantly more patients with sternal fracture were female (37.4% versus 55%), older (30.5 versus 50.6 years), had a lower ISS (median 5 versus 13), a lower mortality (6.56% versus 2.63%), and wore their seatbelts more often

(39.5% versus 70.4%). There was no association between sternal fractures and serious chest visceral injuries (including myocardial contusion and traumatic aortic rupture). There was an association with thoracic spine fractures, but not with fractures elsewhere in the spine or with cord injuries. There were no deaths associated with the occurrence of sternal fractures *per se*. A specific work-up is not indicated but the question of how best to evaluate and monitor for possible blunt myocardia injury remains open.

50. Guth A, Pachter HL, Kim U. Pitfalls in the diagnosis of blunt diaphragmatic injury. *Am J Surg* 1995;**170**:5-9.

    Retrospective review of hospital records and radiographs of patients with blunt diaphragmatic rupture over 18 years (57 patients/11 500 trauma admissions). In 12% the injury was missed initially and the diagnosis delayed from 48 hours to three months. Only 66% of the injuries diagnosed <24 hours were detected on CXR; 22% were found on laparotomy. Fifteen per cent of the patients had a normal CXR overall; this reduced to 4% in isolated left-sided hernias. Eighty-nine per cent of the patients had significant other injuries. DPL was considered unreliable and CT scan was not utilized in sufficient numbers to allow analysis. A brief review of other diagnostic modalities is made.

## Class III references

1. Demling RH, Pomfret EA. Blunt chest trauma. *New Horizons* 1993;**1**:402–21.

   Comprehensive review.

2. Greenberg MD, Rosen CL. Evaluation of the patient with blunt chest trauma: an evidence based approach. *Emerg Med Clin North Am* 1999;**17**(1):41–62.

   Comprehensive review.

7. McLellan BA, Ali J, Towers MJ, Sharkey PW. Role of the trauma-room chest X-ray film in assessing the patient with severe blunt traumatic injury. *Can J Surg* 1996;**39**(1);36–41.

   Retrospective study over two years looking at 37 patients admitted after blunt trauma, who had an admission AP chest X-ray (but no further radiologic or surgical investigation regarding potential chest injuries), who died within 24 hours and had a post-mortem examination performed. In 30% (11 of 37 patients) there was a discrepancy between the injuries diagnosed by the trauma team, the staff radiologist reviewing the chest X-rays (blinded), and the findings on autopsy. None of the missed injuries contributed to the death of the patient.

15. van Wijngaarden MH, Karmy-Jones R, Talwar MK, Simonetti V. Blunt cardiac injury: a 10-year institutional review. *Injury* 1997;**28**(1):51–5.

    A retrospective review of all blunt cardiac injuries (n = 70) at a single institution. The majority of patients were diagnosed on the basis of elevated CK-MB, ST/T wave changes on ECG or arrhythmias. CK-MB elevation was not predictive of arrhythmias, cardiac complications, inotrope requirements or mortality. Cardiac complications requiring treatment occurred in 26% of patients. Only three of 10 deaths were directly attributable to the cardiac injury.

25. Fenton J, Myers ML, Lane P, Casson AG. Blunt cardiac trauma: survival after bichamber rupture. *Ann Thorac Surg* 1993;**55**:1256–7.

    Case report of a 38-year-old male unrestrained passenger in a motor vehicle accident who underwent intubation and bilateral chest tube placement for pneumohemothorax. He had ongoing blood loss from the right chest after initial drainage of 1500 cc hemothorax. After transport to the regional trauma center he underwent CT of head, chest, and abdomen since he was hemodynamically stable. Chest CT revealed bilateral hemothoraces, considerably larger on the right side, and he underwent right posterolateral thoracotomy for drainage of approximately 2000 cc of blood. Pericardial and cardiac lacerations were identified and the right atrial and ventricular injuries were repaired. A total of 25 units of blood (15 units autotransfused) were administered and the patient survived without complication.

30. Beal SL, Pottmeyer EW, Spisso JM. Esophageal perforation following external blunt trauma. *J Trauma* 1998;**28**(10):1425–32.

    Report of five cases and review of literature since 1900 (total of 96 cases). The cervical and upper esophagus was most often involved, a delay in diagnosis was reported in 2/3 of the cases, and a 38% infectious complication rate is related to the delay in diagnosis.

31. Cohn HE, Hubbard A, Patton G. Management of esophageal injuries. *Ann Thorac Surg* 1989;**48**(2):309–14.

    A multiinstitutional study of 39 esophageal injuries treated between 1982 and 1988 and literature review. Prompt diagnosis and aggressive surgical management are reported to improve outcome and lower mortality.

32. Flowers JL, Graham SM, Ugarte MA *et al*. Flexible endoscopy for the diagnosis of esophageal trauma. *J Trauma* 1996;**40**(2):261–5.

    Retrospective analysis of flexible endoscopy performed on 31 patients over four years (24 penetrating, seven blunt). The sensitivity of flexible endoscopy for detecting esophageal injury is reported as 100%, with a specificity of 96% and a diagnostic accuracy of 97%. No complications are reported after esophagoscopy.

33. Shanmuganathan K, Mirvis SE. Imaging diagnosis of nonaortic thoracic injury. *Radiol Clin North Am* 1999;**37**(3):533–55.

    Comprehensive review.

34. Simon RJ, Ivatury RR. Current concepts in the use of cavitary endoscopy in the evaluation and treatment of blunt and penetrating truncal injuries. *Surg Clin North Am* 1995;**75**(2):157–74.
    Comprehensive review.

40. Baumgartner F, Omari B, Lee J *et al.* Survival after trauma pneumonectomy: the pathophysiologic balance of shock resuscitation with right heart failure. *Am Surg* 1996;**62**(11):967–72.
    Retrospective series of nine patients who underwent emergency pneumonectomy for trauma; only two patients survived. Three patients initially survived the surgery but died postoperatively of hypoxemia and right heart failure. Careful attention to preventing volume overloading before and during trauma pneumonectomy may contribute to survival in these patients.

41. Inoue H, Suzuki I, Iwasaki M *et al.* Selective exclusion of the injured lung. *J Trauma* 1993;**34**(4):496–8.
    Retrospective review of 206 consecutive patients over a five-year period with blunt pulmonary trauma who survived five hours or more. In 190 patients (92%) intratracheal bleeding, intrapleural air leakage, and intrapleural bleeding were controllable by conventional therapy, including endobronchial toilet, mechanical ventilation, and tube thoracostomy. In six patients (3%), bleeding and air leaks were controllable by selective pulmonary exclusion using an endotracheal tube with a moveable bronchial occlusion cuff (Univent), avoiding the need for thoracotomy. In 10 patients (5%), thoracotomy was required because of uncontrollable bleeding or air leakage despite selective pulmonary exclusion.

42. Karmy-Jones R, Vallieres E, Kralovich K *et al.* A comparison of rigid versus video thoracoscopy in the management of chest trauma. *Injury* 1998;**29**(9):655–9.
    Retrospective review of 44 thoracoscopic procedures performed in 42 patients following chest injuries over a four-year period. Indications included exploration in 15, retained hemothorax in 10, continued bleeding after chest tube placement in three, air leak in five, and empyema in 11. Video thoracoscopy was used in 24 cases and rigid thoracoscopy in 20. There was no difference in operative times, length of stay or incidence of complications. Rigid thoracoscopy is an effective tool that, in selected cases, increases the utility of thoracoscopy in the management of chest trauma and its complications.

43. Tominaga GT, Waxman K, Scannell G *et al.* Emergency thoracotomy with lung resection following trauma. *Am Surg* 1993;**59**:834–7.
    Over a seven-year period 9443 trauma patients were admitted; 31% (2934) had evidence of chest trauma and, of those, 12% (347) required thoracotomy and 3.5% (12 patients) required emergent pulmonary resections. An overall mortality of 33% with five non-anatomic resections, three lobectomies, and four pneumonectomies is noted. Reviewing the literature, factors potentially responsible for the improved outcomes are discussed (hilar clamping, vasodilators, inotropes).

44. Wagner JW, Obeid FN, Karmy-Jones RC *et al.* Trauma pneumonectomy revisited: the role of simultaneously stapled pneumonectomy. *J Trama* 1996;**40**(4):590–4.
    Twelve patients requiring trauma pneumonectomy were reviewed, comparing simultaneous stapled pneumonectomy versus individual ligation as the surgical method. The overall survival rate was 50% (six patients), with a mean follow-up of $6.5 \pm 1.1$ years. Five survivors were in the stapled group and only one survivor was in the individual ligation group. The stapled group had a significantly shorter operative time.

45. Lie DW, Liu HP, Lin PJ, Chang CH. Video-assisted thoracic surgery in treatment of chest trauma. *J Trauma* 1997;**42**(4):670–4.
    Retrospective study of 50 patients who were treated with VATS. In 12 patients thoracotomy was avoided using VATS. There was no associated morbidity with VATS.

46. Myung Soo Shin, Kang-Jey Ho. Computed tomography evaluation of posttraumatic pulmonary pseudocysts. *Clin Imag* 1993;**17**:189–92.
    Two cases of pulmonary pseudocyst formation after blunt chest trauma are described. The possible pathogenesis of pseudocyst development is discussed. The role of CT in the diagnosis and differentiation of other cavitary lesions of the lung is highlighted.

47. Haenel JB, Moore FA, Moore EE. Pulmonary consequences of severe chest trauma. *Respir Care Clin North Am* 1996;**2**(3):401–24.
    Comprehensive review.

49. Chiu WC, D'Ameilo LF, Hammond JS. Sternal fractures in blunt chest trauma: A practical algorithm for management. *Am J Emerg Med* 1997;**3**:252–5.
    Three-year retrospective review of 33 consecutive adult trauma patients admitted to a level I trauma center with sternal fractures. Clinical indicators drive the search for sternal injury. Most patients were hemodynamically stable and 64% had an ISS <13 and no severe associated extrathoracic injuries. An uncomplicated sternal fracture is not a marker of clinically significant myocardial injury or mediastinal injury and does not warrant extensive work-up and monitoring.

51. Leung JC, Nance ML, Schwab CW, Miller WT Jr. Thickening of the diaphragm: a new computed tomography sign of diaphragmatic injury. *J Thorac Imag* 1999;**14**(2):126–9.
    Retrospective review of imaging findings in eight patients with surgically proven traumatic diaphragmatic rupture. Thickening of the diaphragm was present in six out of eight patients.

52. Lindsey I, Woods SD, Nottle PD. Laparoscopic management of blunt diaphragmatic injury. *Aust NZ J Surg* 1997;**67**(9):619–21.

   Three case reports of management of blunt traumatic diaphragmatic hernias through laparoscopic means.

53. Martin I, O'Rourke N, Gotley D, Smithers M. Laparoscopy in the management of diaphragmatic rupture due to blunt trauma. *Aust NZ J Surg* 1998;**68**(8):584–6.

   Four case reports of diagnosis of traumatic diaphragmatic rupture using laparoscopy.

54. Spann JC, Nwariaku FE, Wait M. Evaluation of video-assisted thoracoscopic surgery in the diagnosis of diaphragmatic injuries. *Am J Surg* 1995;**170**(6):628–30.

   Prospective study on 26 hemodynamically stable patients admitted with blunt or penetrating trauma to the lower chest and upper abdomen that underwent video-assisted thoracoscopy (VATS) followed by celiotomy. VATS identified all eight patients with traumatic diaphragmatic rupture.

55. Shapiro MJ, Heiberg E, Durham M *et al*. The unreliability of CT scans and initial chest radiographs in evaluating blunt trauma induced diaphragmatic rupture. *Clin Radiol* 1996;**51**:27–30.

   Retrospective study of 20 patients with diaphragmatic rupture from blunt thoracoabdominal trauma over a five-year period. The diagnostic accuracy of CXR and CT are compared. Overall 50% (10/20) of diaphragmatic injuries were identified on initial or repeat CXR (all left sided) compared to 42% (5/12) for CT. Positive pressure ventilation significantly reduced the diagnostic accuracy to 33% (4/12) for CXR and 7% (1/7) for CT. Four out of six right-sided hernias were diagnosed in the operating room. Other diagnostic modalities of potential value are briefly discussed.

56. Shah R, Sabanathan S, Mearns AJ, Choudhury AK. Traumatic rupture of the diaphragm. *Ann Thoracic Surg* 1995;**60**(5):1444–9.

   Comprehensive review.

57. Stark P. Imaging of tracheobronchial injuries. *J Thorac Imag* 1995;**10**(3):206–19.

   Comprehensive review.

**Blunt thoracic trauma**

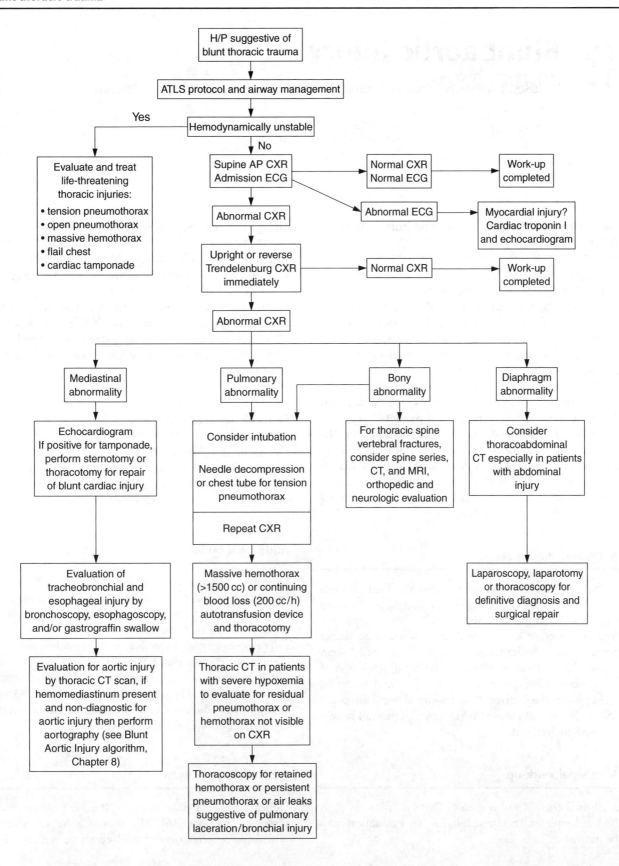

# 8 Blunt aortic injury

*W Joseph Messick, Jennifer Sarafin, Michael A Gibbs, Michael H Thomason*

## History/physical suggestive of blunt aortic injury (BAI)

A mechanism of injury which involves rapid deceleration (high-speed motor vehicle crash or fall from a height) should raise suspicion of BAI. The majority of cases of aortic disruption result from motor vehicle crashes; 24% of the motor vehicle-associated blunt aortic injuries occur from lateral impact rather than head-on impact.[1,2]

There are *no specific signs of traumatic aortic disruption* and the diagnosis cannot be reliably made or excluded clinically. Between 30% and 50% of patients have *minimal external evidence of chest trauma*. In addition, the majority of patients have more clinically impressive concomitant injuries that may detract the clinician from recognition of BAI. Pelvic fractures and thoracic spine fractures have been associated with an increased incidence of concomitant BAI.[3]

## Abnormal chest X-ray

Physician-subjective impression that the mediastinum is widened is the most important finding and occurs in up to 85% in patients with BAI.[4,5] Other suspicious findings on chest X-ray include an obscure or indistinct aortic knob,[4–8] depression of the left main stem bronchus, tracheal deviation to the right, deviation of the nasogastric tube to the right,[4,6,8–10] and widened right paratracheal stripe. Chest X-ray abnormalities are seen in 90–95% of cases of BAI, although they all have a low specificity (5–10%).

## Additional work-up

A normal chest X-ray is seen in 7% of all patients with BAI. If suspicion remains high, further evaluation may be indicated.[4]

## Upright or reverse Trendelenburg chest X-ray

Initial supine AP chest X-ray with poor inspiration often reveals a wide or indistinct mediastinum. An upright or reverse Trendelenburg chest X-ray should be obtained before pursuing further work-up. The X-ray plate should be placed directly beneath the patient and a 72-inch film obtained with the patient (or the technologist, if the patient is mechanically ventilated) holding full inspiration.

## Hemodynamically unstable

Hemodynamic instability is defined as hypotension, tachycardia, base deficit >5 (metabolic acidosis by ABG), low initial or falling hemoglobin, and/or significant fluid resuscitation requirement.

## Additional options

Unstable patients with massive hemothorax require immediate thoracotomy, with consideration of diagnostic peritoneal tap to rule out hemoperitoneum as an additional source of bleeding.

Transesophageal echo has been recommended by some as a diagnostic tool to evaluate the aortic isthmus, but it is very operator dependent.[11–20] If experienced personnel are available, it could be utilized intraoperatively during the course of emergency laparotomy for control of abdominal hemorrhage.

## Helical chest CT scan

Helical chest CT scan may be the best non-invasive screening tool for BAI. The use of a helical scanner with intravenous contrast and continuous 5 mm cuts through the aortic arch and isthmus is essential. If normal, the scan may obviate the need for aortography. Recent prospective studies have shown 100% sensitivity and very good specificity with this technique, without the need for 3D reconstructions.[6,21–23] Some thoracic surgeons will now operate for BAI based solely on the positive helical CT scan, without the added risk and time required for arch aortography.

## Abnormal aortogram

Although the current standard of care remains intra-operative control and repair of BAI,[4,7,24] reports of the use of percutaneous intraluminal stent grafts for definitive therapy have appeared in the literature.[25–28] Other reports describe expectant management of patients with proven BAI, utilizing $\beta$-blocker therapy followed by semielective operative repair or, in some cases, no operative intervention. These alternatives may become more attractive for patients with severe concomitant injuries (such as traumatic brain injury) and comorbid conditions which have a prohibitive risk for surgical repair.[29–34]

Anesthesia should be notified once the diagnosis of BAI is made by helical CT scan or aortography and operative repair is anticipated. The anesthesia team can assist with resuscitation, titration of hemodynamic parameters, and transport to the OR. Recent reports suggest use of $\beta$-blocker therapy (esmolol infusion $\pm$ nitroprusside) to reduce aortic wall stress by titrating to a lower systolic blood pressure and heart rate while maintaining adequate perfusion.[6,29,35]

## Thoracotomy

Current standard of care is urgent/emergent thoracotomy with intraoperative control and repair of BAI. Operative techniques vary (clamp and sew, shunt) and the technique employed should be the one with which the surgeon is most experienced. The most significant postoperative complications are paraplegia and acute renal failure, which are not clearly related to a given technique or cross-clamp time.[4,7]

## Work-up completed

A normal aortogram (read by an experienced radiologist or vascular surgeon)[36] effectively rules out BAI. Helical (spiral) CT of the chest, interpreted by an experienced radiologist, may become the diagnostic study of choice to rule out BAI as larger, prospective studies continue to report 100% sensitivity with no missed injuries.

## Class II references

1. Fabian TC, Richardson JD, Croce MA *et al.* Prospective study of blunt aortic injury: multicenter trial of the American Association for the Surgery of Trauma. *J Trauma* 1997;**42**:374–83.

   Although the data are retrospective, this is the best study on the topic. Obviously, a prospective, randomized study is impossible regarding this injury unless one is examining the impact of one particular diagnostic tool such as helical CT scan compared with TEE. To obtain the type of epidemiological data needed to correlate morbidity and mortality, a population-based study including autopsies on all persons who die at the scene would be required. Short of that, this study by Fabian and associates, including 50 mostly level I or II trauma centers, is the next best thing. They prospectively collected data on 274 patients with blunt aortic injury, focusing on epidemiological factors as well as the influence of timing and surgery type on outcome and morbidity such as paraplegia.

2. Feczko JD, Lynch L, Pless JE, Clark MA, McClain J, Hawley DA. An autopsy case review of 142 non-penetrating (blunt) injuries to the aorta. *J Trauma* 1992;**33**:846–9.

   These are certainly very solid data; however, an autopsy report is somewhat weak unless it includes autopsy results of all deaths in an area. This makes it a true population-based study. This report is not.

3. Ochsner MG Jr, Hoffman AP, DiPasquale D *et al.* Associated aortic rupture–pelvic fracture: an alert for orthopaedic and general surgeons. *J Trauma* 1992;**33**: 429–34.

   This retrospective study from Washington Hospital Center identified a two- to fivefold increase in the incidence of aortic rupture among patients with a pelvic fracture. Conversely 20–45% of patients with aortic rupture had associated pelvic fractures.

4. Fabian TC, Davis KA, Gavant ML *et al.* Prospective study of blunt aortic injury: helical CT is diagnostic and anti-hypertensive therapy reduces rupture. *Ann Surg* 1998;**227**:666–7.

   Helical CT screening may very well be the most reliable non-invasive screening tool that exists. It may even rival aortography, according to this study from Memphis. In this prospective study, 494 patients with possible aortic injury were evaluated with helical CT scans of the thorax. The data show that screening helical CT scan is sensitive enough to perform aortography only when the helical CT suggests aortic injury. For all study patients, sensitivity was 100% for helical CT scan compared with 92% sensitivity for aortography. Specificity was 83% for helical CT compared with 99% for aortography. Accuracy was 86% for helical CT and 97% for aortography. Negative predictive value was 100% for helical CT and 97% for aortography. No patient in this series had spontaneous aortic rupture.

5. Hunt JP, Baker CC, Lentz CW *et al.* Thoracic aorta injuries: management and outcome of 144 patients. *J Trauma* 1996;**40**:547–56.

   A prospective, randomized study to look at issues related to the treatment of patients with torn thoracic aortas would be ideal; however, this study of prospectively collected data from the North Carolina Trauma Registry combined with medical record review answers many questions. It seems to solidify some controversial issues such as shunting versus clamp and sew and whether general surgeons have outcomes as favorable as cardiovascular surgeons (they do). This is a good study with up-to-date epidemiological data.

6. Chirillo F, Totis O, Cavarzerani A *et al.* Usefulness of transthoracic and transesophageal echocardiography in recognition and management of cardiovascular injuries after blunt chest trauma. *Heart* 1996;**75**:301–6.

   This is a prospective study over three years of 134 consecutive patients. Transthoracic and transesophageal echo were compared to aortography or surgery for the detection of aortic injuries sustained from blunt trauma. Transesophageal echo was far better than transthoracic echocardiography ($P < 0.05$), with 93% sensitivity and 98% specificity.

7. Mirvis S, Shanmuganathan K, Buell J, Rodriguez A. Use of spiral computed tomography for the assessment of blunt trauma patients with potential aortic injury. *J Trauma* 1998;**45**:922–30.

   Prospective 25-month study of 1104 blunt chest trauma patients who had contrast-enhanced spiral thoracic CT performed; 118 (10.7%) had mediastinal hemorrhage detected. Direct evidence of aortic injury was detected in 24 (20.3%) of those with mediastinal hemorrhage and 2.2% of all thoracic CT scans. Results were compared with aortography (when performed) , surgery or clinical status at discharge. Based on this, spiral thoracic CT was 100% sensitive, 99.7% specific, and 99.7% accurate for the detection of BAI.

## Class III references

8. Katyal D, McLellan BA, Brenneman FD, Boulanger BR, Sharkey PQ, Waddell JP. Lateral impact motor vehicle collisions: significant cause of blunt traumatic rupture of the thoracic aorta. *J Trauma* 1997;**42**:769–72.

   This is a retrospective review undertaken to examine the relationship between direction of car impact and rupture of the thoracic aorta. Cases over five years were reviewed. Two types of databases were used: a coroner's database and two trauma registries from metropolitan cities. The results confirmed lateral impact is a significant cause of blunt aortic injury, occurring in 48/97 patients with BAI in this series. The 49% incidence of BAI in this series is the highest of any series, showing the significance of lateral impact injuries.

9. Miller FB, Richardson JD, Thomas HA, Cryer HM, Willing SJ. Role of CT in the diagnosis of major arterial trauma after blunt thoracic trauma. *Surgery* 1989;**106**:596–603.

   This is another anecdotal study that confirms clinical judgment in combination with X-ray findings (no matter how subtle) are stronger than either alone. However, lack of a wide mediastinum is again not predictive of a negative aorta. Concern about an obliteration of the aortopulmonary window seems to be the biggest issue here.

10. Mattox KL, Wall MJ. *Trauma: injury to the thoracic great vessels*, 3rd edn. Englewood Cliffs, New Jersey: Appleton and Lange, 1996.

    Good overall review; lots of opinion, some supported by the literature. Well-referenced chapters geared toward surgeons.

11. Poole GV. Fracture of the upper ribs and injury to the great vessels. *Surg Gynecol Obstet* 1989;**169**:275–82.

    This is primarily a review of multiple small series in combination with expert opinion of an experienced trauma surgeon. It is not a metaanalysis.

12. Perchinsky MJ, Long WB, Urman S, Borzatta A. The broken halo sign: a fractured calcified ring as an unusual sign of traumatic rupture of the thoracic aorta. *Injury* 1994;**25**:649–52.

    This anecdotal case report is of two elderly patients with BAI who interestingly had little else on chest X-ray but a calcified aortic ring broken in two separate places with lateral displacement of the ring (displaced by hematoma as noted on aortogram). Conversations I have had with other trauma and thoracic surgeons support this observation. This may represent a sensitive sign of BAI; however, it can serve to alert the trauma surgeon to the possibility of injury. Complete data regarding this unusual sign are missing and may only be available in a large prospective study.

13. Kearney PA, Smith DW, Johnson SB, Barker DE, Smith MD, Sapin PM. Use of transesophageal echocardiography in the evaluation of traumatic aortic injury. *J Trauma* 1993;**34**:696–703.

    Prospectively collected data comparing aortography to transesophageal echo in 69 patients. The chief significance of this paper is the false-positive aortograms and several false-positive transesophageal echoes, suggesting the two modalities might actually complement each other.

14. Vignon P, Rambaud G, Francois B, Preux PM, Lang RM, Gastinne H. Quantification of traumatic

hemomediastinum using transesophageal echo-cardiography: impact on patient management. *Chest* 1998;**113**:1475–80.

This is a case-controlled, retrospective study of 41 patients who had TEE for evaluation of BAI confirmed by another method (aortography, surgery or necropsy). Forty-one age-matched controls who underwent TEE for non-trauma purposes were compared to the study patients. Transesophageal echo had sensitivity of 80%. TEE appeared best used if hemomediastinum was present. If so, then aortography appears required regardless of the status of the aorta by the TEE reading.

15. Ahrar K, Smith DC, Bansal RC, Razzouk A, Catalano RD. Angiography in blunt thoracic aortic injury. *J Trauma* 1997;**42**:665–9.

This is a retrospective review of 89 cases of proven (by surgery or aortography) aortic injuries. Twenty per cent of patients had aortic arch branches involved and at least one patient had a proximal or ascending arch injury that, in the opinion of the radiologists, would have been missed had the TEE alone been used to assess the injury.

16. Nagy K, Fabian TC, Rodman G *et al. Guidelines for the diagnosis and management of blunt aortic injury.* Knoxville, TN: EAST Association for the Surgery of Trauma, 1998.

17. Catoire P, Orliaguet G, Liu N *et al.* Systematic transesophageal echocardiography for detection of mediastinal lesions in patients with multiple injuries. *J Trauma* 1995;**38**:96–102.

This prospective study of 70 patients evaluated 60 patients with TEE-identified abnormalities. The data confirm that TEE is useful not only for confirmatory diagnosis of BAI, but also for assisting with the diagnosis of cardiac contusion.

18. Von Segresser LK, Fischer A, Vogt P, Turina M. Diagnosis and management of blunt great vessel trauma. *J Card Surg* 1997;**12**(suppl):181–92.

This is almost entirely an opinion paper, which was written by thoughtful cardiothoracic surgeons. It is an excellent review of the strengths and weaknesses of aortography and TEE from the operating surgeon's perspective.

19. Pearson GD, Karr SS, Trachiotis GD, Midgley FM, Eichelberger MR, Martin GR. A retrospective review of the role of transesophageal echocardiography in aortic and cardiac trauma in a level I pediatric trauma center. *J Am Soc Echocardiogr* 1997; **10**:946–55.

This was a small retrospective series of patients, all children, who underwent TEE following blunt chest injury. The main thrust of the paper is the large number of cardiac and other thoracic injuries that can be detected using TEE. This paper also reminds us that thoracic aortic injuries occur in children as well as adults.

20. Mirvis SE, Kostrubiak I, Whitley NO, Goldstein LD, Rodrigues A. Role of CT in excluding major aortic injury after blunt thoracic trauma. *Am J Roentgenol* 1987;**149**:601–5.

This is a large retrospective review of 677 patients who had chest X-rays suggestive for BAI. A CT scan was done for all of these patients and reviewed retrospectively. The CT scan was very sensitive for mediastinal hemorrhage (100%) and BAI (90%) and very specific (99% mediastinal hemorrhage, 87% AI).

21. Hiatt JR, Yeatman LA Jr, Child JS. The value of echocardiography in blunt chest trauma. *J Trauma* 1988; **28**:914–22.

This is a prospective study of 73 patients with blunt chest trauma, included in this chapter because of the emphasis on the utility of echocardiography not only to diagnose BAI, but also to assess cardiac dysfunction. Fourteen patients in this series had detectable cardiac dysfunction believed severe enough to have clinical implications.

22. Fernandez LG, Lain KY, Messersmith RN *et al.* Transesophageal echocardiography for diagnosing aortic injury: a case report and summary imaging techniques. *J Trauma* 1994;**36**:877–80.

A report of one successful case and summary of current imaging techniques, as well as summary of the use of transesophageal echocardiography in the management of BAI. There is also a review of other case reports.

23. Franchello A, Olivera G, DiSumma M, Memore L, Scavarda B, Bertoldo U. Rupture of thoracic aorta resulting from blunt trauma. *Int Surg* 1997;**82**:79–84.

This is a small series of 27 consecutive patients who underwent CT scans prior to aortography for suspected BAI based on mechanism of injury or abnormal chest X-rays.

24. Scharrer-Palmler R, Gorich J, Orend KH, Sokiranski R, Sunder-Plassmann L. Emergent endoluminal repair of delayed abdominal aortic rupture after blunt trauma. *J Endovasc Surg* 1998;**5**:134–7.

A single case report of the successful placement of an endoluminal stent for traumatic rupture of the abdominal aorta in a patient with a hostile abdomen. Follow-up was two years.

25. Naude GP, Back M, Perry MO, Bongard FS. Blunt dissection of the abdominal aorta: report of a case and review of the literature. *J Vasc Surg* 1997;**25**:931–5.

Single case report of an endoluminal stent in a 71-year-old woman with traumatic rupture of the aorta following blunt trauma.

26. Vernhet H, Marty-Ane CH, Lesnik A *et al.* Dissection of the abdominal aorta in blunt trauma: management by percutaneous stent placement. *Cardiovasc Intervent Radiol* 1997;**20**:473–6.

This paper describes three patients with blunt aortic injury: one with Palmaz and two with Wallstents.

Follow-up in one patient was two years. All were successful.

27.  Ferko A, Krajina A, Jon B, Lesko M, Voboril Z, Zizka J. Dissection of the infrarenal aorta treated by stent graft placement. *Eur Radiol* 1998;**8**:298–300.

This paper describes two patients with blunt aortic injury treated successfully by stent graft placement. One patient has been followed for 16 months.

28.  Opie LH. *Drugs for the heart*, 4th edn. Philadelphia: WB Saunders, 1997.

This serves as a standard reference for cardiologists and other physicians regarding general dosing for hypertension in aortic aneurysm patients based on standard clinical community practice.

29.  Pate JW, Fabian TC, Walker W. Traumatic rupture of the aortic isthmus: an emergency? *World J Surg* 1995;**19**:119–26.

This is the best and largest review of delayed repair of blunt aortic injuries, albeit a retrospective one. All patients who died of aortic rupture did so within four hours after injury. No patients receiving anti-hypertensives died from rupture. Other operations took priority over the aortic rupture in 33 patients, confirming the belief that abdominal and other significant injuries should in fact take first priority.

30.  Hartford JM, Fayer RL, Shaver TE *et al*. Transection of the thoracic aorta: assessment of a trauma system. *Am J Surg* 1986;**151**:224–9.

This retrospective review merely examined all deaths related to hemorrhage following BAI as a gauge to assess the need for a trauma center six years prior to the writing of this paper. The study supports expeditious transfer to a level I trauma center of patients with transected aortas, since all patients taken to the non-trauma centers died. However, the data are limited and patients are not randomized. Therefore, little else can be deduced from this small study.

31.  Kalmar P, Otto C, Steinjkraus V. Blunt aortic injury: choosing appropriate time for surgery. *Langenbecks Arch Chir Suppl Kongressbd* 1991(suppl):563–70.

This is a small series of 39 patients from Europe where the practice is to delay surgery on patients with BAI for two to eight weeks after injury. This study suggests that waiting (unless pseudoaneurysm is greater than 6 cm) may reduce mortality. Their overall mortality for patients admitted to the hospital alive was 15%. This non-randomized, non-controlled study suggests that occasional waiting (e.g. for concomitant injuries to stabilize) may at least be considered.

32.  Maggisano R, Nathens A, Alexandrova NA *et al*. Traumatic rupture of the thoracic aorta: should one always operate immediately? *Ann Vasc Surg* 1995;**9**:44–52.

This retrospective Canadian study of 59 consecutive patients examined the hypothesis that there may be a selective role for delayed repair of patients with BAI, especially in patients with head trauma and pulmonary and cardiac dysfunction. The subgroup of patients who underwent operations (44 patients) delayed from one day to seven months after injury had a survival rate of 82%. Interestingly, this also includes eight patients who have yet to be operated on, all of whom are still alive. Only two patients in this subgroup died of a ruptured aorta. Both died within the first 72 hours after admission, confirming the observation reported in other series that patients who do not rupture immediately and survive past the first three days have a low incidence of spontaneous rupture if medically treated.

33.  Striffeler H, Leupi F, Kaiser G, Althaus U. Traumatic rupture of the thoracic aorta in childhood with special reference to the therapeutic strategy. *Eur J Pediatr Surg* 1993;**3**:50–3.

This European study suggests a delayed approach may be advised, especially in children with head injuries. This report is a combination of opinion, case report, and anecdotal review supporting the author's bias.

34.  Asaoka M, Sasaki M, Masumoto H, Seki A. Two cases of traumatic aneurysm of the aortic isthmus. *Nippon Kyobu Geka Gakkai Zasshi* 1995;**43**:100–3.

Yet another anecdotal presentation of a patient undergoing successful delayed repair of BAI. This Japanese report confirms European and Canadian data supporting this approach.

35.  Prater SP, Leya FS, McKiernan TL. Post-traumatic pseudoaneurysm of the ascending aorta – an incidental finding two decades later. *Clin Cardiol* 1994;**17**:566–8.

This is a fascinating case report, two decades after the injury of a patient who survived BAI to the ascending aorta. Clearly, survival following BAI is possible without early surgical intervention if the patient does not rupture freely into the pleural space. Although this patient was not managed medically, most who advocate delayed repair of BAI believe medical management for blood pressure is essential.

36.  Fisher RG, Sanchez-Torres M, Whingham CJ, Thomas JW. Lumps and bumps that mimic acute aortic and brachiocephalic vessel injury. *Radiographics* 1997;**17**:825–34.

This is a review by radiologists of anatomic variations to remind trauma surgeons and other radiologists of the pitfalls in assessing potential injuries around the aortic isthmus.

**Evaluation of blunt aortic injury**

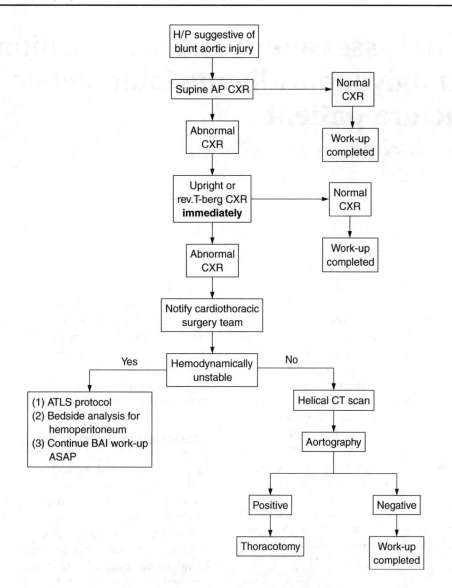

# 9 Initial assessment and stabilization of the hemodynamically unstable pelvic fracture patient

*David G Jacobs, James F Kellam, Michael A Gibbs, Kenneth A Egol*

## Introduction

The hemodynamically unstable pelvic fracture patient presents the clinician with a host of unique challenges in both diagnosis and management. In addition to the sources of life-threatening hemorrhage typically encountered in patients with blunt trauma, retroperitoneal hemorrhage from the fracture itself must also be given serious consideration. Because multiple sources may exist simultaneously in a given patient, and because hemorrhage control may require transport to the operating room or to the angiography suite, a rapid and orderly diagnostic approach is critical to achieve optimal salvage in this highly lethal patient group.[1–4] This chapter outlines the critical decisions that must be kept in mind when encountering patients with complex pelvic fractures, and provides a rationale for the priorities established in the accompanying algorithm.

## Hemodynamic instability

The failure to recognize hemodynamic instability in the multiple trauma patient is a frequent cause of morbidity and even mortality in this patient group. Systolic hypotension is a relatively late finding, and the clinician should be alert to the earlier, and often more subtle, signs such as tachycardia, significant base deficit, unexplained fall in hemoglobin and high intravenous fluid infusion rates and volumes to maintain blood pressure. If any of these adverse indicators are present in the pelvic fracture patient, immediate consultation should be obtained from general surgery and orthopaedic surgery, while aggressive resuscitative efforts are directed at stabilizing the patient's airway, breathing, and circulation. Interventional radiology, if available, should be notified in advance in the event that pelvic angiography and embolization are required. Following definitive control of hemorrhage, all pelvic fracture patients who have manifested hemodynamic instability *at any time*, should be admitted to the intensive care unit (ICU) for ongoing resuscitation and evaluation. It is particularly important to correct any abnormalities involving the "lethal triad" (coagulopathy, hypothermia, and acidosis).

## Life-threatening hemorrhage

Common causes of hemodynamic instability in the trauma patient include tension pneumothorax, and hemorrhagic shock secondary to intrathoracic, intra-abdominal, and external sources. Bleeding from the face and scalp, in particular, can be quite profuse and is often underestimated in terms of its significance. Facial hemorrhage control may require packing and occasionally direct suture ligation (particularly in the case of scalp bleeding) to effect hemostatic control. In patients with pelvic fractures, external bleeding from the pelvic region should alert the physician to the possibility of an open pelvic fracture. External bleeding in association with an open pelvic fracture can be torrential and immediately life-threatening and requires immediate attention. Under these circumstances bleeding is most efficiently controlled with vigorous gauze packing of the bleeding site and non-invasive pelvic stabilization, while definitive hemorrhage control (i.e. angiography and/or external fixation) is pursued. The diagnosis and management of life-threatening intra-abdominal hemorrhage in the context of the pelvic fracture patient is discussed below, while material relating to life-threatening thoracic injuries can be found in Chapter 7.

## Non-invasive pelvic stabilization (NIPS)

Non-invasive pelvic stabilization (NIPS) may be a useful adjunct in the early management of selected patients with pelvic fracture. By reducing mobility of the pelvic fracture fragments, patient discomfort is reduced, especially given the multiple transfers these patients frequently endure. Furthermore, limiting fracture fragment motion may also lead to decreased pelvic fracture-related arterial or venous hemorrhage, and thus contribute to the patient's overall hemodynamic stability.[5–7] NIPS is indicated in those patients whose pelvic fractures are either clinically unstable (bony pelvis is unstable on physical examination), and/or radiologically unstable (any widening of the posterior pelvic ring on the anteroposterior pelvic radiograph). Under these circumstances, NIPS can be achieved by application of any of a number of stabilizing garments. These include the MAST (Military Anti-Shock Trouser),[3] a vacuum splint, or even a standard bedsheet wrapped around the pelvis and secured anteriorly sufficiently to limit movement of the bony pelvis.[8] These techniques may be supplemented by longitudinal skeletal traction of 20–30 lbs on the involved extremity (either femoral or tibial) if an experienced orthopaedic surgeon is immediately available. If the MAST is employed, both lower extremity compartments and the abdominal compartment should be inflated to 30–40 mmHg pressure. Thorough inspection of the abdomen, pelvis, and lower extremities should be carried out prior to NIPS application to identify any sites of significant hemorrhage which must be controlled prior to patient transfer. This information must be relayed to the accepting physician, and these areas immediately reinspected upon arrival at the accepting institution, to ensure adequate and ongoing hemorrhage control.

## Prompt definitive treatment

The prompt availability of *experienced* general surgeons, orthopaedic surgeons, and interventional radiologists is mandatory to achieve optimal salvage of these critically injured patients. Ideally, the general surgeon and orthopaedic surgeon should be present upon patient arrival. Interventional angiography should be available within 30 minutes of notification. If none of these resources can be brought to bear in this time frame, the patient should be transferred to an institution of higher capability. However, if *life-threatening* intra-abdominal hemorrhage is present, and an experienced general surgeon is promptly available, emergent laparotomy should be carried out to control abdominal

cavitary hemorrhage. If life-threatening pelvic-related hemorrhage is identified at laparotomy, the extraperitoneal space of the true pelvis should be packed,[1] NIPS applied, and the patient transferred to an institution where experienced trauma surgeons, orthopaedic surgeons, and angiographers are available.

## Determining the presence of life-threatening intraabdominal hemorrhage

Determining the presence of *life-threatening* intra-abdominal hemorrhage is perhaps the most critical step in the evaluation and management of hemodynamically unstable pelvic fracture patients, as this will determine whether the patient is triaged to the operating room for emergent laparotomy, or perhaps to the radiology suite for attempted pelvic embolization. An error at this step can result in needless, non-therapeutic laparotomy (with all of its attendant morbidity and mortality), or perhaps worse, in exsanguination from controllable intraabdominal sources while undergoing ill-advised angiography. The clinician must therefore quickly determine whether there exists sufficient hemoperitoneum to be the sole cause of, or contribute significantly to, the patient's ongoing hemodynamic instability. Given the inadvisability of abdominal CT in hemodynamically unstable patients,[9] and the well-documented inaccuracy of DPL (diagnostic peritoneal lavage) in patients with pelvic fracture,[2,7,10–14] the diagnostic test of choice in this situation is the performance of a DPT (diagnostic peritoneal tap). This test should be performed using an open supraumbilical approach to reduce the chances of a false-positive aspirate. Aspiration of 5–10 cc of gross blood is considered a positive tap, and an indication for emergent laparotomy. An alternative to DPT is abdominal ultrasonography, performed by the radiologist, surgeon, or emergency physician at the patient's bedside in the emergency department, *but only if it is immediately available, and reliably interpreted*. If the results of the abdominal ultrasound are in any way equivocal, a DPT *must* be done. Refer to related material on the evaluation of abdominal injury in Chapter 6.

## Role of early skeletal stabilization

Application of an external fixation device may be a useful adjunct in the management and hemodynamic stabilization of patients with hemorrhagic pelvic fractures.[15–18] Like the MAST garment, the principle behind external fixation is rapid and reliable stabilization of the fracture fragments thus, theoretically, reducing ongoing hemorrhage secondary to repeated injury to the smaller arteries and veins bridging the fracture fragments.[7,10,19,20] Unlike the MAST garment, however, external fixation devices do allow for continued access to the patient's abdomen, groin, perineum, and lower extremities for laparotomy, if indicated, as well as vascular or urinary catheter insertion and application of distal femoral traction. Not all patients with pelvic fractures will benefit from early skeletal fixation, and the various fixation techniques do have their own complications.[21,22] Therefore, early involvement of an experienced orthopaedic surgeon is critical in determining whether skeletal stabilization should be employed, as well as the particular type of stabilization (external fixator, internal fixation, skeletal traction).[11,23–28] *Definitive* pelvic fracture fixation should be accomplished when the patient is hemodynamically stable, pelvic fracture-related hemorrhage has been controlled, and the nature of the instability of the pelvic ring has been ascertained.[8,11,23,29–34]

## Role of angiography

Pelvic angiography can be life-saving in *selected* patients with pelvic fracture-related arterial hemorrhage.[35] Although the timing of angiography relative to early skeletal fixation remains quite controversial,[7,18,36–38] most authorities would agree that this adjunct should be considered for patients who remain hemodynamically unstable after all other sources of hemorrhage have been controlled, as well as for those who require blood transfusion in excess of 5 units within 24 hours or 8 units within 48 hours of admission.[10,14,39] Pelvic fracture anatomy does not seem to correlate well with the need for pelvic angiography.[39–42] Radiology should be notified as soon as the need for angiography is identified in order to ensure their prompt availability. Likewise, angiography should not be delayed by the performance of non-life-threatening diagnostic and therapeutic procedures. Contrast studies of the genitourinary tract should be delayed until after angiography has been completed, as these may obscure the angiographic field and delay/prevent angiographic control of pelvic hemorrhage. The patient should remain in a monitored environment (ED or ICU) while awaiting angiography. In the setting of pelvic fracture-related hemorrhage, pelvic angiography should be carried out with a flush aortogram with bilateral runoff, followed by bilateral selective injections into the iliac vessels. If arterial hemorrhage is documented, control of this should be obtained via conventional embolization techniques, using non-resorbable emboli. Under certain

circumstances (vessel spasm or abrupt cutoff of a named vessel without frank extravasation), pre-emptive embolization should be performed to reduce the likelihood of recurrent arterial hemorrhage. Occasionally, a given patient's initial pelvic angiogram will be falsely negative due to arterial spasm or hypotension. Such patients, if they remain hemodynamically unstable, or have excessive transfusion requirements, may benefit from a second attempt at pelvic angiography and embolization. Every effort should be made to correct hypotension prior to this second attempt to reduce the chances of another false-negative examination.

## Treatment of life-threatening intraabdominal hemorrhage

In the hemodynamically unstable patient, laparotomy should be directed towards life-saving maneuvers, i.e. the damage control laparotomy. Hemorrhage should be controlled rapidly by organ resection if possible (i.e. spleen, kidney) or by other means of hemostasis, including packing, if resection is not feasible (i.e. liver). Enteric spillage is controlled grossly by ligation, oversewing, or stapling with no attempt to re-establish bowel continuity. Definitive organ injury repair is accomplished at subsequent laparotomy once control of pelvic-related hemorrhage has been achieved and the patient is no longer acidotic, coagulopathic, or hypothermic. If hemodynamic stability is *rapidly* restored during laparotomy, definitive repair of organ injury (including diverting colostomy for selected patients with open pelvic fractures) may be undertaken provided other extraabdominal life-threatening conditions (including expanding retroperitoneal hematoma) are not present. A large and/or expanding retroperitoneal hematoma seen at the time of laparotomy is an indication for pelvic angiography immediately following completion of the laparotomy, regardless of the hemodynamic stability of the patient.[14] When life-threatening pelvic-related hemorrhage is identified at laparotomy, the extraperitoneal space of the true pelvis should be packed prior to angiography.[1] Radiology should be notified as soon as the need for angiography is identified in order to ensure its immediate availability at the completion of the laparotomy. In patients with evidence of *severe* closed head injury (GCS < 8, unilateral dilated pupil, lateralizing neurologic signs), *rapid* CT scanning of the head, if not already performed, should *precede* pelvic angiography in order to ensure a noncontrasted head CT.

The timing of the initial skeletal stabilization (if indicated) relative to the laparotomy (simultaneous vs before/after) should be mutually agreed upon by the attending traumatologist and orthopaedic surgeon. There is, however, some evidence to suggest that laparotomy may cause further destabilization of the pelvic retroperitoneal compartment, resulting in a significant increase in the space into which retroperitoneal hemorrhage can occur.[43,44] Thus, in those situations where both emergent laparotomy and external pelvic fixation are required, some consideration should be given to applying the external fixation device *prior* to proceeding with laparotomy, if this can be accomplished without undue delay.

## Initial management of open pelvic fractures

An open pelvic fracture is one in which the fracture site communicates directly with the external skin or with an adjacent mucosal surface (i.e. vagina, bladder, or rectum). It is imperative to determine the exact site of communication between the fracture site and the skin or mucosal surface. This is critical because patients whose fractures communicate with lacerations of the *anterior* abdominal wall or flank do not require fecal diversion, while those with lacerations involving either the buttock or the perineum will require a completely diverting colostomy. This should be performed within 48 hours of injury as the incidence of pelvic-related sepsis increases dramatically beyond this point.[45] These wounds should also be subjected to serial irrigation and debridement (sometimes as frequently as daily), until a clean and granulating surface is obtained. Prior to performing the colostomy, the general surgeon should consult with the orthopaedic surgeon so as not to place the colostomy in a site which would preclude the orthopedic surgeon from obtaining optimal exposure for open reduction and internal fixation (ORIF) of the pelvic fracture if required.

## Summary

The successful management of the hemodynamically unstable pelvic fracture patient requires the early and aggressive input from a multidisciplinary team with specific expertise in shock resuscitation, emergent skeletal stabilization, and angiographic control of pelvic fracture-related arterial hemorrhage. Errors in diagnostic sequencing can lead to delays in definitive treatment and subsequent morbidity and mortality. Continued aggressive resuscitation with warmed blood products is mandatory whether the patient is in the emergency department, operating room, angiography suite, or the intensive care unit. Frequent clinical re-evaluation is critical in order that patients with

previously unrecognized or recurrent sources of hemorrhage are promptly identified and appropriate therapy initiated prior to the development of irreversible end organ collapse and death.

## Class II references

7.  Moreno C, Moore EE, Rosenberger A, Cleveland HC. Hemorrhage associated with major pelvic fracture: a multispecialty challenge. *J Trauma* 1986;**26**:987–94.

    A retrospective review of 92 patients with pelvic fractures who required greater than six units of packed cell transfusion within 24 hours of injury. Several important findings were noted.

    (1) High incidence of non-therapeutic laparotomy in patients with a negative peritoneal tap and a microscopically positive peritoneal lavage.
    (2) The application of external fixation devices was successful in 95% of patients in whom it was used as evidenced by a 50% reduction in blood transfusion requirement following fixator application.
    (3) A 71% success rate in the control of pelvic fracture-related hemorrhage associated with the use of MAST.
    (4) A large number of patients died as a result of uncontrolled pelvic fracture-related hemorrhage. Angiography was reserved for patients who did not respond to MAST, external fixation or laparotomy. Perhaps more aggressive use of early angiography would have resulted in salvage of some of the patients who exsanguinated from their injuries. The article concludes with an excellent summary algorithm that, despite being 14 years old, addresses many of the controversial areas concerning the management of these difficult patients.

9.  Cerva DSJ, Mirvis SE, Shanmuganathan K, Kelly IM, Pais SO. Detection of bleeding in patients with major pelvic fractures: value of contrast-enhanced CT. *Am J Roentgenol* 1996;**166**:131–5.

    This is a retrospective analysis of 30 patients with blunt trauma and pelvic fractures who underwent both pelvic angiography and preangiographic CT. Overall, accuracy of CT for determining the presence or absence of bleeding was 90%. However, three patients (10%) had no contrast extravasation demonstrated by CT but had bleeding demonstrated by angiography. Furthermore, it must be emphasized that CT scan should only be obtained in hemodynamically stable patients (which will not be the case for many patients with fracture-related arterial hemorrhage requiring embolization).

10. Evers BM, Cryer HM, Miller FB: Pelvic fracture hemorrhage. Priorities in management. *Arch Surg* 1989;**124**:422–4.

A retrospective review of 245 consecutive patients with pelvic fractures with the intent of determining the appropriate roles of external fixation, angiography, and laparotomy in these patients. The study reinforces the high incidence of negative and non-therapeutic laparotomies when the decision for laparotomy is based upon a microscopically positive DPL. Though not a randomized comparison, the study suggests that external fixators are perhaps more effective at controlling pelvic fracture-related hemorrhage than the use of the MAST (Military Anti-Shock Trousers). Arteriography was reserved for patients with continued hemodynamically instability after laparotomy and/or pelvic stabilization, which, in this series, occurred at an average of four hours after admission. The 89% mortality in patients with pelvic arterial injuries suggests that earlier and more liberal use of pelvic angiography may lead to improved outcomes.

13. Hubbard SG, Bivins BA, Sachatello CR, Griffen WOJ. Diagnostic errors with peritoneal lavage in patients with pelvic fractures. *Arch Surg* 1979;**114**:844–6.

A retrospective review of 222 patients with pelvic fractures, 61 of whom underwent diagnostic peritoneal lavage. Approximately 30% of the positive peritoneal lavages proved to be false positive. Several other authors have documented this finding of the lack of specificity of microscopically positive DPL in patients with pelvic fracture. These particular authors also advocate a modification of the typical infraumbilical DPL approach. They recommend supraumbilical open DPL in patients who have sustained pelvic fractures.

14. Panetta T, Sclafani SJ, Goldstein AS, Phillips TF, Shaftan GW. Percutaneous transcatheter embolization for massive bleeding from pelvic fractures. *J Trauma* 1985;**25**:1021–9.

A retrospective analysis of the role of angiography with embolization for patients with massive bleeding from pelvic fractures. Indications for angiography were well defined and included: (1) four or more units of blood transfused within 24 hours; (2) six or more units of blood transfused within 48 hours; (3) negative or borderline peritoneal tap and lavage in an unstable patient; or (4) large pelvic retroperitoneal hematoma discovered at the time of celiotomy. Thirty-one patients were treated over a $7\frac{1}{2}$ year period. External fixation was not employed in this patient series and open reduction internal fixation and MAST were used infrequently. Overall mortality in this select patient group was 35% but mortality rate related to bleeding was approximately 13%. Four patients died as a result of embolization and one wonders whether mortality could have been reduced with either earlier angiography or the addition of external fixation to the treatment algorithm. Also of note in this paper is the high percentage of false-positive peritoneal lavage related to anterior dissection of the retroperitoneal hematoma.

20. Moss MC, Bircher MD. Volume changes within the true pelvis during disruption of the pelvic ring – where does the haemorrhage go? *Injury* 1996;**27** (suppl):21–3.

A very meticulously done study using 10 cadaveric pelves and measuring serial changes in pelvic volume brought on by increased widening of the pubic symphysis and the SI joint. This paper challenges the commonly accepted notion that pelvic fractures and dislocations result in a significant increase in pelvic volume. In this paper, a 1 cm widening of the pubic symphysis was associated with a 4.6% increase of the true pelvis. Likewise, a 1 cm displacement of the SI joint was associated with a 3.1% increase in pelvic volume. The authors therefore conclude that the increasing blood and fluid requirements associated with pelvic fracture must be due to hemorrhage outside the true pelvis and that the role of external fixation may be to limit migration of blood out of the pelvis.

22. Ghanayem AJ, Stover MD, Goldstein JA, Bellon E, Wilber JH. Emergent treatment of pelvic fractures. Comparison of methods for stabilization. *Clin Orthop* 1995;**318**:75–80.

The authors employed a cadaveric model to compare the effect on pelvic volume of three methods of stabilization of pelvic fractures. Each device (external fixator, pelvic stabilizer, pelvic C-clamp) performed similarly in terms of their application time and their ability to restore pelvic volume and reduce pubic diastasis. Complications associated with the actual application of the device were of least clinical significance for the external fixator.

26. Vrahas MS, Wilson SC, Cummings PD, Paul EM. Comparison of fixation methods for preventing pelvic ring expansion. *Orthopedics* 1998;**21**:285–9.

This study compares three methods of internal fixation and three methods of external fixation in six human cadaveric pelves subjected to simulated, unilateral, vertically unstable pelvic disruptions. External fixation provided the most reliable and practical control of pelvic expansion.

32. Pennal GF, Tile M, Waddell JP, Garside H. Pelvic disruption: assessment and classification. *Clin Orthop* 1980;**151**:12–21.

Original description of mechanism-based classification of pelvic fracture. Reference also includes concise discussion of pelvic fracture imaging in the acute setting.

36. Bassam D, Cephas GA, Ferguson KA, Beard LN, Young JS. A protocol for the initial management of unstable pelvic fractures. *Am Surg* 1998;**64**:862–7.

A prospective study in which 15 pelvic fracture patients were managed according to a pelvic fracture algorithm in which patients with primarily anterior pelvic ring fractures underwent emergency external fixation for control of hemorrhage, whereas those with primarily posterior pelvic ring fractures underwent emergency angiography to control hemorrhage. Blood product requirements and hospital stay were similar in each group. However, 50% of the patients in the external fixation group ultimately required angiography because of failure of the external fixator to control hemorrhage. None of the patients initially treated with angiography required external fixation for hemorrhage control. The authors conclude that hemodynamically unstable patients with anterior-posterior compression Type II and Type III (APC-2, APC-3), lateral compression Type II and Type III (LC-2, LC-3) or vertical shear (VS) injuries should undergo immediate angiography if laparotomy is not indicated.

38. Huittinen VM, Slatis P. Postmortem angiography and dissection of the hypogastric artery in pelvic fractures. *Surgery* 1973;**73**:454–62.

    A classic paper describing postmortem angiography carried out on patients with pelvic fracture. Evidence of contrast extravasation was noted in 23 of 27 patients, with evidence of injury to a major named branch of the hypogastric artery in only three of these. This, the authors suggest, indicates that the majority of pelvic fracture-related bleeding is caused by bleeding from cancellous bone at the fracture site itself and not from associated arterial injury. This, in turn, perhaps suggests that reapproximation and stabilization of the fracture site itself may be a more efficacious approach to controlling pelvic fracture-related hemorrhage than pelvic angiography and embolization.

43. Ghanayem AJ, Wilber JH, Lieberman JM, Motta AO. The effect of laparotomy and external fixator stabilization on pelvic volume in an unstable pelvic injury. *J Trauma* 1995;**38**:396–400.

    *Ex vivo* study carried out in five cadaveric specimens examining the effect of laparotomy and external fixator stabilization on pelvic volume. APC3 "injuries" were created using this cadaveric model and then the pelvic volume measured using CT scan images with and without stabilization of the fracture with an external fixation device. The authors conclude that laparotomy in patients with pelvic fractures further destabilizes the pelvis, resulting in a significant increase in pelvic volume. Therefore, they recommend that, where feasible, external fixation of the fractured pelvis precede laparotomy in order to avoid this destabilizing effect. The dangers inherent in applying this sort of *ex vivo* data to the clinical situation are appropriately discussed in the text.

44. Grimm MR, Vrahas MS, Thomas KA. Pressure-volume characteristics of the intact and disrupted pelvic retroperitoneum. *J Trauma* 1998;**44**:454–9.

    Examines the role of external fixation in pelvic fractures using nine cadaveric specimens and measures intrapelvic pressures with and without external

fixation applied to an open book pelvic model. Open book fractures resulted in a significant increase in retroperitoneal capacitance, which was only modestly controlled with external fixation. In addition, laparotomy resulted in a significant decrease in retroperitoneal pressure, which was not improved with reapplication of external fixation.

## Class III references

1. Bosse M. The acute management of pelvic ring injuries. In: Levine AM, ed. *Orthopedic knowledge update: trauma*. Rosemont, Ill: American Academy of Orthopedic Surgeons, 1996:217–26.

   This chapter provides the reader with a comprehensive discussion of all of the important aspects of pelvic fracture diagnosis and management, from the perspective of an orthopaedic surgeon. This chapter concludes with a helpful summary algorithm detailing the approach to the hemodynamically unstable patient with pelvic fracture.

2. Gilliland MD, Ward RE, Barton RM, Miller PW, Duke JH. Factors affecting mortality in pelvic fractures. *J Trauma* 1982;**22**:691–3.

   This is a retrospective review of 100 consecutive patients with pelvic fractures. Several important findings were noted:

   (1) The presence of hypotension on admission significantly increased mortality.
   (2) Patients with posterior pelvic fractures had lower blood pressure and initial hemoglobin levels and required more packed cells.
   (3) There was a high incidence of false-positive peritoneal lavage in patients with pelvic fractures.

3. Mucha PJ, Welch TJ. Hemorrhage in major pelvic fractures. *Surg Clin North Am* 1988;**68**:757–73.

   An excellent overall review of the various adjuncts that can be helpful in hemorrhage control in patients with major pelvic fractures. Good discussion of the authors' specific protocol for use of MAST in patients with pelvic fractures.

4. Nerlich M, Maghsudi M. Algorithms for early management of pelvic fractures. *Injury* 1996;**27**(Suppl):37.

   A reasonable discussion of the issues surrounding the initial evaluation and resuscitation of hemodynamically unstable patients with pelvic fracture. Unfortunately, the accompanying algorithms are less useful than the discussion and do not adequately address many of the critical branch points in the management of this particular type of patient.

5. Batalden DJ, Wichstrom PH, Ruiz E, Gustilo RB. Value of the G suit in patients with severe pelvic fracture. Controlling hemorrhagic shock. *Arch Surg* 1974;**109**:326–8.

A retrospective descriptive study of 10 patients in whom the MAST (Military Anti-Shock Trousers) were used to control pelvic fracture-related hemorrhage. The authors concluded that, compared to historical controls, the MAST decreased hemorrhage and contributed to the restoration of blood pressure.

6. Flint LMJ, Brown A, Richardson JD, Polk HC. Definitive control of bleeding from severe pelvic fractures. *Ann Surg* 1979;**189**:709–16.

    A retrospective review of 40 patients with "severe" pelvic fractures managed over an approximate 10-year period. Twenty-two of these patients were managed according to a specific protocol, which included the use of MAST. MAST appeared to control hemorrhage in nine of 10 patients in whom they were used. Patients managed according to the protocol had a statistically significant reduction in overall mortality and in deaths attributed to shock, compared to non-protocol patients. Specific details regarding the protocol for MAST use are provided in the text. Based upon their experience, the authors feel that the use of MAST is justified in patients with pelvic fracture, and that failure to respond promptly to MAST suggests the need to proceed immediately to pelvic angiography. The strength of the authors' recommendation is obviously compromised somewhat by the use of historical controls.

8. Routt MLJ, Simonian PT, Swiontkowski MF. Stabilization of pelvic ring disruptions. *Orthop Clin North Am* 1997;**28**:369–88.

    Extensive review of the treatment of pelvic fractures, with greatest emphasis upon the technical aspects of bony stabilization. Includes a brief discussion of emergent stabilization of the bony pelvis employing such techniques as a vacuum bean bag, a large circumferential sheet or MAST.

11. Flint L, Babikian G, Anders M, Rodriguez J, Steinberg S. Definitive control of mortality from severe pelvic fracture. *Ann Surg* 1990;**211**:703–6.

    A retrospective review of 60 consecutive patients with "severe pelvic fracture bleeding", managed according to a well-defined protocol. MAST (Military Anti-Shock Trousers) were used to control pelvic hemorrhage for periods of time exceeding 24 hours with good success. External fixation and angiography used infrequently. No non-therapeutic laparotomies performed for a positive peritoneal aspirate, but 50% non-therapeutic laparotomy rate in patients operated on for a microscopically positive lavage. Employing this protocol, the vast majority of patients were ready for open reduction internal fixation within 24 hours of injury and an overall 5% mortality rate was achieved in the protocol group. In the discussion section of this paper, JD Richardson cites a prospective randomized control trial of MAST versus external fixation carried out at his institution. Although this experience was never published,

Richardson indicates that this study was stopped after 16 months because it seemed as though the results with external fixation were superior to those with MAST.

12. Gilliland MG, Ward RE, Flynn TC, Miller PW, Ben-Menachem Y, Duke JHJ. Peritoneal lavage and angiography in the management of patients with pelvic fractures. *Am J Surg* 1982;**144**:744–7.

    A retrospective descriptive study of 100 patients with pelvic fractures evaluated by peritoneal lavage and abdominal pelvic angiography. This paper describes a relatively early experience in the management of patients with pelvic fractures, predating the use of CT scan and external fixation. Therefore, visceral angiography, in addition to pelvic angiography, was used along with peritoneal lavage to identify intraabdominal hemorrhage. This paper highlights the low specificities associated with the positive peritoneal lavage in patients with pelvic fractures, in that 47% of the DPLs in this series were falsely positive. Furthermore, a 50% mortality was noted in patients who underwent non-therapeutic laparotomy. The authors therefore advocate the use of arteriography to improve the low specificity associated with peritoneal lavage in hemodynamically stable patients with pelvic fracture. Currently, abdominal CT scan would provide a better alternative to visceral angiography to reduce the incidence of non-therapeutic laparotomies in this patient population.

15. Gylling SF, Ward RE, Holcroft JW, Bray TJ, Chapman MW. Immediate external fixation of unstable pelvic fractures. *Am J Surg* 1985;**150**:721–4.

    This is a retrospective descriptive study of 66 patients with double pelvic ring fractures comparing morbidity and mortality in patients treated with external fixation with those treated with bedrest. Forty stable patients were treated with bedrest whereas 26 patients with "unstable fractures", as determined by the attending orthopedist, were treated with the application of external fixation within 24 hours of injury. Morbidity and mortality in the two groups are similar, suggesting (according to the authors) that the early application of external fixation reduces morbidity and mortality in patients with unstable pelvic fractures to levels seen in patients with stable pelvic fractures. However, the design of this particular study as well as the use of historical controls seriously limits the validity of these conclusions.

16. Riemer BL, Butterfield SL, Diamond DL *et al.* Acute mortality associated with injuries to the pelvic ring: the role of early patient mobilization and external fixation. *J Trauma* 1993;**35**:671–5.

    A retrospective review of 600 patients attempting to demonstrate the efficacy of early external fixation in patients with pelvic fractures. Using well-defined criteria for placement of external fixation, these authors demonstrated a reduction in overall mortality in hypotensive patients as well as in patients with traumatic brain injury when early external fixation was employed. Although historical controls are used, a decreased mortality was not observed in a consecutive group of patients without pelvic ring fractures suggesting that the improved survival might indeed be due to early external fixation. Unfortunately, the authors never define exactly what they mean by "early".

17. Wild JJ, Hanson GW, Tullos HS. Unstable fractures of the pelvis treated by external fixation. *J Bone Joint Surg (Am)* 1982;**64**:1010–20.

   A description of 45 patients with "unstable" fractures of the pelvic ring treated with external fixation. The timing of external fixation would have to be considered delayed by modern standards in that the first 20 patients had their fixators placed in an average of $6\frac{1}{2}$ days, whereas the final 25 patients had their fixators placed in an average of 2.2 days. Despite this apparent delay in the use of external fixation, the authors describe a "dramatic decrease in bleeding" for patients following fixator placement. Furthermore, no patient required "extensive" blood transfusion after fixator placement, although the term "extensive" was never defined.

18. Young JW, Burgess AR, Brumback RJ, Poka A. Pelvic fractures: value of plain radiography in early assessment and management. *Radiology* 1986;**160**:445–51.

   Classic paper discussing the anatomic foundation of pelvic fractures and the mechanism-based classification thereof. The article is well illustrated. These authors advocate "rapid external surgical immobilization" with the external fixator and claim that this has vastly reduced the need for emergent pelvic angiography.

19. Eastridge BJ, Burgess AR. Pedestrian pelvic fractures: 5-year experience of a major urban trauma center. *J Trauma* 1997;**42**:695-700.

   A retrospective review of 111 patients with "high energy pelvic ring disruptions" over a five-year period. Overall mortality in this patient group was 23.4%. Their results are organized according to mechanism-derived fracture type, with the vast majority of their patients having sustained LC1-type fractures. None of these fractures require pelvic fixation. The authors documented a reduced transfusion requirement and lower mortality for patients with LC2 fractures managed with external fixation compared to those managed without external fixation. However, overall numbers of patients were small and historical controls were used.

21. Ganz R, Krushell RJ, Jakob RP, Kuffer J. The antishock pelvic clamp. *Clin Orthop* 1991;**267**:71–8.

   Original description of the antishock pelvic shock clamp and its use in five patients. In this series, two of the five patients in whom it was used had hemodynamic improvement. No complications were noted.

23. Failinger MS, McGanity PL. Unstable fractures of the pelvic ring. *J Bone Joint Surg (Am)* 1992;**74**:781–91.

   No new information here but a well-referenced and concise summary of the state of the art as it relates to pelvic fracture management.

24. Simonian PT, Routt MLJ, Harrington RM, Tencer AF. Anterior versus posterior provisional fixation in the unstable pelvis. A biomechanical comparison. *Clin Orthop* 1995;**310**:245–51.

   In this study, APC3 pelvic fractures were created in six cadaveric pelves in order to determine whether a single pin external fixator or the pelvic C-clamp was superior at reducing pelvic fracture-induced motion. Neither modality reduced motion to levels comparable to the intact specimen. The anterior external fixator was more effective at decreasing anterior pelvic motion, while the pelvic C-clamp was more effective at decreasing posterior pelvic motion. However, both devices brought about comparable reductions in overall pelvic motion.

25. Tile M. Pelvic ring fractures: should they be fixed? *J Bone Joint Surg (Br)* 1988;**70**:1–12.

   This helpful review article briefly discusses some of the advantages and disadvantages of various fixation methods for patients with pelvic fracture. The author advocates the use of the external fixator or pelvic C-clamp for patients with open book type injuries or unstable vertical shear fractures. External fixation devices may also be used for definitive stabilization in selected circumstances. Symphyseal plating provides more stable fixation than an external fixator and may be indicated in the treatment of open book pelvic fractures, especially immediately following laparotomy in patients in whom there has been no fecal or urinary contamination.

27. Wolinsky PR. Assessment and management of pelvic fracture in the hemodynamically unstable patient. *Orthop Clin North Am* 1997;**28**:321–9.

   This recent review article provides a concise, yet complete, summary of the epidemiology, anatomy, classification, and treatment of pelvic fractures in patients who are hemodynamically unstable. The author provides well-defined indications for acute placement of external fixation devices in trauma patients. These include fractures with increased pelvic volume (the Tile type B or the Young and Burgess type APC2 or LC3 injuries) and completely unstable injuries (the Tile type C or Young and Burgess type APC3 or VS fractures).

28. Yang AP, Iannacone WM. External fixation for pelvic ring disruptions. *Orthop Clin North Am* 1997;**28**:331–44.

   This helpful article reviews the assessment and classification of pelvic injuries and discusses the indications for, and techniques involved in, the placement of external fixation devices in pelvic fracture patients.

29. Burgess AR, Eastridge BJ, Young JW *et al*. Pelvic ring disruptions: effective classification system and treatment protocols. *J Trauma* 1990;**30**:848–56.

   This is a retrospective review of 210 consecutive patients with pelvic fractures, the majority of whom had sustained lateral compression I (LC-1) injuries. The authors claim that a classification-based treatment protocol reduces morbidity and mortality. However, although this mechanism-based protocol was provided, the authors describe several clinical situations that were exempted from adhering to the protocol. Furthermore, the overall mortality in this series, 8.6%, is not significantly different from other published series. Finally, the large number of LC-I type pelvic fractures in this series (49%) may, in part, be responsible for their overall low morbidity and mortality.

30. Goldstein A, Phillips T, Sclafani SJ *et al*. Early open reduction and internal fixation of the disrupted pelvic ring. *J Trauma* 1986;**26**:325–33.

   A retrospective descriptive study of 33 patients who underwent open reduction internal fixation for pelvic fractures. Fifteen of these were arbitrarily defined as early fixation (less than 72 hours), while the remaining 18 patients were defined as late fixation. The early group was more "seriously injured" than the late group but had similar outcomes suggesting, according to the authors, that early fixation is superior to late fixation. However, insufficient information is supplied to precisely determine the relative severity of injury of the two groups and the two groups are clearly not equivalent with respect to their injury mechanisms. Furthermore, no statistics were supplied in the paper to determine the significance of the reported outcomes. Finally, there was a high postoperative wound complication rate in the early group, negating its purported beneficial effect.

31. Latenser BA, Gentilello LM, Tarver AA, Thalgott JS, Batdorf JW. Improved outcome with early fixation of skeletally unstable pelvic fractures. *J Trauma* 1991;**31**:28–31.

   This is a retrospective review of the authors' experience with two different approaches to pelvic fracture management, attempting to demonstrate improved outcome with pelvic fracture fixation (internal or external) within eight hours of patient arrival in the emergency department. However, in addition to the timing of fracture fixation, other aspects of pelvic fracture management differed between the two groups, most notably the failure to perform diverting colostomies for open pelvic fracture patients in the "delayed" fixation group. Thus, although the concept of early pelvic fracture fixation may have validity, this particular study provides no support for this practice. Carefully controlled studies will need to be performed before this approach can be recommended.

33. Rafii M, Firooznia H, Golimbu C, Waugh TJ, Naidich D. The impact of CT in clinical management of pelvic and acetabular fractures. *Clin Orthop* 1983;**178**:228–35.

   A retrospective descriptive study of 38 consecutive patients with pelvic and acetabular fracture who underwent CT scan examination of the pelvis. In addition to providing enhanced anatomic delineation of the *known* pelvic fracture, CT scanning also resulted in the identification of a number of *unsuspected* fractures, thus demonstrating the integral role of CT scanning in the complete evaluation of hemodynamically stable patients with pelvic fracture.

34. Tile M. Pelvic fractures: operative versus non-operative treatment. *Orthop Clin North Am* 1980;**11**:423–64.

   A classic article with the initial description of the mechanism-based classification of pelvic fractures into anterior-posterior compression (APC), lateral compression (LC), and vertical shear (VS). The article is well illustrated and accompanied by numerous appropriate radiographs.

35. Matalon TS, Athanasoulis CA, Margolies MN *et al*. Hemorrhage with pelvic fractures: efficacy of transcatheter embolization. *Am J Roentgenol* 1979;**133**:859–64.

   A retrospective descriptive study of 30 patients who underwent angiography for control of pelvic fracture-related arterial hemorrhage. Blood transfusion requirements were markedly reduced in the successfully embolized patient group, averaging 32 units in the 48 hours preceding angiography and five units in the 48 hours postangiography. However, there was a similar reduction in transfusion requirement in patients in whom no pelvic site of bleeding was demonstrated on angiography, thus casting some doubt on the contribution made by angiography in controlling hemorrhage. The mortality rate was actually higher in patients who underwent angiography with embolization compared to those whose angiography was negative.

37. Gruen GS, Leit ME, Gruen RJ, Peitzman AB. The acute management of hemodynamically unstable multiple trauma patients with pelvic ring fractures. *J Trauma* 1994;**36**:706–11.

   A retrospective review of 36 multiply injured patients with pelvic fractures and admitting blood pressure less than 90 mmHg. The patients were managed according to a well-defined protocol that did not employ external fixation. Pelvic angiography was used in 10 patients (28%) but only three of 10 required embolization. Overall, series mortality was 11% which is generally consistent with other series where external fixation was used. A large number of patients were excluded from the final statistical analysis and the discussion following this paper was generally negative and questioned whether their results (particularly their low yield of therapeutic angiography) could have been improved with the use of external fixation.

39. O'Neill PA, Riina J, Sclafani S, Tornetta P. Angiographic findings in pelvic fractures. *Clin Orthop* 1996;**329**:60–7.

This paper presents a retrospective review of 39 patients with pelvic fractures who underwent angiography for hemodynamic instability or ongoing blood loss. Indications for arteriography were well defined. No correlation was observed between the blood transfusion requirements and fracture type or between blood transfusion requirements and findings on angiography. As all patients in the study underwent angiography, the study is not helpful in defining appropriate criteria for identifying those patients who would benefit from angiography. Though external fixation was used only rarely in this series of patients, the authors' more recent experience has led them to advocate emergent external pelvic fixation in the emergency department for all APC2, APC3, LC3, and vertical shear injuries.

40. Cryer HM, Miller FB, Evers BM, Rouben LR, Seligson DL. Pelvic fracture classification: correlation with hemorrhage. *J Trauma* 1988;**28**:973–80.

The authors propose a "new" classification scheme for pelvic fractures which they claim allows for reasonably accurate predictions of who will require greater than four units of transfusion within 48 hours of injury. These patients, whom they term "unstable", include those with greater than 0.5 cm displacement or gap at any pelvic fracture site as well as those with open book fractures. All patients with pelvic fracture-related arterial injuries were in this "unstable", patient group. However, somewhere between 15% and 26% of "stable" pelvic fracture patients (i.e. those predicted to bleed less than four units within 48 hours of injury) will actually bleed four or more units. Therefore, the overall efficacy of this classification scheme is questionable.

41. Kam J, Jackson H, Ben-Menachem Y. Vascular injuries in blunt pelvic trauma. *Radiol Clin North Am* 1981; **19**:171–86.

A retrospective review of 63 pelvic fracture patients who underwent angiography. An attempt was made to correlate angiographic findings with findings on plain film and injury mechanism. In this series, the superior gluteal artery was the artery injured most frequently, followed by the internal pudendal obturator and lateral sacral arteries. *Bleeding*, however, most often originated in the internal pudendal, followed by the superior gluteal, lateral sacral, and obturator arteries. Most importantly, the authors were unable to predict the presence, site or severity of vascular injuries from the patterns of pelvic fracture on plain films. Likewise, the precise mechanisms of injury are not helpful in predicting the presence or severity of vascular injury detected at arteriography. These data, therefore, suggest that pelvic arteriography should be obtained early on in the course of the hemodynamically unstable patient with pelvic fractures, regardless of the injury mechanism or the findings on plain radiography.

42. Klein SR, Saroyan RM, Baumgartner F, Bongard FS. Management strategy of vascular injuries associated with pelvic fractures. *J Cardiovasc Surg (Torino)* 1992; **33**:349–57.

The authors review their experience with 429 pelvic fracture patients. External fixation was employed in a small number of patients, with decreased bleeding noted in 77%. Angiography was also performed in a limited number of patients but was associated with a 66% negative angiography rate. Patients with posterior pelvic fractures, in general, required more blood transfusions and all pelvic fracture-related arterial hemorrhage was found exclusively in this patient group.

45. Richardson JD, Harty J, Amin M, Flint LM. Open pelvic fractures. *J Trauma* 1982;**22**:533–8.

A retrospective review of 37 patients with open pelvic fractures managed according to a standardized protocol that included use of MAST and angiography, but not external fixation. Overall survival was approximately 95% in the series. The role and timing of diverting colostomy for open pelvic fracture are presented. The authors conclude that diverting colostomy is unnecessary in patients whose fracture site communicates with the anterior abdominal wall, but is required in those whose fracture site communicates with either the buttocks or perineum. Furthermore, diverting colostomy should be completed within 48 hours of injury in order to avoid pelvic sepsis, the incidence of which begins to increase at this time.

**Initial assessment and stabilization of the hemodynamically unstable patient with pelvic fracture**

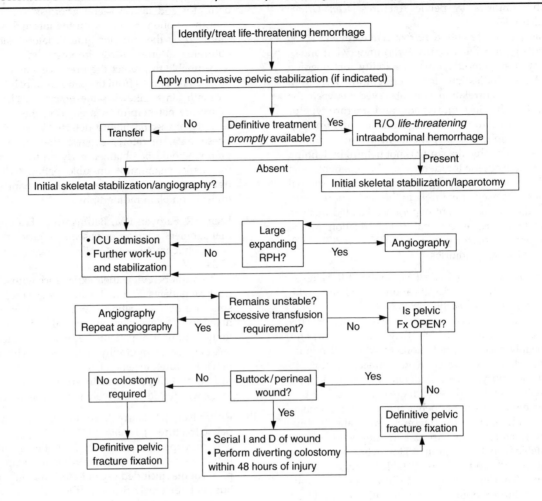

# 10 Hematuria in blunt trauma

*Karen J Brasel, Edmund J Rutherford*

## Blood at urethral meatus, scrotal hematoma, high-riding prostate

Evaluation of hematuria in the blunt trauma patient begins with visual inspection. Blood at the urethral meatus or a scrotal hematoma/perineal ecchymoses suggest a urethral injury and mandate a retrograde urethrogram. Other findings suggestive of a urethral injury include inability to void, an unstable pelvic fracture or a high-riding prostate on rectal examination. A retrograde urethrogram should be performed before inserting a urinary catheter. Treatment of a disrupted urethra may require placement of a suprapubic cystostomy by an experienced surgeon. If the retrograde urethrogram is negative for a urethral injury, a urinary catheter is inserted and evaluation continues (see below).

## Urethral injury

An experienced surgeon should treat a documented urethral injury. Attempted placement of a urinary catheter may convert a partial transection to a complete transection. The preferred initial management of a urethral injury is suprapubic cystostomy. Most incomplete and anterior urethral injuries heal with minimal stricture formation. Some have recommended initial urethral alignment for posterior injuries to prevent the formation of long strictures, but this results in a higher rate of impotence.[1]

## Hematuria

Hematuria is categorized as either gross or microscopic. Gross hematuria is defined as red- or pink-tinged urine and has too numerous to count (TNTC) red cells microscopically. Not all microscopic hematuria with TNTC red cells presents as gross hematuria (see below). Gross hematuria is evaluated by a cystogram.

## Cystogram

Since the abdominal CT scan is frequently performed before cystography, it is tempting to try to exclude bladder injuries by clamping the Foley catheter in an attempt to distend the bladder. Because of inadequate distension, the absence of extravasation does not rule out an injury. A minimum of 250–300 ml of contrast instilled into the bladder is necessary for a properly performed cystogram. Therefore, an abdominal CT scan cannot replace a cystogram.[2,3]

## Intraperitoneal bladder rupture

Intraperitoneal bladder rupture requires surgical repair. Repair should be accomplished in two layers of 3-0 absorbable suture. The first layer should incorporate the mucosa and bladder muscle and the second the bladder muscle and peritoneum. The bladder neck should be meticulously repaired and the ureteral orifices visualized. Five milliliters of indigo carmine IV will be visualized within 10 minutes if additional enhancement is necessary. Catheter drainage should be maintained for 7–10 days.[4,5]

## Extraperitoneal bladder rupture

The management of extraperitoneal bladder rupture may depend on other injuries but catheter drainage is usually sufficient. The urine must be sterile at the time of injury. Drainage is maintained for 14 days, at which time a cystogram is obtained. If there is continued extravasation, catheter drainage is maintained and cystography repeated weekly.[4–6]

## Abdominal CT scan

Abdominal CT scan has supplanted IVP in the evaluation of urologic trauma. In addition to improved evaluation of renal injuries, abdominal CT scan offers the benefit of evaluating other abdominal organs and is often used in evaluating the blunt trauma patient. The sensitivity of CT scan in detecting ureteral injuries is not known.[7]

## Microscopic hematuria

Urine dipstick is an accurate and reliable screening test for microscopic hematuria.[8] Other causes for a positive urine dipstick, such as myoglobinuria, must be kept in mind. All patients with microscopic hematuria and shock (usually defined as a systolic blood pressure <90 mmHg) should be evaluated for urologic injuries. In the absence of shock, it has been suggested that microscopic hematuria does not require any further evaluation.[5,9–17] At least one report noted that this approach would miss a few cases of severe renal injury.[5] Other larger series included the absence of major associated injuries as a prerequisite to forego further urologic evaluation.[18]

## Pelvic fracture

The necessity of radiographic evaluation of microscopic hematuria in the presence of a pelvic fracture is controversial. Pelvic fracture fragments have correlated to the site of bladder injury, particularly with extraperitoneal ruptures. Given the low incidence of bladder rupture with pelvic fracture (10%), it has been suggested that cystography be reserved for patients at high risk for such an injury, such as those with significant pubic arch involvement.[19,20]

## Work-up completed

Simultaneous injuries to both the upper and lower urinary tract are rare (0.6%).[21] Therefore, evaluation should be focused on the site of maximal injury. In addition, severe urologic injuries may be present without hematuria. In a review of 65 cases of renal artery thrombosis, 27% presented without hematuria.[8] Other late complications include late hematuria and hypertension.[22,23]

## Class II references

8. Kennedy TJ, McConnell JD, Thal ER. Urine dipstick vs. microscopic urinalysis in the evaluation of abdominal trauma. *J Trauma* 1988;**28**:615–17.

A large retrospective comparison of dipstick and microscopic urinalysis in 1485 patients. Blunt trauma accounted for 1347 (91%) of the patients. Only 276 (18.6%) were dipstick positive. False-negative readings (dipstick negative and >1 RBC/hpf) occurred in 100 (6.9%) patients. The degree of microscopic hematuria was between 2 and 10 RBC/hpf in 99 and 11 RBC/hpf in the remaining patient. There were no cases of missed injury in the 100 false negatives. False-positive readings (dipstick positive and <2 RBC/hpf) occurred in 64 (4.3%) patients. The authors conclude that urine dipstick is accurate and reliable as a screening test for the presence or absence of hematuria. No explanation for the 64 false positives is offered.

11. Hardeman SW, Husman DA, Chinn HKW, Peters PC. Blunt urinary tract trauma: identifying those patients who require radiological diagnostic studies. *J Urol* 1987;**138**:99–101.

A prospective, non-randomized series of 506 patients with blunt trauma and hematuria. All patients had microscopic urinalysis, IVP, and cystogram. CT, arteriography, and retrograde urethrogram were used when indicated. There were 25 patients with urologic injuries. Twenty-one patients had gross hematuria, one had microscopic hematuria and shock, and three had microscopic hematuria without shock. There were 11 renal injuries, eight bladder injuries, and two urethral injuries in the patients with gross hematuria. The single patient with microscopic hematuria and shock had a vascular injury; the three patients with microscopic hematuria without shock had minor renal contusions (2) or laceration (1). The authors conclude that the presence of microscopic hematuria without shock does not require further evaluation. The presence or absence of a pelvic fracture in these patients was not noted and the number of patients with bladder rupture is small. Therefore, no recommendations regarding the work-up of patients with microscopic hematuria and a pelvic fracture can be made solely from the data in this paper.

12. McAndrew JD, Corriere JN Jr. Radiographic evaluation of renal trauma: evaluation of 1103 consecutive patients. *Br J Urol* 1994;**73**:352–4.

Retrospective review of 1103 consecutive patients. An abnormal IVP was found in 10% of normotensive patients with microscopic hematuria. Only one of 60 blunt trauma patients with an abnormal IVP had a significant renal injury. This normotensive patient, with a positive DPL and lethal head injury, was found at exploration to have a major renal laceration. The degree of microscopic hematuria was not stated. None of the 605 blunt trauma patients with microscopic hematuria without shock or significant associated injuries required operative intervention solely for the renal injury. The authors conclude that, in the absence of injuries suggestive of renal damage such as lower rib fractures, flank or abdominal abrasions, etc., microscopic hematuria without shock does not require radiographic evaluation.

13. Mee SL, McAninch JW, Robinson AL *et al*. Radiographic assessment of renal trauma: A 10-year prospective study of patient selection. *J Urol* 1989;**141**:1095–8.

    A prospective, non-randomized series of 738 patients with blunt trauma and either gross or microscopic hematuria. One-hundred and fifteen patients with either gross hematuria or microscopic hematuria and systolic blood pressure <90 were evaluated with IVP, CT, and/or angiography. There were 94 contusions, seven minor lacerations, 11 major lacerations, and three vascular injuries in this group. Of the 623 patients with microscopic hematuria and no shock, 408 had no imaging study and 215 patients underwent radiographic evaluation to evaluate other injuries. No significant renal injuries were found in any of these patients, with follow-up from five days to four years. The authors confirm the findings of the next authors: patients who have microscopic hematuria without shock do not need further urologic workup. It should be noted that this series is restricted to patients with renal injuries, so the presence of a pelvic fracture in a patient with microscopic hematuria is not addressed.

14. Nicolaisen GS, McAninch JW, Marshall GA *et al*. Renal trauma: re-evaluation of the indications for radiographic assessment. *J Urol* 1985;**133**:183–7.

    Prospective evaluation of 359 consecutive patients with renal trauma. Indications for radiographic assessment and therefore inclusion were (1) >5 RBC/hpf, (2) retroperitoneal hematoma at celiotomy for associated injuries, or (3) flank tenderness or ecchymosis, a rapid deceleration injury or an entrance wound in the vicinity of the kidneys in patients with <5 RBC/hpf. Patients with pelvic fractures, hematuria, and normal findings on IVP were excluded since the source of hematuria was believed to be the bladder. There were 306 blunt and 53 penetrating injuries. Three groups were identified: group 1 included 85 patients with gross hematuria or microscopic hematuria and shock; group 2, 221 patients with microscopic hematuria without shock; and group 3, 53 patients with penetrating trauma. Group 1 included 23 (27%) patients with significant renal injuries. All patients in group 2 had renal contusions, were managed non-operatively, and experienced no complications. The authors conclude that excretory urography can be avoided in blunt trauma patients with microscopic hematuria without shock.

18. Miller KS, McAninch JW. Radiographic assessment of renal trauma: our 15 year experience. *J Urol* 1995;**154**:352–5.

    Another large retrospective series of 2024 blunt trauma patients with suspected renal trauma includes the series reported by Mee *et al*. detailed above. Four hundred and twenty-two patients with gross hematuria or microscopic hematuria and shock were evaluated, finding 344 contusions, 25 minor lacerations, 30 major lacerations, and 23 vascular injuries. Thirty-four of these patients underwent renal repair. One thousand five hundred and eighty-eight patients had microscopic hematuria and no shock. One thousand and four of these patients were not imaged. Five hundred and eighty-four patients were imaged at the discretion of the emergency department physician or to evaluate associated injuries. Five hundred and eighty-one renal contusions, one minor laceration, and one major laceration were found and managed non-operatively. One major laceration was found at the time of exploratory celiotomy done for associated injuries and this was repaired. Long-term (time unspecified) follow-up was available for 51% of the patients not imaged, with one patient having hypertension, one infection, hematuria in 24, flank pain in eight, and a "chronic problem" in one. The sheer size of this series makes it worthy of consideration as Class II data.

22. Maling TJB, Little PJ, Maling TMJ, Guneskera A, Bailey RR. Renal trauma and persistent hypertension. *Nephron* 1976;**16**:173–80.

    A well-designed retrospective case-control study to evaluate the prevalence of hypertension in a cohort of patients with previous renal trauma (6–138 months before the study) and no hypertension compared to age- and gender-matched controls. There were 63 patients in each group. Hypertension was defined as a diastolic pressure above 90. All patients had serum creatinine, electrolytes, and urinalysis at the time of evaluation. Hypertensive patients also had an intravenous urogram. The prevalence of hypertension was equal in each group (13 with previous renal trauma, 12 controls). Unequal kidney size was found in three of 13 hypertensive patients in the group with previous renal trauma and none of the controls. The authors concluded that previous renal injury was not associated with an increased risk of permanent hypertension. Unfortunately, the degree of the initial renal injury in the majority of these patients is unknown and 10 patients with renal trauma were excluded due to incomplete follow-up.

## Class III references

1. Cass AS. Urethral injury in the multiple-injured patient. *J Trauma* 1984;**24**:901–6.

   Retrospective study of 74 patients with urethral injury, 48 posterior and 26 anterior. All 48 posterior injuries had associated injuries including a fractured pelvis in 46. The management of posterior urethral injury has changed from primary realignment to suprapubic cystostomy followed by later urethral surgery. The impotence rate is significantly lower with suprapubic cystostomy. It is unclear whether the impotence is due to the injury itself, type of pelvic fracture or the surgical dissection to reconstruct the urethra.

2. Mee SL, McAninch JW, Federle MP. Computerized tomography in bladder rupture: diagnostic limitations. *J Urol* 1987;**137**:207-9.

    A case report of two patients with bladder ruptures not definitively diagnosed by abdominal CT. Both patients had gross hematuria and underwent abdominal CT with 120 cc of IV contrast with the Foley clamped. One patient had a filling defect in the bladder interpreted as clot and the other had intra-abdominal fluid with a density less than blood. Intraperitoneal bladder rupture was definitively diagnosed by cystogram. The authors conclude that cystography remains the most reliable method of diagnosing bladder rupture, although it should again be noted that neither abdominal CT scan was normal.

3. Rehm CG, Mure AJ, O'Malley KF, Ross SE. Blunt traumatic bladder rupture: the role of retrograde cystogram. *Ann Emerg Med* 1991;**20**:845-7.

    A retrospective series of 21 patients with bladder rupture over a 39-month period, attempting to delineate the correct radiographic evaluation for bladder rupture. Seventeen patients had gross hematuria and all four patients with microscopic hematuria had unstable pelvic fractures. Seven of the 21 were hypotensive at the time of evaluation and all seven had unstable pelvic fractures. The degree of hematuria in these seven patients was not described. Bladder rupture was not definitively diagnosed by CT in all seven patients undergoing CT scan (20 patients underwent cystogram and the method of definitive diagnosis was not described in the remaining patient). Five patients had free fluid on abdominal CT scan and the scans of the other two were normal. The method of obtaining the CT scan (whether or not a Foley catheter was in place and if it was clamped) was not described. There are significant problems with this paper, including questions about correct abdominal CT scan technique to evaluate potential bladder rupture and the correct interpretation of an abdominal CT scan that shows intraperitoneal fluid without other injury.

4. Cass JA, Luxenberg M. Features of 164 bladder ruptures. *J Urol* 1987;**138**:743-5.

    A retrospective case series of 164 bladder ruptures primarily from blunt trauma over a 26-year period. Ninety-five patients had gross hematuria, 16 had microscopic hematuria, 37 had hematuria recorded as present (degree not known), and 16 had no hematuria. A pelvic fracture was present in 13 of the 16 patients without hematuria. The hemodynamic status of the patients was not reported. Three of 31 patients with extraperitoneal rupture managed with catheter drainage had complications, including clot

retention, pseudodiverticulum formation, and pelvic sepsis. Follow-up cystograms were obtained at 10–14 days postinjury; the number of patients healed at this time is not specified.

5. Corriere JN, Sandler CM. Management of the ruptured bladder: Seven years of experience with 111 cases. *J Trauma* 1986;**26**:830-3.

    This retrospective case series includes 95 bladder ruptures secondary to blunt trauma. All intraperitoneal ruptures, combined injuries, and nine extraperitoneal ruptures were managed operatively. Nine patients with extraperitoneal ruptures died before therapy, and the remaining 39 were treated with catheter drainage. Follow-up cystograms demonstrated healing by 10–90 days postinjury; 87% were healed by 10 days.

6. Kotkin L, Koch MO. Morbidity associated with non-operative management of extraperitoneal bladder injuries. *J Trauma* 1995;**38**:895-8.

    This retrospective case series describes the results of non-operative management in 29 of 36 patients with extraperitoneal injuries secondary to blunt trauma over 10 years. Four of 27 surviving patients developed significant complications, including three vesicocutaneous fistulae and one patient with bladder calculi.

7. Cass AS, Vieira J. Comparison of IVP and CT findings in patients with suspected severe renal injury. *Urology* 1987;**29**:484-7.

    Review of 22 patients thought to have a severe renal injury by clinical examination and initial IVP. CT scans were performed from two to four hours after the IVP in most cases. The IVP showed an indefinite diagnosis in 18 patients and a definite diagnosis in four patients. CT scan showed a definite diagnosis in all 22 patients, although CT scan identified no discrete renal injury in four patients.

9. Barlow B, Gandhi R. Renal artery thrombosis following blunt trauma. *J Trauma* 1980;**20**:614-17.

    A case report of a single patient with blunt renal injury and no history of hematuria who presented two days postinjury with severe flank pain, nausea, and vomiting, still without hematuria. IVP demonstrated non-visualization of the left kidney, confirmed by arteriogram. The patient underwent nephrectomy without complications. A review of 65 cases reported at that time revealed that 30% presented with gross hematuria, 43% with microscopic hematuria, and 27% with no hematuria.

10. Eastham JA, Wilson TG, Ahlering TE. Radiographic assessment of blunt renal trauma. *J Trauma* 1991;**31**:1527-8.

    Retrospective review of 337 patients with microscopic hematuria but no shock following blunt trauma. All patients were assessed with an IVP. There were 30 (9%) patients with an abnormal IVP, 28 renal contusions, one ureteropelvic junction disruption, and one non-functioning kidney. Thus, only one (0.3%) significant urologic injury would have been missed. The authors conclude that blunt trauma patients with microscopic hematuria without shock do not require radiographic evaluation.

15. Cass AS, Luxenberg M, Gleich P, Smith CS. Clinical indications for radiographic evaluation of blunt renal trauma. *J Urol* 1986;**136**:370–1.

    A large retrospective series during an eight-year period of 831 patients with blunt renal injury and hematuria. Patients with other urologic injuries were excluded. Two patients had microscopic hematuria without shock and significant renal injury – one pedicle injury and one rupture. Management is not described. The authors conclude that a very small number of patients with significant renal injury have microscopic hematuria only and are hemodynamically normal.

16. Chandhoke PS, McAninch JW. Detection and significance of microscopic hematuria in patients with blunt renal trauma. *J Urol* 1988;**140**:16–18.

    This relatively large retrospective series of 339 patients with blunt renal trauma and microscopic hematuria was reviewed to establish the accuracy of urine dipstick compared with microscopic analysis. All patients had urine dipstick, urinalysis, and renal imaging with IVP, CT, and/or angiography. The specificity and sensitivity of urine dipstick were greater than 97.5% for detecting hematuria, although the ability to quantify degree of hematuria was poor. Five patients had vascular injury and two had renal lacerations; the remaining 332 had renal contusions. All patients with a diagnosis other than contusion were in shock at presentation. The authors concluded that, since the degree of hematuria is not important, the urine dipstick is an adequate way to screen for the presence of microscopic hematuria. Also of note is that no patient in this group of 339 had a significant renal injury with microscopic hematuria alone without the presence of shock.

17. Herschorn S, Radomski SB, Shoskes DA, Mahoney J, Hirshberg E, Klotz L. Evaluation and treatment of blunt renal trauma. *J Urol* 1991;**146**:274–7.

    A retrospective series of 126 patients with blunt renal trauma. Renal injuries were classified as major (pedicle injury or shattered kidney), moderate (deep lacerations through corticomedullary junction or extending into the collecting system) or minor (contusion, subcapsular hematoma, superficial laceration). All patients with major injuries had gross hematuria and three were in shock. Twenty of 21 patients with moderate injuries had gross hematuria (six with

shock) and one had microscopic hematuria and shock. Of the 91 patients with minor injuries, 52 had gross hematuria, 36 had microscopic hematuria, and three had no hematuria (one with shock). The authors concluded that patients with microscopic hematuria and without shock do not need further urologic evaluation.

19. Fallon B, Wendt JC, Hawtrey CE. Urological injury and assessment in patients with fractured pelvis. *J Urol* 1984;**131**:712–14.

    A retrospective series of 199 patients with blunt pelvic fracture, including 32 patients with urologic injury. A urine specimen was not obtainable in two patients; 29 patients had gross hematuria; and one patient had microscopic hematuria alone. The hemodynamic status of the patient with microscopic hematuria alone was not described. The authors conclude that, in the absence of gross hematuria or clinical signs of a lower tract injury, urologic evaluation of patients with pelvic fractures is unnecessary.

20. Hochberg E, Stone NN. Bladder rupture associated with pelvic fracture due to blunt trauma. *Urology* 1993;**41**:531–3.

    A retrospective series of 103 patients with pelvic fracture who underwent cystography, documenting an incidence of bladder rupture in patients with pelvic fracture of 10%. All patients with bladder rupture had gross hematuria. The authors conclude that since the incidence of bladder rupture in patients with pelvic fracture is relatively low, routine cystography is not indicated and can be reserved for patients with gross hematuria or hemodynamic abnormalities.

21. Peterson NE, Schulze KA. Selective diagnostic uroradiography for trauma. *J Urol* 1987;**137**:449–51.

    A retrospective case series of 225 patients with blunt urologic injury over a 15-year period. One hundred and ninety-nine patients had renal injuries, 24 had lower tract injuries, and two had simultaneous upper and lower tract injuries. The authors conclude that simultaneous upper and lower tract injury is rare, therefore urologic evaluation may cease after a single urologic injury is identified.

23. Teigen CL, Venbrux AC, Quinlan DM, Jeffs RD. Late massive hematuria as a complication of conservative management of blunt renal trauma in children. *J Urol* 1992;**147**:1333–6.

    A case report of two pediatric patients with blunt renal injury and massive hematuria weeks after initial non-operative treatment. Both cases of pseudoaneurysm were successfully treated with percutaneous transcatheter embolization.

## Hematuria in the blunt trauma patient

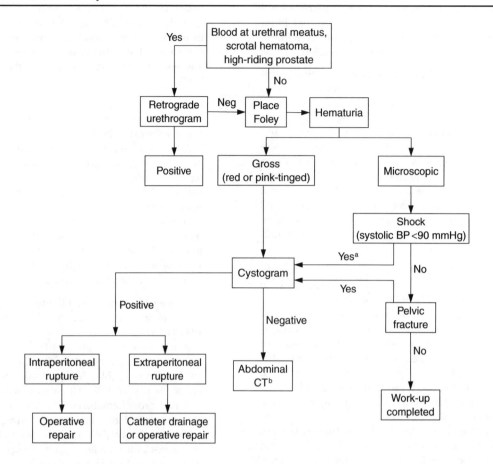

[a] Need for celiotomy may delay or preclude need for cystogram

[b] Abdominal CT is frequently done before cystogram to evaluate for other intraabdominal injuries, *but cannot replace cystogram*

# 11 Penetrating chest trauma

*Eddy H Carrillo, Christopher D Wohltmann, J David Richardson*

Chest trauma is very common, accounting for 25–50% of traumatic injuries.[1] Penetrating chest injuries are seldom isolated in the chest cavity. Rodriguez and associates reported an incidence of 43% of extrapulmonary injuries in 67 patients.[2] The etiology of penetrating chest trauma varies; however, most institutions report an incidence of approximately 55% for stab wounds and 45% for gunshot wounds.[1,3] Observation or placement of tube thoracostomy, adequate volume resuscitation, occasional need for respiratory support, serial chest roentgenograms, and observation are the only treatments required in 80–85% of patients.[4–6] Historically, only a small number of patients will require urgent thoracotomy for control of bleeding, repair of tracheobronchial disruptions, relief of cardiac tamponade or control of associated injuries.[3]

## Hemodynamic stability and initial clinical presentation

The extent of the initial management of any patient with penetrating chest trauma is dictated by their initial hemodynamic stability. The initial therapy is aimed at restoring both adequate oxygenation and perfusion of vital structures and includes: airway assessment and control; adequate ventilation; intravenous access; hemorrhage control; resuscitation with management of associated shock; and initial cardiorespiratory monitoring. When measures are undertaken to establish a patent airway, the cervical spine must be protected. The secondary assessment follows and finally, in the definitive care phase, all the patient's injuries are treated and plans for final disposition are made.[7] Much of the significant care will be provided during the early acute phase. Temporary closure of chest wall defects, removal of blood from the pericardial sac, drainage of blood and air from the chest cavities, and restoration of circulating volume deficits are life-saving procedures that must be performed during the initial resuscitation.[4,7,8]

## Chest X-ray

Despite some limitations, the initial anteroposterior (AP) chest X-ray remains the single most important and expeditious test to initially determine the extent of injuries after penetrating chest trauma. It frequently detects potentially life-threatening injuries that require immediate treatment. X-rays should not delay patient resuscitation or immediate treatment and should be deferred in unstable patients. Radiopaque markers should be used to document the entry and exit site of projectiles. Finally, the radiograph is extremely useful to identify the position of tubes and intravascular devices placed during the initial resuscitation.[7,8]

It has also been suggested that in stable patients, after a careful history and physical examination, normal vital signs, unremarkable AP chest X-ray, no evidence of intrathoracic penetration, and no other reason for admission, outpatient management can be entertained if the patient remains asymptomatic after a 3–4 hour observation period and a normal repeat chest X-ray.[9]

## Thoracostomy chest tube

The purpose of thoracostomy chest tube placement is to promote air or fluid evacuation, lung reexpansion, and restoration of intrapleural negative pressure. Because air has low density, it tends to accumulate in the upper half of the pleural space, while fluids with a higher density tend to collect in the posterior lower half of the thoracic cavity when the patient is in the supine position. The ideal site of tube insertion is the third or fourth intercostal space in the anterior or mid-axillary line immediately behind the pectoralis major fold. In this location the scar is hardly visible and the technique of tube insertion is easier because there are no muscles, other than intercostals, to traverse. In this location the tube is more comfortable and less restrictive. In most trauma patients, large tubes (36 to 40 French) are preferred because they facilitate drainage of hemothorax.[10]

A chest X-ray should always be obtained immediately after tube insertion to document lung reexpansion and tube position, retained hemothorax, large hematomas or cavitation injuries in pulmonary parenchyma, missile tract if possible, and to evaluate missile proximity to vital structures (e.g. cardiac, esophagus, great vessels, diaphragm, intraabdominal). Output from the chest tube is also extremely useful to determine the need for an urgent thoracotomy. Most authors currently agree that an output from the thoracostomy tube exceeding 11 at the time of placement, or more than 150–200 cc/hour for more than four hours, indicates the need for a thoracotomy.[1,2,6,11] The specific numbers are subject to institutional guidelines or the managing surgeon's preference; however, there is no disagreement that large hemothoraces or ongoing hemorrhage, especially in the presence of hemodynamic instability, are an indication for immediate thoracotomy.

The role of prophylactic antibiotics for tube thoracostomy is extremely controversial with either blunt or penetrating trauma. In a metaanalysis, Fallon[12] suggested that the use of antibiotics for the duration of the tube thoracostomy, and not just around the time of insertion, lowered the incidence of thoracic empyema. In a previous report from our institution, the incidence of empyema was 2% in patients where antibiotics were administered within 24 hours of placement of their initial chest tube and 2% in patients who received no antibiotics within 24 hours of placement of their initial chest tube.[13] Because of this small incidence of thoracic empyema, it is difficult to detect those factors that may predispose patients to infectious complications. Currently, we follow a policy of selective use of antibiotics after chest tube placement.

## Cardiac tamponade

With rapid and improved non-invasive diagnostic modalities, the use of and indications for pericardiocentesis have decreased. Patients with cardiac tamponade often show significant hemodynamic improvement with volume infusion alone. However, if deterioration occurs instead, urgent pericardial decompression by pericardiocentesis or thoracotomy is indicated. Pericardiocentesis works best in those patients where a critical tamponade has progressed slowly and liquid blood may be present. Pericardiocentesis is less useful in those

patients who present with massive or rapid hemopericardium.[14,15]

While most patients with cardiac wounds present in profound shock with severe tamponade or few signs of life, some arrive at a hospital with "compensated" tamponade. These cardiac injuries require rapid diagnosis and treatment to prevent sudden deterioration. A pericardial window provides a rapid and safe means of diagnosing cardiac injuries in patients with equivocal signs of cardiac injuries.[16]

## Resuscitation thoracotomy

This is a procedure that is indicated to resuscitate trauma victims who present *in extremis*. The results are poor in the majority of patients, but occasional survivors have been documented in patients with signs of life and the presence of cardiac tamponade or ongoing pulmonary hemorrhage. Survival rates are extremely low for patients with associated abdominal injuries or in the absence of vital signs or signs of life in the field.[17–20]

The objectives of resuscitative thoracotomy are very well defined and entail:

- maintenance of cardiac and cerebral perfusion by relief of cardiac tamponade and/or restoration of efficient cardiac contractility
- control of hemorrhage by cardiorrhaphy, compression of bleeding intrathoracic vessels, and/or reduction of intraabdominal blood losses by temporary vascular control of the descending thoracic aorta
- improving survival while minimizing complications and avoiding unnecessary risks to the operating team.[19,20]

## Location of the injury and clinical relevance

After the immediate life-threatening injuries are excluded, the surgeon should focus on the site of the thoracic injury as the next step in determining priorities.[21] To facilitate work-up, diagnosis, and overall management, penetrating thoracic wounds are divided in the following anatomical areas:

- unilateral
- parasternal or precordial
- thoracoabdominal
- transmediastinal.

It is again important to emphasize the value of the initial chest X-ray to help determine the best course of action following the principles described above.

## Unilateral and peripheral chest wounds

These wounds are anatomically defined as being lateral to the midclavicular line. As for any penetrating thoracic wound, their management will be dictated by hemodynamic stability. The incidence of cardiac and major vascular injuries is lower, compared to central wounds. Instability in this setting is usually due to hemorrhage above or below the diaphragm or tension pneumothorax. Most of these patients are managed with a thoracostomy chest tube. Further care will be determined by output from the chest tube, as well as by findings from subsequent chest X-ray or other ancillary tests.[21] Stable patients with stab wounds and peripheral gunshot wounds with a normal initial chest X-ray can be safely observed and should have a repeat hematocrit and chest X-ray. If these are normal, the patient can be discharged safely.[9]

## Parasternal wounds

If a patient is hemodynamically unstable with a parasternal wound, the decision to operate immediately is relatively straightforward.[11] If signs suggest cardiac injury in a patient who is relatively stable, the decision becomes more difficult. In this scenario, most institutions use one of two alternatives: subxyphoid pericardial window and/or pericardial sonography.[4,16,18,23] Ultrasonography is safe, portable, expeditious, and can be repeated as indicated. Emergency department sonography with a subxyphoid view is intended to determine the presence of fluid within the pericardial sac. A normal-appearing sonogram does not completely rule out the presence of a cardiac injury and these patients should be observed. If the surgeon still suspects injury, ultrasound is followed by another examination (e.g. pericardial window, TEE).[23]

## Thoracoabdominal wounds

These are lower chest wounds that traverse the diaphragm, inflicting injury to retroperitoneal or intraperitoneal structures.[21] Trajectory is important in determining the presence of associated abdominal injuries. The evaluation of patients with lower chest wounds should begin as previously described. However, additional measures should be taken to determine the presence or absence of diaphragmatic injuries. There is no consensus on how best to proceed. Patients with peritoneal penetration or with clear signs and symptoms of intraabdominal injury require laparotomy.[21] Computed tomography (CT) of the chest and abdomen has been shown to be useful as an initial screen for low-suspicion abdominal, torso, and flank gunshot wounds;[24–26] however, CT is not reliable to identify diaphragmatic injuries.[25] Cavitary endoscopy is the diagnostic test of choice to identify diaphragmatic injuries in this subset of patients.[27,28]

Routine exploratory laparotomy for gunshot wounds to the right thoracoabdominal region has been challenged. Currently, it is recommended that:

- stable patients with gunshot wounds to the right thoracoabdominal area and no signs of peritonitis can be managed non-operatively
- selected patients with documented injuries to the liver can be managed non-surgically
- thoracoabdominal CT is a non-invasive and comprehensive means of detection and follow-up when non-surgical management is chosen.[25]

Injuries to the left thoracoabdominal region are more controversial. The incidence of diaphragmatic injuries in these patients is higher and if a diaphragmatic injury is missed in the initial evaluation, it does have the potential to present in a delayed fashion with strangulation of abdominal contents. The value and limitations of chest X-ray, CT, and peritoneal lavage are well known. Currently, cavitary endoscopy (laparoscopy or thoracoscopy) is the diagnostic test of choice in stable patients with penetrating injuries to the left thoracoabdominal region.[27–29]

## Transmediastinal gunshot wounds

Transmediastinal wounds can present major management problems for two reasons:

(1) multiple injuries to vital structures are common
(2) the operative approach to control hemorrhage may not afford the optimum exposure to repair the various structures injured.[11] These structures include the heart, tracheobronchial tree, and esophagus as well as the spinal cord. A bullet may cross from one hemithorax to the other and no vital structures may have been injured. This has been observed in 37% of patients that arrive hemodynamically stable or regain hemodynamic stability soon after arrival.[29] Presumably, these missiles traverse the retrosternal clear space. A tube thoracostomy may be needed but no major operative treatment is required.

Our trauma unit has reported a protocol whereby patients in hemodynamic unstable condition undergo immediate operation and patients in stable condition undergo a rapid work-up (including angiography, esophagography, esophagoscopy, bronchoscopy, and pericardial window) to evaluate the organs at risk for injury. This approach has functioned well for the past two decades.[29] Currently, we are evaluating the use of dynamic CT scanning of the chest in hemodynamically stable patients. Preliminary results suggest that hemodynamically stable patients can be safely evaluated initially with CT of the chest.

If no injuries are identified by the various diagnostic techniques, it is advisable to monitor these patients continuously for 24 hours. We have had no deaths or serious complications as a result of this approach. In addition, it shortens hospital stay and eliminates the risk of a major operative procedure. When injuries to specific anatomical structures are demonstrated, this approach has allowed for careful planning of incisions to treat the specific injuries diagnosed.[11,28]

The decision for operative management of the stable patient with penetrating thoracic injuries is based on many variables, including location of the injury, gunshot versus stab wounds, the potential for intraabdominal or retroperitoneal injuries, and concern for occult injuries that may cause delayed morbidity. Currently, there are some new alternatives available to the clinician to facilitate the diagnosis of potentially life-threatening complications.

## Ultrasonography

Abdominal transthoracic or transesophagic ultrasonography helps in the evaluation of trauma patients, especially at the bedside.[23,30] In penetrating chest trauma, it is not intended to provide specific anatomical diagnosis but rather to determine the presence of hemopericardium and to decrease the time required to reach a decision to perform definitive surgery.[30]

## Cavitary endoscopy

Video-assisted thoracoscopic surgery (VATS) and laparoscopy are widely available to evaluate stable patients with penetrating injuries. Although they were introduced decades ago, recent interest has been increased with the onset of advanced video technology.[28,31,32] At this time the data support the use of cavitary endoscopy in *hemodynamically stable* patients with penetrating injuries of the lower chest and upper abdomen for the diagnosis of occult diaphragmatic lacerations, to identify peritoneal penetration in tangential gunshot wounds of the abdomen, to evaluate small or low-grade liver or splenic lacerations, and as a complement to CT of the chest, abdomen, back, and flank.[24,25,27,28,31]

## Thoracic computed tomography

Computed tomography plays a prominent diagnostic role in penetrating chest trauma. It can unmask subtle or unsuspected injuries and may be used serially to monitor various pathological processes. An increasing number of associated thoracic injuries, such as trajectory or location of missiles, pneumomediastinum, and pericardial effusions or hemopericardium can be easily identified with CT scanning of the chest.[24,25] The chest CT also has a significant value in the evaluation of retained hemothorax or persistent pneumothorax.[33]

According to Mattox and Wall, much of the literature on thoracic CT scanning for trauma patients was acquired using the first- or second-generation CT scanners. Currently, third-generation, high-speed scanners are available and provide resolution much improved over former models and allow for computerized reconstructions of anatomical structures within the chest.[22] The CT scan has, however, distinct disadvantages, since critically ill patients must be transported, demanding continuous monitoring to avoid complications.

New endovascular procedures have generated tremendous interest in the use of endovascular stented grafts in a wide variety of vascular conditions such as small intimal defects[34] or for the endovascular removal of foreign bodies (most often bullets) which become lodged in the heart or pulmonary vessels. These have, in the past, required thoracotomy, cardiotomy, and other more invasive procedures. Use of these new endovascular procedures will increase with advancing improvements in technology.[22]

## Indications for thoracotomy

The indications for emergency department thoracotomy have been previously described. Urgent thoracotomy usually is indicated for:

- location of the entrance wound in the chest (70% in the upper mediastinum)
- blood pressure less than 90 mmHg systolic
- initial thoracostomy output greater than 1000 ml
- radiographic evidence of a large retained hemothorax
- large air leaks
- documented injuries to mediastinal structures
- clinical evidence of pericardial tamponade.[4,6,7,26]

A small number of patients will require a delayed thoracotomy, usually for initially missed injuries, retained thoracic collections or documented empyema. VATS has become extremely useful in this particular setting and its indications and benefits in this subset of patients continue to expand.[27,30,33,36]

## Further care and monitoring

Most patients with penetrating injuries to the chest, especially those who have required an operation, are best served if further care and monitoring are provided in an intensive care unit setting. The initial goals of management include, but are not limited to:

- support and monitoring of the cardiovascular and respiratory systems to optimize oxygen delivery and tissue perfusion
- management of fluids
- drainage and obliteration of the pleural cavity
- monitoring hourly output from the chest cavity
- pain control
- management of secretions.[8,10]

Orders for mechanical ventilation and cardiovascular medications are immediately transcribed and changed as indicated by arterial blood gas determinations and cardiovascular stability. All connections should be checked, secured, and wrapped with adhesive tape to prevent dislodgement or leaks. All tubes should be labeled and output documented on arrival at the intensive care unit. A chest X-ray should be obtained as soon as possible, to document:

- position of endotracheal and pleural tubes
- position of monitoring lines
- pneumothorax
- retained collections in the pleural space
- atelectasis or infiltrate
- foreign bodies in the heart or pulmonary circulation
- degree of shift or width of the mediastinum.[8,10]

## Conclusion

Penetrating chest trauma causes a broad spectrum of injuries that requires an organized and systematic approach to minimize complications and optimize initial care. Prompt resuscitation and surgical management are indicated for patients that present *in extremis*. In patients who present in a more stable condition, a thorough initial assessment, diagnostic evaluation, and appropriate observation are determined by the location of the injury and initial findings on the plain chest X-ray. Clinical skills and sound judgment, along with the initial radiographic findings, provide the basis for an adequate initial treatment in most patients, with more sophisticated imaging procedures indicated in very few patients.

## Class I references

29. Rozycki GS, Feliciano DV, Ochsner G, Knudson MM. The role of ultrasound in patients with possible penetrating cardiac wounds: a prospective multicenter study. *J Trauma* 1999;**46**:543–52.

Prospective study of the value of ultrasonography for the diagnosis of hemopericardium in 261 patients. There were 225 (86.2%) true-negative, 29 (11.1%) true-positive, no false-negative, and seven (2.7%) false-positive examinations, resulting in a sensitivity of 100%, specificity of 96.9%, and overall accuracy of 97.3%.

## Class II references

1. Tominaga GT, Waxman K, Scannell G, Annas C, Ott RA, Gazzaniga AB. Emergency thoracotomy with lung resection following trauma. *Am Surg* 1993; **59**:834–7.

Large retrospective study of 2934 patients requiring emergency thoracotomy in a level I trauma center. Of these, 12 required emergency lung resection. This review emphasizes the value of emergency lung resection to control hemorrhage in penetrating trauma.

3. Mandal AK, Oparah SS. Unusually low mortality of penetrating wounds of the chest. *J Thorac Cardiovasc Surg* 1989;**97**:119–25.

Extensive retrospective review from an inner-city hospital, where an organized and comprehensive approach to penetrating chest injuries demonstrates a very low mortality and minimal morbidity. The authors emphasize that in the 39% of patients who required an associated laparotomy, there was no increase in complications.

5. Carrillo EH, Block EFJ, Zeppa R, Sosa JL. Urgent lobectomy and pneumonectomy after penetrating thoracic trauma. *Eur J Emerg Med* 1994;**1**:126–30.

Review of 259 patients who underwent urgent thoracotomies for penetrating chest trauma. Forty-three patients (17%) required some type of pulmonary resection to control bleeding or major tracheobronchial disruptions. Emphasis is placed on the timing of these pulmonary resections and its value for definitive control of bleeding or air leaks.

9. Ordog GJ, Balasubramanium S, Wasserberger J. Outpatient management of 357 gunshot wounds to the chest. *J Trauma* 1983;**23**:832–5.

Retrospective review of 357 patients with gunshot wounds to the chest. The authors describe their experience and emphasize that following the basic principles of management of penetrating chest trauma and an in-house protocol, a select group of patients can be safely managed on an outpatient basis.

12. Fallon WF Jr. Post-traumatic empyema. *J Am Coll Surg* 1994;**179**:483–92.

Based on a detailed meta-analysis, this study suggests that the use of antibiotics lowers the incidence of thoracic empyema in trauma patients. The author emphasizes that to reduce the incidence of posttraumatic empyema effectively, chest tube prophylaxis with antibiotics should be used for the duration of the tube thoracostomy and not just around the time of insertion.

13. Etoch SW, Bar-Natan MF, Miller FB, Richardson JD. Tube thoracostomy. Factors related to complications. *Arch Surg* 1995;**130**:521–6.

The authors reviewed 426 trauma patients who underwent tube thoracostomy to determine the complication rate. Thoracic empyema was observed in 2% of patients who received prophylactic antibiotics and in 2% of those who did not receive any type of antimicrobial prophylaxis. Based on those findings, the authors do not recommend routine use of prophylactic antibiotics in patients undergoing chest tube placement.

16. Miller FB, Bond SJ, Shumate CR, Polk HC, Richardson JD. Diagnostic pericardial window. *Arch Surg* 1987;**122**:605–9.

Five-year review of 104 patients who underwent a pericardial window to document hemopericardium. The authors conclude that in stable patients with highly suspicious precordial wounds, pericardial window provides a rapid and safe alternative to diagnose cardiac injuries in patients with equivocal signs of heart injury.

17. Schwab CW, Adcock OT, Max MH. Emergency department thoracotomy (EDT): a 26 month experience using an "agonal" protocol. *Am Surg* 1986;**52**:20–5.

Following a strict protocol, the authors report a survival rate with emergency department thoracotomy of 13 of 14 agonal patients with stab wounds to the heart.

18. Moreno C, Moore EE, Majure JA, Hopeman AR. Pericardial tamponade: a critical determinant for survival following penetrating cardiac wounds. *J Trauma* 1986;**26**:821–7.

The presence of cardiac tamponade appears to be a favorable condition in patients undergoing emergency department thoracotomy. In their patients who underwent emergency department thoracotomy, the survival rate was 73% in patients with cardiac tamponade and only 11% in those without cardiac tamponade.

19. Branney SW, Moore EE, Feldhaus KM, Wolfe RE. Critical analysis of two decades of experience with postinjury emergency department thoracotomy in a regional trauma center. *J Trauma* 1998;**45**:87–94.

Retrospective review of 950 emergency department thoracotomies over a 23-year span. The authors report an overall survival rate of 4.4%, with 3.9% surviving functionally intact. Stab wounds to the chest and gunshot wounds to the abdomen were the two mechanisms of injury most likely to be survived.

24. Grossman MD, May AK, Schwab CW *et al*. Determining anatomic injury with computed tomography in selected torso gunshot wounds. *J Trauma* 1998;**45**:444–56.

The authors report a six-year retrospective review of 50 patients who sustained gunshot wounds and underwent CT scan solely to determine trajectory or to rule out intracavitary penetration. This diagnostic test supplemented the standard approach to management of such wounds and was performed only in stable patients.

25. Ginzburg E, Carrillo EH, Kopelman T *et al*. The role of computed tomography in selective management of gunshot wounds to the abdomen and flank. *J Trauma* 1998;**45**:1005–9.

Retrospective review of 83 patients where abdominal computed tomography was used as the intial screening to identify intraabdominal injuries. When the protocol described by the authors was followed closely, this technique was extremely useful to document peritoneal violation or intraabdominal injuries.

27. Sosa JL, Markley M, Sleeman D, Carrillo EH. Laparoscopy in abdominal gunshot wounds. *Surg Lap Endosc* 1993;**3**:417–19.

This is one of the early reports of the value of diagnostic laparoscopy to document peritoneal penetration in hemodynamically stable patients with low-suspicion abdominal gunshot wounds.

29. Richardson JD, Flint LM, Snow NJ, Gray LA, Trinkle JK. Management of transmediastinal gunshot wounds. *Surgery* 1981;**90**:671–6.

The authors analyze the management of penetrating mediastinal trauma and propose an orderly work-up based on hemodynamic stability to determine any sites of potential injury. The authors also point out that 40% of patients with transmediastinal gunshot wounds do have associated intraabdominal injuries. Following an organized protocol, the authors report that 20% of their patients did not require an operation.

33. Heniford BT, Carrillo EH, Spain DA *et al*. The role of thoracoscopy in the management of retained thoracic collections after trauma. *Ann Thorac Surg* 1997;**63**:940–3.

The authors report an overall success rate of 76% of thoracoscopy to drain retained thoracic collections after trauma. When thoracoscopy was performed less than seven days after admission, no cases of empyema were noted at operation.

35. Siemens R, Polk HC, Gray LA, Fulton RL. Indications for thoracotomy following penetrating thoracic injury. *J Trauma* 1977;**17**:493–500.

Some of the classic indications for thoracotomy are well described in this publication. The authors present their experience with 53 patients who required urgent thoracotomy.

36. Carrillo EH, Schmacht DC, Gable DR, Spain DA, Richardson JD. Thoracoscopy in the management of posttraumatic persistent pneumothorax. *J Am Coll Surg* 1998;**186**:636–40.

Report of 11 patients with posttraumatic persistent pneumothorax. Thoracoscopy succesfully identified the source of the air leak and a segemental stapled resection was performed with complete success to resolve the air leak. Length of hospital stay was dramatically reduced when compared with non-operative management with chest tubes.

## Class III references

2. Rodriguez A, Thomas MD, Shilinglaw WRC. Lung and tracheobronchus. In: Ivatury RR, Cayten CG, eds. *The textbook of penetrating trauma*. Media: Williams and Wilkins, 1996:531–52.

Extensive review of tracheobronchial and thoracic injuries. Extensive personal experience by the authors, some supported by current literature. In general, a very well-referenced chapter.

4. Richardson JD, Miller FB, Carrillo EH, Spain DA. Complex thoracic injuries. *Surg Clin North Am* 1996;**76**:725–48.

Review article with extensive references and occasional personal observations, most supported by the literature available.

6. Richardson JD. Indications for thoracotomy in thoracic trauma. *Curr Surg* 1985;**42**:361–6.

This paper describes the principles of the management of patients with complex thoracic injuries, delineating in a very organized fashion the indications for emergent thoracotomy. The author supports his observations with publications on this topic by the trauma program at the University of Louisville and with his personal experience.

7. American College of Surgeons Committee on Trauma. *Advanced life support for doctors. Instructor course manual.* Chicago: American College of Surgeons, 1997:147–63.

This manual sets the standard of initial trauma care and presents established treatment methods. A systematic, concise approach to the early care of the trauma patient is the hallmark of the ATLS™ program.

8. Carrillo EH, Williams MJ. Thoracic surgery. In: Civetta JM, Taylor RW, Kirby RR, eds. *Critical care*. Philadelphia: Lippincott-Raven, 1997:1131–46.

This chapter describes the principles of initial management, essential diagnostic tests and procedures, and initial therapy in critically injured patients with thoracic trauma. Emphasis is placed on the initial management and resuscitation, as well as the principles of critical care after urgent thoracic surgery.

10. Gregoire J, Deslauriers J. Closed drainage and suction systems. In: Pearson FG, Deslauriers J, Ginsberg RJ *et al. Thoracic surgery.* New York: Churchill Livingstone, 1995:1123–7.

Excellent review on indications for chest tube drainage and suction systems.

11. Richardson JD. Thorax. In: Ivatury RR, Cayten CG, eds. *The textbook of penetrating trauma*. Media: Williams and Wilkins, 1996:273–9.

Review of the initial management of patients with penetrating chest trauma. The author is a well-known authority on the topic and describes current clinical management based on his extensive personal experience, with a well-referenced biliography.

14. Buckman RF, Buckman PD, Badellino MM. Heart. In: Ivatury RR, Cayten CG, eds. *The textbook of penetrating trauma*. Media: Williams and Wilkins, 1996:500–1.

Good overall review of penetrating cardiac injuries. The authors describe at length the different indications for pericardiocentesis or pericardial window in precordial wounds and cardiac tamponade.

15. Ivatury RR, Rohman M. The injured heart. *Surg Clin North Am* 1989;**69**:93–110.

Excellent review with extensive bibliographic documentation.

20. Ivatury RR. Resuscitative thoracotomy. In: Ivatury RR, Cayten CG, eds. *The textbook of penetrating trauma*. Media: Williams and Wilkins, 1996:207–14.

Updated review of indications, contraindications, and potential benefits of emergency department thoracotomy. The author has dedicated the last two decades to understanding the benefits and limitations of this procedure. This chapter is well written and presents a wealth of first-class statistics.

21. Jorden RC. Penetrating chest trauma. *Emerg Med Clin North Am* 1993;**11**:97–107.

The author presents the approach to patients with penetrating chest trauma based on anatomic location of the injury.

22. Mattox KL, Wall MJ. Newer diagnostic measures and emergency management. *Chest Surg Clin North Am* 1997;**7**:213–26.

This review article presents the diagnostic alternatives used clinically in patients with trauma to the chest. The authors discuss the pros and cons of 1997 technology.

23. Johnson SB, Kearney PA, Smith MD. Echocardiography in the evaluation of thoracic trauma. *Surg Clin North Am* 1995;**75**:193–205.

Review of the current role of echocardiography in thoracic trauma, mostly supported by personal opinion and some current literature.

26. Pezzella AT, Silva WE, Lancey RA. Cardiothoracic trauma. *Curr Probl Surg* 1998;**35**:647–790.

This monograph is divided into three parts: the general aspects of cardiothoracic trauma; specific injuries of the thorax and its contained organs; and special problems of cardiothoracic injury. The monograph is particularly well illustrated with abundant tables and figures; the references are complete and current.

28. Carrillo EH, Heniford BT, Etoch SW *et al.* Video-assisted thoracic surgery in trauma patients. *J Am Coll Surg* 1997;**184**:316–24.

Extensive review article of the indications, benefits, and potential limitations of video-assisted thoracoscopic surgery in trauma patients. There are several illustrations and extensive references.

31. Sosa JL, Puente I, Lemasters L *et al.* Video thoracoscopy in trauma: early experience. *J Laparoendosc Surg* 1994:**4**:295–300.

One of the early reports of the value of video thoracoscopy in trauma. The authors demonstrate that this is a safe and truly minimally invasive alternative in trauma.

32. Namias N, McKenney M, Sosa JL. Laparoscopic repair of a gunshot wound to the diaphragm: a case report. *J Laparoendosc Surg* 1995;**5**:59–61.

Case report of an endoscopic repair of a diaphragmatic laceration secondary to a gunshot wound of the chest.

34. Ginzburg E, Cohn S, McKenney M *et al.* The use of percutaneously placed endovascular stents for vascular trauma. *J Trauma* 1998;**45**:1120.

The authors describe the value of percutaneously placed vascular stents in seven patients with acute vascular injuries (four traumatic, three iatrogenic). Excellent early patency rate was obtained; however, the authors caution that long-term follow-up will be required to accept this as an alternative to conventional surgical management.

## Penetrating chest trauma

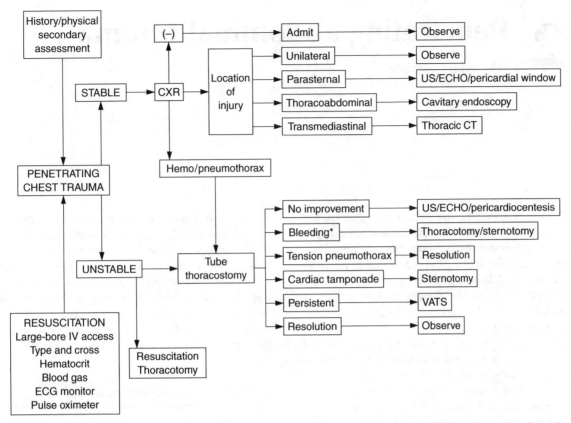

* >1 l or 200 cc/hour for 4 hours. CXR = chest radiograph; VATS = video-assisted thoracoscopic surgery; ECHO = cardiac echocardiography; CT = computed tomography; US = ultrasound.

# 12 Penetrating abdominal trauma

*Edward E Cornwell*

The hallmark of managing the patient with penetrating abdominal trauma lies in balancing the responsibility to minimize unnecessary or non-therapeutic operations, while completely eliminating the occurrence of preventable death due to delays in potentially life-saving surgical intervention. Even the experienced examiner is occasionally humbled by the barrier that the abdominal wall represents in this regard.

Injuries secondary to stab wounds occur as a result of direct penetration of visceral structures. Gunshot injuries may occur as a result of direct penetration of the missile, as well as transfer of energy from a wave of thermal injury created around the path of the bullet. In this regard, patients can conceivably have an injury to an intraabdominal structure without direct penetration of the peritoneal cavity.

## Physical examination

The examination begins with documentation of the vital signs (pulse, blood pressure, respiration, temperature). Close attention should be paid to the pulse pressure and the pulse rate. While patients with gross hypotension and intraabdominal exsanguination are easily identified by vital signs, a diagnostic dilemma may be posed by the young, previously healthy victim of abdominal trauma who presents with a moderate rate of ongoing hemorrhage. Such a patient, for example, with a preinjury pulse of 60 and blood pressure of 130/70 (a pulse pressure of 60), may have a delayed diagnosis if the unsuspecting clinician does not realize that a blood pressure of 110/90 (a pulse pressure of 20) and a pulse rate of 90 may represent a loss of 25% of circulating blood volume.

The abdominal examination begins with inspection of abdominal contour (flat, scaphoid, distended). Careful inspection should also be undertaken to assess for tenderness away from the stab or bullet wound site or eviscration of omentum or other intraabdominal structures. Defects in the abdominal wall, which may represent entrance and/or exit wounds, should also be looked for. While these wounds may give valuable information regarding potential structures that have been injured, it should be remembered that bullets may bounce off structures and take non-direct paths so that the path of a bullet is not necessarily represented by a straight line between entrance and exit wound.

## Controversies in management

In previous decades the list of management options in the treatment of patients with abdominal gunshot wounds would be brief ... surgical exploration.[1–3] In suggesting an alternative treatment algorithm (where gunshot wounds in clinically stable patients are managed selectively, as would be done with stab wounds), it is important to consider the reasons for this time-honored but only recently questioned approach.

### Assumptions supporting mandatory explorations for abdominal gunshot wounds

It has been traditionally taught that:

- abdominal gunshot wounds carry an extremely high rate of visceral injuries requiring repair (as high as 98%)[3]
- laparotomy is the only way to reliably rule out an intraabdominal injury
- a delay in therapeutic laparotomy in an initially asymptomatic patient increases morbidity and mortality
- negative laparotomy causes minimal morbidity.

In suggesting an alternative algorithm of selective management of gunshot wounds to the abdomen (reserving laparotomy for those patients with hemodynamic

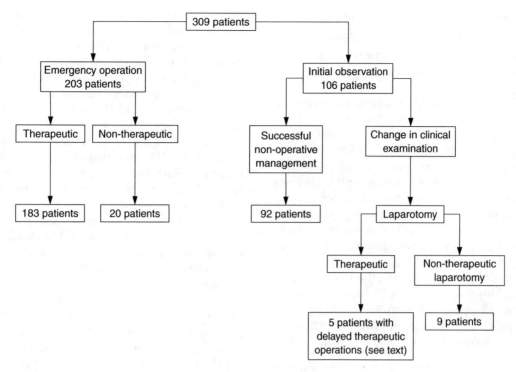

**Figure 12.1** Results of a protocol of selective management of abdominal gunshot wounds.[9]

instability, peritonitis or visceral evisceration),[4-6] each of these assumptions will be addressed by highlighting large prospective series of selectively managed patients.[7-9]

It must be emphasized at the outset that selective management of abdominal gunshot wounds can only be safely pursued if each of the following conditions is met:

- on-site availability of an experienced examiner performing serial clinical evaluations of the patient
- an acute care setting where patients can be closely monitored for changes in their initial clinical presentation
- continuous operating room availability for patients who show changes in their clinical signs.

Patients admitted to trauma centers that cannot offer these resources are better served by immediate surgical exploration.

A prospective protocol-guided study of 309 selectively managed patients with gunshot wounds of the anterior abdomen was reported by Demetriades and colleagues from the Los Angeles County + University of Southern California (LAC + USC) Medical Center.[9] The admitting and subsequent physical findings were carefully recorded as well as the results of laparotomy and of non-operative observation. In addition, an assessment of "likely" or "unlikely" peritoneal penetration was made on the basis of bullet entrance and exit

wounds (or entry wounds and X-rays). Ninety-two patients (29.8%) were successfully managed non-operatively and the overall non-therapeutic laparotomy rate was 10.8 %, but would have been >40% had a policy of mandatory exploration been in place (Figure 12.1) and >24% even if only patients with "likely" peritoneal penetration were explored.

The most important patients in this series are the five who were initially observed, and underwent a delayed therapeutic laparotomy. This includes one patient who, in violation of the protocol, was observed for 48 hours despite developing abdominal distension and a drop in hematocrit and receiving transfusions of 6 units of blood. This patient was operated on for liver and kidney injuries and experienced a long, complicated postoperative course (ARDS, abdominal hypertension, candidiasis) before ultimately being discharged from the hospital. This dramatically demonstrates the hazard of pursuing non-operative management to excess.

The remaining four patients with delayed diagnosis developed fever and abdominal tenderness after between six and 14 hours of observation. All four patients had right colon injuries managed by primary repair. One developed a psoas abscess managed by percutaneous aspiration and was discharged on the ninth postoperative day. The other three had no postoperative complications.

The results of this and other studies suggest that:

- when all patients are included and carefully followed, the non-therapeutic laparotomy rate with a policy of mandatory exploration for abdominal GSWs is higher than previously accepted[9–11]
- initial clinical evaluation by experienced examiners identifies the need for surgical intervention in the vast majority of patients (198 of the 203 patients in the LAC + USC study – 97.5%)
- there are not enough patients (12 patients in two studies) with delayed therapeutic laparotomies from a carefully monitored circumstance to support or refute long held assumptions regarding added morbidity. The four appropriately observed patients in the LAC + USC series who underwent delayed therapeutic operations all had right colon injuries; an intraabdominal postoperative infection developed in one (25%). This rate is consistent with the 27% intraabdominal infection rate seen in a subsequently reported article from the same institution on patients with colon injuries who had immediate surgery.[12]

Finally, the suggestion that non-therapeutic laparotomy following abdominal GSWs carries minimal morbidity is similarly refuted by prospective studies. Renz *et al.* reported a >40% morbidity rate when complications were carefully reported prospectively.[13] The aforementioned series from LAC + USC had a complication rate of 27.6% among non-therapeutic laparotomies and an average length of stay of 6.4 days (versus a 5.5% complication rate and a 3.3 days length of stay for successfully observed patients). The mean hospital charges were about $18 100 for the therapeutic laparotomy group and $8600 for the observed group.

In summary, the algorithm of selective management of abdominal gunshot wounds questions, with Class II data, the assumptions behind the long-accepted policy of mandatory exploration. There remains no substitute for a careful clinical examination, which is to be serially repeated for patients not undergoing immediate laparotomy.

## Diagnostic adjuncts

Even when thoroughly performed, the abdominal examination may be compromised by the presence of alcohol, other drugs or concomitant injuries to the head or other regions. Therefore, other diagnostic modalities are frequently employed in patients with abdominal trauma.

### Diagnostic peritoneal lavage

Diagnostic peritoneal lavage (DPL) can be performed in the emergency department.[10,14,15] Since its introduction by Root in 1967 DPL has been considered the diagnostic procedure of choice to detect intraabdominal hemorrhage in an unstable trauma patient.

The technique is performed under local anesthesia with a low midline linear abdominal incision performed after decompression of the bladder and stomach with a nasogastric tube. Dissection through the midline linea alba and down to the peritoneum allows for direct observation of the insertion of a dialysis catheter and infusion of one liter of crystalloid solution. (It should be noted that aspiration of gross blood, bile or intestinal contents is considered a ''positive tap'' and an indication for emergent abdominal exploration without infusion of the liter of crystalloid.) Patients with penetrating trauma have criteria for positivity that vary from institution to institution, from as low as 1000[14] to as high as 100 000 RBCs per cubic mm.[15] Employing the lower number increases the chances for performing non-therapeutic laparotomy, while raising the threshold for positivity runs the risk of missed or delayed diagnosis of injuries requiring surgical intervention.

DPL has the advantages of being useful in the early minutes after admission and has high sensitivity to identify intraperitoneal hemorrhage. Its drawbacks are its inability to assess the retroperitoneum and its occasional oversensitivity in patients with minimal bleeding.

### Ultrasonography

In many trauma centers ultrasonography of the abdomen is available in the emergency department and has all but supplanted DPL because of its ability to rapidly detect intraabdominal hemorrhage non-invasively in the unstable patient. The focused abdominal sonogram for trauma (FAST) has been described as a rapid survey to assess for blood in the hepatorenal recess of Morrison, the pericardial sac, the perisplenic region, and the pelvis around the bladder.[16] In a study of 371 patients, Rozycki and colleagues found ultrasound to have an 83.8% sensitivity and a 97.4% specificity in detecting blood in the subset of patients with penetrating injuries.[17] A smaller pilot study has analyzed sonographic evaluation of wound tracts.[18] The abdominal ultrasound is quickly gaining popularity as a portable, low-cost, non-invasive, and repeatable modality to allow rapid assessment of the abdominal trauma patient.

### CT

The CT scan has a proven track record in detecting hemoperitoneum, injuries to solid organs, retroperitoneal hemorrhage, and bowel wall thickening. The recent advent of helical CT scanners allows for rapid imaging of patients with multiple system injuries, who require evaluation of other body regions (i.e. head and chest). In patients with penetrating trauma, CT may establish or rule out peritoneal penetration when there are tangential trajectories.[19] The disadvantage of CT is the requirement for patients to be transported to the radiology suite, which makes it an inappropriate test for the hemodynamically unstable or underresuscitated patient.

### Wound exploration

Wound exploration is offered as a diagnostic adjunct in patients with abdominal stab wounds.[14,15] The goal of the procedure (performed under local anesthesia in the emergency department) is to ascertain whether the stab wound tract could have caused peritoneal penetration. As it is difficult in many patients to ascertain the exact depth of stab wounds which course through multiple muscle layers, the practicality is that the procedure is completed once it is clear whether or not the wound tract penetrates the anterior fascial layers of the abdominal wall (anterior sheath medially and external oblique aponeurosis laterally). If an operator familiar with the procedure determines that there was no fascial penetration, then the wound may be treated as an abdominal wall laceration and the patient discharged.

Each of these diagnostic modalities is offered as an option in the selective management of penetrating abdominal trauma. Theoretically, modalities such as these are worth the time and expense only if they improve the sensitivity of serial physical examination. If the 98% sensitivity previously described can be routinely duplicated, one is hard pressed to recommend any of these diagnostic modalities as a routine screen.

### Special consideration: diagnostic laparoscopy

Delayed diaphragmatic hernias secondary to penetrating injuries are potentially lethal entities.[20] Their clinical challenge lies in the fact that their presentation may range from asymptomatic to the presence of signs due to obstruction, ischemia, strangulation, and perforation of incarcerated viscera. Three prospective studies suggest that the incidence of left hemidiaphragm injury following left penetrating thoracoabdominal trauma (wounds between nipples and costal margins) is about 25% in asymptomatic patients (i.e. no other indication for emergency laparotomy).[21–23] With the advent of minimally invasive techniques (laparoscopy, thoracoscopy), diaphragmatic injuries can be effectively ruled out in the early posttraumatic period, thus preventing delayed complications of diaphragmatic hernia.[21–24] Laparoscopy is recommended over thoracoscopy as it allows concomitant evaluation of the abdomen for hemoperitoneum or other suspicious findings. Similarly, it can be performed without the anesthetic challenge of inserting a double lumen endotracheal tube.

In summary, under appropriate circumstances selective management is advocated both for stab wounds[25] and gunshot wounds to the abdomen. The overall implication of the algorithm offered is that, while intraabdominal injuries requiring surgical intervention routinely cause signs and symptoms, diaphragmatic injuries frequently present in an asymptomatic fashion. Thus, serial physical examination is recommended for patients with true abdominal entry wounds (between costal margins and inguinal ligaments), while laparoscopy is advised for those patients with thoracoabdominal entry sites.

### Class II references

3. Liebenberg ND, Maasch AJ. Penetrating abdominal wounds: A prospective trial of conservative treatment based on physical signs. *S Afr Med J* 1988;**74**:231–3.

   A prospective study of 105 patients reporting positive laparotomy findings in 103 (98%), concluding that virtually all patients with abdominal gunshot wounds require laparotomy.

4. Huizinga WKJ, Baker LW, Mtshali ZW. Selective management of abdominal and thoracic stab wounds with established peritoneal penetration: the eviscerated omentum. *Am J Surg* 1987;**153**:564–8.

   This prospective study from South Africa of 276 patients with truncal stab wounds and omental evisceration reaches a different conclusion from American reports. Fifty-nine percent of the patients had intraabdominal injury, prompting a recommendation of omental amputation and observation in these patients.

7. Muckart DT, Abdool AT, King B. Selective conservative management of abdominal gunshot wounds: a prospective study. *Br J Surg* 1990;**77**:652–5.

   This is a series of 111 patients, 22 (20%) of whom were successfully managed non-operatively for abdominal gunshot wounds.

8. Demetriades D, Charalambides D, Lakhoo M, Pantanowitz D. Gunshot wound of the abdomen: role of selective conservative management. *Br J Surg* 1991;**78**:220–2.

   This prospective study of 146 patients with gunshot wounds to the abdomen is the larger of two prospective South African analyses of selective management. Forty-two patients (28%) were initially observed.

Seven of these patients subsequently required delayed laparotomy (17%) without mortality or serious morbidity.

9. Demetriades D, Velmahos G, Cornwell EE III *et al*. Selective nonoperative management of gunshot wounds of the anterior abdomen. *Arch Surg* 1997; **132**:178-183.

   This is the largest prospective analysis of patients selectively managed for gunshot wounds to the abdomen (309 patients; see text and Figure 8.1).

10. Keleman JJ III, Martin RR, Obney JA *et al*. Evaluation of diagnostic peritoneal lavage in stable patients with gunshot wounds to the abdomen. *Arch Surg* 1997;**132**:909–13.

    This is a prospective trial involving two urban trauma centers which evaluated 44 patients who were hemodynamically stable and were undergoing laparotomy. Injuries were present in 32 patients (73%), which parenthetically points to a 27% non-therapeutic laparotomy rate in this series. The negative predictive value (78.6%) of DPL at 100 000 red cells/mm$^3$ suggests that the test is not sensitive enough to avoid serial physical examinations.

12. Cornwell EE III, Velmahos GC, Berne TV *et al*. The fate of colonic suture lines in high-risk trauma patients: a prospective analysis. *J Am Coll Surg* 1998;**187**:58–63.

    A prospective study of 56 patients with traumatic colon injuries and other comorbid factors for the development of septic complications. Fifteen of the 56 patients developed postoperative intraabdominal infections (27%).

13. Renz BM, Feliciano DV. Unnecessary laparotomies for trauma: a prospective study of morbidity. *J Trauma* 1995;**38**:350–6.

    This is a prospective case series of 254 patients with non-therapeutic laparotomy for trauma (98%). The morbidity rate was 41.3% including atelectasis (15.7%), perioperative hypertension requiring therapy (11%), pleural effusion (9.8%), pneumothorax (5.1%), prolonged ileus (4.3%), and pneumonia (3.9%). This is a major contribution from a well-known trauma center that feels secure enough in its reputation to identify the higher than expected morbidity when complications are carefully followed prospectively.

14. Oreskovich MR, Carrico CJ. Stab wounds of the anterior abdomen. *Ann Surg* 1983;**198**:411–19.

    This prospective study of 572 patients analyzed an algorithm using local wound exploration and DPL for stable patients without peritonitis and stab wounds to the anterior abdomen. It employed a positive DPL criteria of 100 000 red cells/mm$^3$. Three hundred and eighty seven patients without obvious need for emergency surgery underwent wound exploration; 151 had negative explorations and were discharged without complications. The remaining 236 patients underwent diagnostic peritoneal lavage followed by laparotomy in 196 (40 patients towards the end of the study with DPL red counts less than 1000 were observed for 24 hours and discharged without complications). One hundred and eighty three of 185 patients going directly to surgery (99%) underwent a therapeutic laparotomy. The overall non-therapeutic laparotomy rate was 22% coming predominantly from patients with fewer than 50 000 red cells/mm$^3$ in their DPL. The authors thus recommend an algorithm including wound exploration and DPL with the "positive" criteria being 1000 cells/mm$^3$, the figure below which no patient had an injury.

15. Feliciano DV, Bitondo CG, Steed G *et al*. Five hundred open taps or lavages in patients with abdominal stab wounds. *Am J Surg* 1984;**148**:772–7.

    This is a four-year prospective study of 500 patients with stab wounds to the anterior abdomen who had no obvious indication for emergency surgery. A treatment algorithm of local wound exploration and DPL for patients with peritoneal penetration (positive criteria 100 000 red cells/mm$^3$) led to laparotomy in 224 patients (45%). The non-therapeutic laparotomy rate was 12.6%. Among the remaining 276 patients who were initially observed due to negative DPLs, five underwent a subsequent therapeutic operation (1.8%), with one death.

16. Rozycki GS, Ochsner MG, Feliciano DV *et al*. Early detection of hemoperitoneum by ultrasound examination of the right upper quadrant: a multicenter study. *J Trauma: Injury Infect Crit Care* 1998;**45**:878–83.

    This is a report generated from the trauma registries of the four Level I trauma centers utilizing ultrasound in trauma patients. Two hundred and seventy five patients, of whom 55 had penetrating abdominal trauma, were reported in the process of determining that hemoperitoneum after trauma is most frequently detected in the right upper quadrant. This is a retrospective evaluation of prospectively collected information stored in trauma registries.

17. Rozycki GS, Ochsner MG, Schmidt JA *et al*. A prospective study of surgeon-performed ultrasound as the primary adjuvant modality for injured patient assessment. *J Trauma: Injury Infect Crit Care* 1995;**39**:492–500.

    This is a prospective study of 371 patients (76 with penetrating injuries). The sensitivity for the detection of hemoperitoneum was 83.8% and the specificity was 97.4%.

18. Fry WR, Smith RS, Schneider JJ, Organ CH Jr. Ultrasonographic examination of wound tracts. *Arch Surg* 1995;**130**:605–8.

    This is a prospective pilot study of 29 patients with penetrating thoracoabdominal trauma. Five wounds were assessed to be penetrating and were subsequently confirmed by surgery or subsequent chest X-ray. The remaining 24 patients had a diagnosis of non-penetration which was reportedly confirmed by clinical course. The authors thus reported a positive and negative predictive accuracy of 100% for the technique. Absolute validation of the assessment of superficial tracts is lacking, as peritoneal penetration and benign abdominal examination can go hand-in-hand, as is confirmed by other reports.

21. Murray JA, Demetriades D, Cornwell EE III *et al*. Penetrating left thoracoabdominal trauma: the incidence and clinical presentation of diaphragm injuries. *J Trauma: Injury Infect Crit Care* 1997;**43**:624–6.

A prospective study of 107 patients including those with and without indications for emergency surgery. The 26% diaphragmatic injury rate among those patients without other indications for surgery prompted subsequent published analysis exclusively of stable patients with no indications for emergency surgery.

22. Murray JA, Demetriades D, Asensio JA *et al*. Occult injuries to the diaphragm: prospective evaluation of laparoscopy in penetrating injuries to the left lower chest. *J Am Coll Surg* 1998;**187**:626–30.

This is a prospective evaluation of 110 consecutive clinically stable patients presenting with penetrating injuries to the thoracoabdominal region. The 24% incidence of diaphragmatic injuries is credible since all patients underwent laparoscopic evaluation strictly for the presence of the wound without any other indications for emergency surgery.

23. Ivatury RR, Simon RJ, Stahl WM. A critical evaluation of laparoscopy in penetrating abdominal trauma. *J Trauma* 1993;**34**:822–8.

This is a prospective report of 100 penetrating abdominal trauma patients (65 stab wounds, 35 gunshot wounds) who were hemodynamically stable without immediate indications for laparotomy. Sixty of the wounds were in the thoracoabdominal region and 17 of these patients (28%) had diaphragmatic injuries. The authors conclude that laparoscopy is excellent for evaluating the diaphragm and thoracoabdominal wounds and urge caution in attempting to exclude hollow viscous injuries. Peritoneal penetration is easily ruled out in the case of tangential wounds as well.

24. Ochsner MG, Rozycki GS, Lucente F *et al*. Prospective evaluation of thoracoscopy for diagnosing diaphragmatic injury in thoracoabdominal trauma: a preliminary report. *J Trauma* 1993;**34**:704–10.

This is a prospective analysis of 14 patients with penetrating thoracoabdominal trauma. In this early report the accuracy of thoracoscopy was 100% for identifying or ruling out diaphragmatic injuries (positive in nine patients, positive in five patients). A small preliminary study.

## Class III references

1. Moore EE, Moore JB, Van-Duzer-Moore S *et al*. Mandatory laparotomy for gunshot wounds penetrating the abdomen. *Am J Surg* 1980;**140**:847–51.

This study of 245 patients with gunshot wounds identified some abnormality in 235 patients (96%). This paper does not distinguish between therapeutic laparotomy and abnormalities such as minor solid organ injuries which may not require a therapeutic procedure.

2. Moore EE, Marx JA. Penetrating abdominal wounds: rationale for exploratory laparotomy. *JAMA* 1985;**253**:2705–8.

A review article.

5. Granson MA, Donovan AJ. Abdominal stab wound with omental evisceration. *Arch Surg* 1983;**118**:57–9.

A retrospective report of 100 patients. A 69% rate of intraabdominal injury prompted a recommendation of surgical exploration for omental evisceration.

6. Burnweit CA, Thal ER. Significance of omental evisceration in abdominal stab wounds. *Am J Surg* 1986;**152**:670–3.

This is a retrospective study of 115 patients presenting with omental evisceration following abdominal stab wounds. Injuries were present in 86 patients (75%). The discussion of this paper, presented at the Southwestern Surgical Conference in April 1986, is most interesting. It centered around the acceptance of a 25% non-therapeutic laparotomy rate for patients with omental evisceration and a >30% unnecessary laparotomy rate in those patients with omental evisceration and hemodynamic stability.

11. Nance FC, Wennar MH, Johnson LW *et al*. Surgical judgement in the management of penetrating wounds of the abdomen: experience with 2212 patients. *Ann Surg* 1974;**179**:639–46.

A retrospective report that includes 432 patients with gunshot wounds. The paper identifies a 16.4% negative laparotomy rate and is the first large series of patients with gunshot wounds to the abdomen managed by observation. Fifty-two such patients were managed without complications.

19. Ginzburg E, Carrillo EH, Kopelman T *et al*. The role of computed tomography in selective management of gunshot wounds to the abdomen and flank. *J Trauma: Injury Infect Crit Care* 1998;**45**:1005–9.

This retrospective study of 83 patients who had abdominal CT scans as part of a protocol of selective management of gunshot wounds to the abdomen included 38 patients with wounds to the flank. Fifty-three patients had CT scans which confirmed the lack of peritoneal penetration and apparently did not change the non-operative management. The CT scan appeared to change the management in 11 patients who had positive peritoneal penetration and underwent surgery.

20. Murray J, Demetriades D, Ashton K. Acute tension diaphragmatic herniation: case report. *J Trauma: Injury Infect Crit Care* 1997;**43**:698–700.

A case report of a patient who had a benign stab wound to the thoracoabdominal region followed 23 months later by an incarcerated diaphragmatic hernia with stomach and left chest causing mediastinal shift and cardiac arrest and ultimately death.

25. Shorr RM, Gottlieb MM, Webb K *et al*. Selective management of abdominal stab wounds: importance of the physical examination. *Arch Surg* 1988;**123**:1141–5.

This is a study of 330 patients presenting with stab wounds to the true abdomen. All patients were evaluated with physical examination. One hundred and seven patients underwent therapeutic laparotomy (32%), 47 patients (14%) had non-therapeutic or negative laparotomy, and 176 patients (53%) were observed for 24 hours and discharged. There were three missed injuries in the last group (1.7%).

**Alternative treatment for penetrating abdominal trauma**

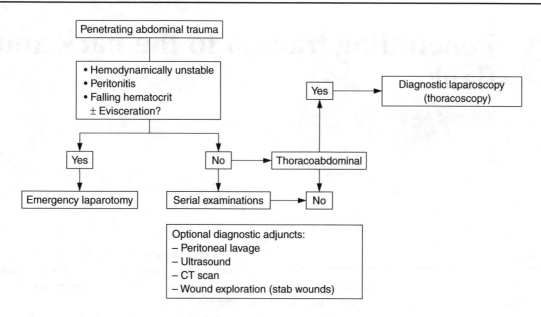

# 13 Penetrating trauma to the back and flank

*William S Miles*

## Introduction

Significant intraabdominal and retroperitoneal injuries can occur after penetrating injuries to the flank or back. This anatomical area encompasses a wide expanse of the torso that may be associated with many solid organs and other vital structures. Controversy still exists as to the appropriate evaluation and management of these lateral and posterior torso wounds.

Historically, patients sustaining flank or back penetrating wounds underwent mandatory celiotomy.[1–4] Though this diagnostic and management modality rarely missed injuries, it resulted in a high number of non-contributory celiotomies, not to mention potentially significant morbidity. Over the past 10–15 years, there has been a rapid explosion in technology and the availability of other diagnostic modalities for the more rapid detection of injuries with less morbidity and costs. These will be discussed based on the algorithms presented. With the advancement of technology, the diagnostic management of these patients will be further streamlined.

## Initial assessment

The first step in managing penetrating trauma to the back or flank is to adhere to the Advanced Trauma Life Support (ATLS) standard guidelines.[5] Airway, breathing, and circulation should be assessed and managed. Volume resuscitation should be undertaken if hemodynamics warrant. Then following certain guidelines, the diagnostic evaluation can be undertaken with high accuracy and patient safety.

A complete physical exam is done to assess the body for all wounds and injuries, including the perineum and scalp.[6] Care should be undertaken to evaluate the full lung exam, looking specifically for decreased lung sounds from a pneumothorax. The abdominal exam should assess for involuntary guarding and rebound tenderness.

A chest X-ray should be performed for all injuries since the trajectory of injury cannot be ascertained from the entrance wound.[5,7] For gunshot wounds, an anteroposterior view and a lateral view should be performed with markers at entrance and exit wounds.

## General approach to back and flank injuries

The back and flank have defined landmarks, separate from the true abdomen. The flank has landmarks that encompass the space from the posterior to anterior axillary lines, the iliac crest inferiorly and the sixth intercostal space superiorly. The back's landmarks include the space from the bilateral posterior axillary lines laterally to the tip of the scapula superiorly and the sacroiliac crests inferiorly.[8,9]

Any penetrating injuries within these anatomic landmarks warrant some type of evaluation based on associations of organ injury. The evaluation may vary depending on the ballistic mechanism involved (gunshot or knife wounds).

## Gunshot wounds

### Shotguns

These injuries warrant a separate discussion since, depending on the distance between the muzzle and the skin, different approaches may have to be undertaken. Close-range (<10 yards) shotgun wounds involve significant tissue destruction, since the missiles are clumped together and the wadding component of the shell may penetrate the wound. These wounds generally involve operative intervention since they behave like high-velocity gunshot wounds, causing significant dead tissue. If the patient has a normal clinical exam and is hemodynamically stable, additional diagnostic modalities should be undertaken to determine degree of pellet penetrance and associated injuries. Most of the wounds will involve the peritoneal or vital retroperitoneal structures, depending on the trajectory. If this additional exam is negative, the wound created by close-range shotgun blasts should be debrided, with careful removal of any wadding.[2–4,9,10]

Long-range (>10 yards) shotgun wounds tend to involve a wider body area since the shotgun pellets spread to a wider pattern. The pellet penetrance into soft tissues is significantly less due to the rapidly declining velocity but these pellets can still cause significant damage. The majority of these patients tend to be hemodynamically stable and therefore the managing physician has a finite time period to explore more organ-specific diagnostic procedures.

## Handguns

The majority of gunshot wounds are caused by low-velocity handguns shot at relatively close range (7 meters). Though the kinetic energy is significantly less compared to higher velocity rifle wounds, the specific characteristic of the missile itself can still have significant destructive capabilities as compared to stab wound penetration. Gunshot victims with flank and back wounds may have significantly more associated injuries, greater hemodynamic instability, and the potential for peritoneal signs.[11] However, a significant number of patients with penetrating gunshot wounds to the flank and back have tangential injuries and are hemodynamically stable with normal abdominal exams; in these patients, a more organ-directed diagnostic approach may be warranted, as seen in the algorithm.[4,11–19]

## Stab wounds

Location and mechanism of injuries are important in determining the diagnostic and therapeutic approaches to penetrating flank and back stab wounds. The majority of significant injuries in hemodynamically stable patients tend to be retroperitoneal rather than intraperitoneal. Therefore signs of peritonitis may be delayed due to the tamponade effects of tissues and organs. There are several approaches for the diagnostic evaluation of these injuries; these include clinical observation, selective management, operative exploration, radio-graphic imaging studies, laparoscopy, and diagnostic peritoneal lavage.[1,7,8,16,18,20–23] Depending on institutional availability and physician abilities, each has its own level of accuracy, false-positive and false-negative results, and potential morbidity.

Historically, most of these injuries were managed by mandatory exploration.[1–4] Over the last two decades, the trend has been away from aggressive management to organ-specific protocols to address financial and morbidity constraints.

Wounds above the costal margin may include the pleural cavity and/or the diaphragm, causing a hemothorax or pneumothorax and a diaphragmatic rent, allowing bowel to be entrapped and causing bowel ischemia.[8,14,18,20]

## Diagnostic modalities

### Clinical exam

Historically, patients with flank and back wounds underwent mandatory celiotomy. Due to higher morbidity, hospital charges, and costs, the recent trend has been away from this. Ideally a selective management policy allows for early identification of significant injury and decreased incidence of non-therapeutic celiotomy. The physical exam does not stop at admission. To approach a high diagnostic accuracy, serial physical exam must be performed and documented in a chronologic order. With this approach, an accuracy of 95% can be achieved.[3,6,8] Most studies include an arm of clinical examination for patients with a higher risk of potential injury. Serial clinical exams alone have been shown to cause a longer delay in the identification of some retroperitoneal injuries when compared to other more specific radiologic evaluations.[4,7,8,11,19]

### Ultrasound

Ultrasonography has been a relatively recent introduction in the diagnosis of flank and back penetrating injuries. The focused assessment for the sonographic examination of the trauma patient (FAST) has replaced diagnostic peritoneal lavage (DPL) as a rapid diagnostic procedure in most patients, including pregnant patients, obese patients, and those with prior abdominal surgery. It is a non-invasive test and in trained hands it is extremely rapid, cost effective, and can be performed serially.[9] It can evaluate the peritoneum, the thorax, and selective organs in the retroperitoneum. Its disadvantages include the requirement for at least 70 cc of peritoneal fluid for a positive study and a 20% incidence of failure to detect injury to solid organs such as the liver and spleen. Most of the studies have been on ultrasound use in blunt abdominal injury, but several have shown the advantages of this modality in the quick identification of organ injury with penetrating flank and back trauma. If available, it can be a useful adjunct to identify area-specific abnormalities, such as fluid in the peritoneum or thorax, and renal trauma such as injury to the kidney. This modality can identify those patients with injuries that require celiotomy earlier and those patients where a more organ-specific work-up could be utilized such as arteriography or contrast-enhanced computed tomography scan (see below).[8,9,21]

## Diagnostic peritoneal lavage

Most published studies have standardized the accepted results for DPL in blunt trauma, but the results that signify a positive study in penetrating trauma remain controversial. In one study a red blood cell count of 5000/mm$^3$ is considered positive due to a high specificity and sensitivity. In most studies, DPL is only 2–4% less accurate when used in penetrating back and flank wounds as compared to blunt abdominal trauma. It may not allow early discharge of patients, but may more rapidly identify the need for earlier celiotomy for some patients.[1,11,19,22,23] Results for a positive study are listed in Box 13.1.[1]

## Local wound exploration

This diagnostic modality may be used to screen those hemodynamically stable patients without peritoneal abdominal findings who appear to have superficial wounds. This technique may identify those patients at low risk for potential injury caused by penetrating knife wounds.[4,6] Using local anesthetics and under sterile conditions, wound exploration may determine if the retroperitoneal or peritoneal cavities have been violated by identifying whether the muscle/fascia layers were penetrated. When identified, a more selective diagnostic management can be utilized. If the wounds are determined to be superficial, then the patient could be observed or discharged depending on physician judgment. Local wound exploration should

only be considered for stab wounds to the flank and back that are below the costal margin since there is a greater possibility of iatrogenic pneumothorax if wounds above the costal margin are explored.[4] The physician should remember that different tissue layers may be penetrated at different levels due to torso rotation and movement of the victim at the time of injury.

This modality can reduce the potential costs and morbidity associated with other diagnostic modalities and decrease the expense of a hospital stay for observation. This technique was shown in one study to accurately identify the depth of penetration in hemodynamically stable patients with flank and back stab wounds.[4]

## Laparoscopy

The potential for laparoscopy to be used for the selective management of patients with penetrating wounds to the flank and back has only recently come to the fore. Multiple studies show the potential benefits of laparoscopic evaluation of abdominal contents including avoiding non-therapeutic celiotomies in 34% of stab wounds and 60% of gunshot wounds in the patient population studied. This decreased the hospital length of stay and costs.[14,18,24,25] Laparoscopy in hemodynamically stable patients with stab or gunshot wounds may determine peritoneal penetration, hemoperitoneum, and isolated diaphragmatic lacerations and confirm the presence of retroperitoneal or pericolic hematomas. Surgeons can then make the judgment for or against surgical exploration. Pitfalls for laparoscopy continue to be evaluating and identifying hollow viscus injuries and the overall costs of equipment.

Laparoscopic technology has improved tremendously and now with the presence of needlescopic (2 mm side viewing) cameras and equipment such as non-crushing bowel graspers, etc., a more thorough evaluation of the intestinal tract can be undertaken without much difficulty. This technique has eliminated the need for general anesthesia and the laparoscopic evaluation can be performed in the emergency department or a monitored setting.[18,24,25]

The cost of laparoscopy may be a concern for some institutions for there is a significant start-up cost as well as maintenance costs. In one study comparing laparosopy with non-therapeutic laparotomy, laparoscopy reduced overall costs (charges by $1500). Length of stay and total costs were also reduced.[18,24]

Laparoscopy should be considered only by experienced surgeons for use as an adjunct in identifying those patients with a higher risk for cavitary injury. Other diagnostic modalities such as contrast-enhanced computed tomography may reduce the need for invasive procedures such as laparoscopy.

---

**Box 13.1** Criteria for a positive diagnostic peritoneal lavage in penetrating trauma

| | |
|---|---|
| RBC | 10 000 RBC/cc$^3$ |
| WBC | 500 WBC/cc$^3$ |
| Bile | Present |
| Food particles | Present |
| Amylase | Elevated |

---

## Contrast-enhanced computed tomography (CECT)

With the improvement in CT technology over the last decade, this modality has been used more frequently in this patient population. It is non-invasive, relatively rapid, and has been shown in many studies to have a high diagnostic accuracy. The inclusion of rectal contrast in addition to the oral and vascular contrast has greatly improved the diagnosis of peritoneal and retroperitoneal injuries. In one study comparing CECT with other more conventional modalities (such as wound exploration, abdominal roentgenograms, DPL, and angiography), CT scan was shown to have a negative predictive value of 100% and a positive predictive value significantly higher than any of the other modalities.[23] Studies have shown that if the CT scan evaluation shows no gross injury but the patient has a higher risk for potential injury, such as blast effect, multiple wounds, etc. or whose abdominal exam is unreliable, a short hospital stay for observation may be necessary.[1,7–9,11–13,16,17,20,23,26]

This diagnostic modality is perhaps the most utilized in this population of patients since it is non-invasive, relatively rapid, and most physicians managing patients with penetrating wounds to the back and flank have direct access to it.

## Class I reference

7. Easter DW, Shackford SR, Mattry RF. A prospective, randomized comparison of computed tomography with conventional diagnostic methods in the evaluation of penetrating injuries to the back and flank. *Arch Surg* 1991;**126**:1115–19.

   The only prospective randomized study comparing CT with other conventional diagnostic methods – wound exploration, abdominal X-ray, intravenous pyelography, DPL, and arteriography – depending on physician judgment. Studying 85 patients in two years, the authors determined that in hemodynamically stable patients without peritoneal signs, CT took slightly longer to determine disposition, but there were no missed injuries. A normal CT scan adequately excludes substantial injury.

## Class II references

1. Boyle EM, Maier RV, Salazar JD *et al*. Diagnosis of injuries after stab wounds to the back and flank. *J Trauma* 1997;**42**(20):260–5.

   This retrospective study reviewed 203 patients over 10 years. It showed that on changing from mandatory celiotomy to selective management and diagnosis, the celiotomy rate decreased from 100% to 24% and the therapeutic celiotomy rate increased from 15% to 80%. Stable patients had a DPL and if this was negative, they then had a triple contrast CT scan. The authors determined that the threshold for a positive DPL was 10 000 RBC/mm$^3$.

2. McCarth MC, Lowdermilk GA, Canal DF *et al*. Prediction of injury caused by penetrating wounds to the abdomen, flank, and back. *Arch Surg* 1991;**126**:962–6.

   Retrospective review of 392 patients with torso injuries of abdomen, back, and flank. A limited study in clarifying extremes. Based on their data, the authors felt that all gunshot wounds should have mandatory exploration. Ninety per cent of their patients had significant injuries (10% non-therapeutic celiotomy). Separate analysis of gunshot wounds into abdominal, flank, and back was not undertaken.

6. Demetriades D, Rabinowitz B, Sofianos C. The management of penetrating injuries of the back. *Ann Surg* 1987;**207**(1):72–4.

   This study looked expressly at abdominal examination as an indicator for surgical exploration. The authors observed all patients without peritoneal signs. They determined that abdominal examination is reliable in detecting clinically significant intra-abdominal injuries even with penetrating injuries to the back.

8. Kirton OC, Wint D, Thrasher B *et al*. Stab wounds to the back and flank in the hemodynamically stable patient: a decision algorithm based on contrast-enhanced computed tomography with colonic opacification. *Am J Surg* 1997;**173**:189–93.

   Prospectively collected data using contrast-enhanced CT in evaluation of stab wounds to the back and flank. Categorized each as low risk (penetration beyond deep fascia) or high risk (penetration beyond deep fascia). The algorithm, however, used this modality as the primary initial screening tool. With this designation the authors were able to discharge many patients earlier.

12. Benz BM, Feliciano DV. Gunshot wounds to the right thoracoabdomen – a prospective study of nonoperative management. *J Trauma* 1994;**37**(5):737–44.

    A prospective study of 13 patients with small caliber gunshot wounds to the thoracoabdomen. Hemothorax was treated with a chest tube. Twelve of 13 patients with hemodynamically stable presentations and no peritonitis (just local wound tenderness) underwent CT scan within eight hours of admission. These patients had a shorter length of stay (5.1 days). The authors reported successful non-operative management in this limited patient population.

13. Benz BM, Bott J, Feliciano DV. Failure of non-operative treatment of gunshot wound to the liver predicted by computed tomography. *J Trauma* 1996;**41**(1):171.

    Follow-up results of initial study. Authors reviewed subsequent failures of non-operative management in penetrating injuries of the thoracoabdomen. They felt that patients whose initial CT showed a vascular blush in the liver parenchyma should undergo celiotomy. A vascular blush on CT could not be reliably managed non-operatively.

14. Ditmars ML, Bongard F. Laparoscopy for triage of penetrating trauma: the decision to explore. *J Laparoendoscopic Surg* 1996;**6**(5):285–91.

    The authors evaluated laparoscopy in 106 hemodynamically stable patients with abdominal wounds. They used laparoscopy as a screening tool for peritoneal penetrance. They still had a non-therapeutic laparotomy rate of 24%. A significant number (39%) of patients had positive findings. Not all required laparotomy. The authors suggest that laparoscopy could be a useful screening tool.

15. Nagy KK, Brenneman FD, Krosner SM *et al*. Routine preoperative "one-shot" intravenous pyelography is not indicated in all patients with penetrating abominal trauma. *J Am Coll Surg* 1997;**185**:530–3.

    This prospectively collected study of 240 laparotomies was performed over 15 months. It assessed all abdominal wounds including back and flank wounds. It showed that IVP is indicated only in stable patients and did not reliably exclude renal trauma. IVP is useful in a small group of patients with gross hematuria or injury in renal proximity.

16. Meyer DM, Thal ER, Weigelt JA *et al*. The role of abdominal CT in the evaluation of stab wounds to the back. *J Trauma* 1989;**29**(9):1226–30.

    Prospective study evaluating 250 patients with stab wounds to the back. The authors found that abdominal CT with IV and oral contrast had a 89% sensitivity, 98% specificity, and an accuracy of 97%; a reliable study to evaluate this patient population.

17. Phillips T, Sclafani JJ, Goldstein A *et al*. Use of contrast-enhanced CT enema in the management of penetrating trauma to the flank and back. *J Trauma* 1986;**26**(7):593–601.

    This prospectively collected, retrospectively reviewed study showed that in the evaluation of the peritoneum and retroperitoneum in penetrating trauma, an enema was a useful adjunct to identify injuries and reduce the number of non-therapeutic laparotomies.

18. Ivatury RR, Simon RJ, Stahl WM. A critical evaluation of laparoscopy in penetrating abdominal trauma. *J Trauma* 1993;**34**(6):822–7.

    Prospective non-randomized study evaluating 100 hemodynamically stable patients with penetrating abdominal wounds. Twenty-five per cent had injuries in the flank and lower abdomen. The authors concluded that the diagnostic accuracy of laparoscopy is excellent for hemoperitoneum, solid organ injuries, diaphragmatic lacerations, and retroperitoneal hematomas. Discordant results were usually due to flank

and lower abdominal wounds. They emphasized the poor, experience-dependent results in evaluating hollow viscus injuries.

20. Armenakas NA, Duckett CP, McAninch JW. Indications for nonoperative management of renal stab wounds. *J Urol* 1999;**161**(3):768–71.

    Authors at a level I trauma center evaluated 200 renal stab wounds retrospectively. Over half (54%) had non-operative management with only three failures. They cite management criteria based on aggressive radiologic data and clinical exam. Simple stab wounds to the kidney without extravasation could be closely observed, depending on reliable serial examinations and follow-up.

21. Albrecht RM, Vigil A, Schermer CR *et al*. Stab wounds to the back and flank in hemodynamically stable patients: evaluation using triple-contrast computed tomography. *Am Surg* 1999;**65**:683–8.

    This retrospective review evaluated 141 patients over a two-year period. It determined that triple-contrast CT could be used to safely triage patients with stab wounds to the back and flank. The authors showed that patients with a low-risk scan (penetration into subcutaneous abdominal wall or retroperitoneum but not near vital structures) and no associated injuries could be safely discharged. Other patients with a potentially high-risk scan (penetration near organ or vessel or active extravasation) could be observed for 24 hours unless symptoms changed.

22. Peck JJ, Berne TV. Posterior abdominal stab wounds *J Trauma* 1981;**21**(4):298–306.

    Retrospective study of 1776 patients with abdominal-posterior and thoracoabdominal wounds. It showed that adjunct diagnostic studies (DPL, IVP, arteriography) can be useful and determined that observation could be useful in the selective management of these patients.

23. Himmelman RG, Martin M, Gilkes S *et al*. Triple-contrast CT scans in penetrating back and flank trauma. *J Trauma* 1991;**31**(6):852–5.

    Prospective study evaluating 88 patients with hemodynamic stability and penetrating trauma to the back and flank. The authors used DPL and observation liberally and separated the scans into high and low risk. The negative predictive value of a low-risk or moderate-risk CT scan was 100% ± 11%.

24. Marks JM, Youngelman DF, Buk T. Cost analysis of diagnostic laparoscopy vs laparotomy in the evaluation of penetrating abdominal trauma. *Surg Endosc* 1997;**11**:272–6.

    Retrospective chart review. The authors conclude that total costs and length of stay were significantly lower with laparoscopy compared to laparotomy. There were 37 patients evaluated; they received either laparotomy or laparoscopy or both. No other diagnostic modality was included in the analysis.

## Class III references

3. Vanderzee J, Christenberry P, Jurovich GJ. Penetrating trauma to the back and flank: a reassessment of mandatory celiotomy. *Am Surg* 1987;**5**:220–2.

   A retrospective review based on a change in management from mandatory celiotomy to selective management. The authors reviewed 34 patients with stab wounds and gunshot wounds. They felt stab wounds in hemodynamically stable patients should have selective management but all gunshot wound patients should have celiotomy.

4. Berne TV. Management of penetrating back trauma. *Surg Clin North Am* 1990;**70**(3):671–6.

   Short review on this subject. Explains the limited but still useful modality of local wound exploration in a small subgroup of patients – superficial-appearing stab wounds – that may reduce the need for further, more expensive diagnostic modalities or observation.

5. American College of Surgeons Committee on Trauma. *Advanced trauma life support for doctors.* Chicago: American College of Surgeons, 1997.

   This expert consensus opinion of the American College of Surgeons Committee on Trauma on current research and clinical practice in trauma care outlines one safe method of initial care for the injured patient.

9. Feliciano DV. Diagnostic modalities in abdominal trauma: peritoneal lavage, ultrasonography, computed tomography scanning, and arteriography. *Surg Clin North Am* 1991;**71**(2):241–56.

   An excellent review of all diagnostic modalities useful in the management of abdominal trauma, including flank and back injuries. The section on penetrating trauma emphasizes the improvement of accuracy, specificity, and sensitivity of contrast-enhanced CT scans in the diagnosis and management of these patients.

10. Moore EE, Marx JA. Penetrating abdominal wounds: rationale for exploratory laparotomy. *JAMA* 1985;**253**(18):2705–8.

    Basic review of multiple mechanism penetrating wounds to anterior and posterior abdomen and flank. The authors advocated selective management with individualized patient evaluation for hemodynamically stable penetrating wounds to the flank and back. They liberally used retroperitoneal contrast studies to evaluate these patients. They also believe that the safest policy is to explore the abdomen if there is any question of visceral injury.

11. McConnell DB, Trunkey DD. Nonoperative management of abdominal trauma. *Surg Clin North Am* 1990;**70**(3):677–88.

    The authors stress that all gunshot wound victims should have mandatory celiotomy, but that there should be selective management with the use of observation in stab wound patients. They advocate the use of CT scans for flank and back wounds where results may determine operative versus non-operative management decisions.

19. Henneman PL. Penetrating abdominal trauma. *Emerg Clin North Am* 1989;**7**(3):647–66.

    Basic review of mechanisms of injuries and diagnostic approaches to abdominal penetrating injuries.

25. Villavicencio RT, Aucar JA. Analysis of laparoscopy in trauma. *J Am Coll Surg* 1999;**189**(1):11–20.

    An outcome analysis of 37 studies using over 1900 trauma patients. Laparoscopy was analyzed as a diagnostic, screening, and therapeutic tool. As a screening tool, laparoscopy missed 1% of injuries, but helped 63% avoid non-therapeutic celiotomy. As a diagnostic tool, there were 41–77% of missed injuries per patient and a 1% procedure-related complication rate. The authors felt that its use as a therapeutic tool is limited and more studies are required on the use of laparoscopy in this context.

26. Baniel J, Schein M. The management of penetrating trauma to the urinary tract. *J Am Coll Surg* 1994;**178**:417–25.

    Collective review of management for this patient population. The authors extensively evaluate all diagnostic modalities including IVP, CT, arteriography, and laparotomy as well as specific organ (bladder, kidney, etc.) evaluation. They stress the value of CT in the diagnostic management of these patients.

## Penetrating wounds to back and flank: gunshot wounds

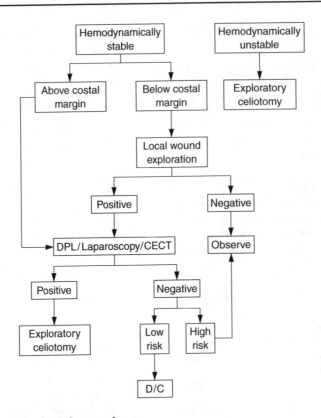

## Penetrating wounds to back and flank: stab wounds

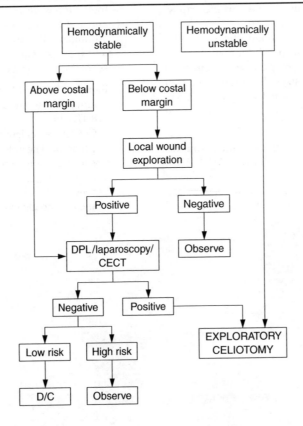

# 14 Evaluation of gluteal gunshot wounds

*J Christopher DiGiacomo, Gerald W Shaftan*

## Introduction

The gluteal region overlies the posterior pelvis and is defined as that area bounded superiorly by the posterior iliac crests (approximately the level of the spinous process of L4), laterally by the greater trochanter/midaxillary line, and inferiorly by the inferior border of the gluteus maximus, which forms the gluteal crease. The majority of muscle mass of the gluteal region is formed by the gluteus maximus, which directly overlies the sciatic nerve and the remainder of the muscles: gluteus medius, piriformis, superior gemellus, obturator internus, inferior gemellus, quadratus femoris, and adductor magnus. Deep to the gluteus medius lies the gluteus minimus which occupies the gap between the greater trochanter of the femur and the posterolateral aspect of the iliac wing. The musculature is supplied by the anterior and posterior divisions of the internal iliac artery. These vessels are large in diameter but short in length and enter the gluteal region from the pelvis through the greater sciatic foramen superior (the superior gluteal artery) and inferior (the inferior gluteal and internal pudendal arteries) to the piriformis along with the sciatic nerve, which enters deep to the piriformis.

This chapter focuses on isolated gluteal gunshot entrance wounds. Additional gunshot wounds involving the torso, including gluteal exit wounds, are not discussed, since trajectories cannot be accurately assessed.

## Hemodynamic instability

Hemodynamic instability is hypotension, tachypnea or tachycardia which either does not respond or transiently responds to the initial fluid resuscitation. Additional signs of hypovolemia may include altered sensorium in the absence of head injury or neuroactive compounds, hypoxemia, cool mottled skin, persistent or recurrent tachycardia, inadequate urine output, and persistent lactic acidosis.

## Resuscitation

Resuscitation in preparation for the operating room includes two large-bore peripheral IVs (18 gauge or larger), with blood drawn for at least basic laboratory studies and type and crossmatch. Portable anterior–posterior X-ray studies of the chest, abdomen, and pelvis should be performed if time and the patient's condition allow. Nasogastric and urinary catheters should be inserted unless contraindicated and a first-generation cephalosporin should also be given intravenously if time permits.

## Trajectory

The sentinel issue in gluteal gunshot wounds is whether the projectile traversed the bony ring of the pelvis and therefore entered the abdominal cavity.[1] There is a 97% incidence of injury requiring operative intervention for abdominal gunshot wounds. Obviously, however, the projectile will not produce an intraabdominal injury if it remains outside the bony ring of the pelvis.

## History

The details of the event should be discerned to help determine trajectory. If the patient was standing stationary, the gluteal gunshot wound most likely extends inferiorly. If the patient was running away from the assailant, the trajectory is more likely to track anteriorly, given the normal forward inclination of the torso when running. If the patient was in the prone position when shot, as may be the case if discovered from behind by a jealous lover or spouse, the trajectory more likely will track superiorly.

## Physical examination

The findings of an anterior gunshot wound, peritoneal signs or gross blood in the urine or on digital rectal exam all warrant prompt celiotomy. The absence of abdominal tenderness or blood in the urine or rectum does not rule out injury and further diagnostic work-up is warranted.[1-13] Given the intimate proximity of the sciatic nerve to the superior and inferior gluteal arteries and internal pudendal artery in the greater sciatic foramen, a thorough neurovascular assessment of the lower extremities is essential. A neurologic deficit should raise concern for an associated vascular injury.[14-16]

## Diagnostic studies

If operation is not indicated by the above positive findings, trajectory should be determined. This can be done most easily with portable X-ray anterior–posterior abdomen/pelvic, lateral pelvic, and oblique pelvic views. The gunshot wound should be marked with a radiopaque marker or paperclip. The oblique pelvic X-ray is performed with the film under the patient with the X-ray beam angled 45° to the side of the entrance wound. This allows the ipsilateral iliac wing to be viewed on end. The projectile, if still present in the patient, will be seen either outside the bony ring of the pelvis, which rules out intraabdominal injury, or across the bony ring of the pelvis, in which case it is an abdominal gunshot wound and warrants prompt celiotomy.[1]

If there is concern that the trajectory passes through the pelvis below the peritoneal reflection, it is appropriate to evaluate the rectum and bladder. The rectum can be visualized with rigid proctosigmoidoscopy and a retrograde cystogram with bladder overdistension can rule out an injury to the urinary bladder. If the patient is entirely stable from the hemodynamic standpoint and computed tomography is readily available, triple-contrast CT of the abdomen and pelvis can provide an accurate evaluation of both trajectory and organ injury.[5]

## Class II references

1. DiGiacomo JC, Schwab CW, Rotondo MF *et al.* Gluteal gunshot wounds: who warrants exploration? *J Trauma* 1994;**37**:622–8.

    A large retrospective study of patients with isolated gluteal gunshot wounds which demonstrated that peritoneal irritation or gross blood in the urine or at

digital rectal exam has a 90% sensitivity for predicting injuries which required operative repair. The absence of these findings did not rule out significant injury. The triage criterion of trajectory across the bony ring of the pelvis, however, was 93% accurate overall and no patients with an extrapelvic trajectory had missed injuries. The authors suggest an algorithm of physical examination and plain film X-rays which include an oblique pelvic X-ray to help determine an extrapelvic or transpelvic trajectory.

2. Duncan AO, Phillips TF, Scalea TM, Maltz SB, Atweh NA, Sclafani SJA. Management of transpelvic gunshot wounds. *J Trauma* 1989;**29**:1335–40.

    A large retrospective study of patients with transpelvic gunshot wounds. Nearly 60% of patients had injuries which required celiotomy. The evaluation algorithm for stable patients required physical, digital rectal, and rigid protoscopic examination. Peritoneal lavage, CT scan, and angiography were used liberally to further assess the patients. Patients with positive studies went to the operating room and those with negative studies progressed to the next study in the algorithm. All four missed injuries were retroperitoneal, pointing out the fallibility of all preoperative diagnostic studies and the importance of trajectory determination in injury identification.

3. Fallon WF, Reyna TM, Brunner RG, Crooms C, Alexander RH. Penetrating trauma to the buttock. *South Med J* 1988;**81**:1236–8.

    Retrospective study of gluteal gunshot and stab wounds which emphasizes the need for trajectory determination and the use of protoscopy in addition to digital rectal examination to assess the rectum.

4. Ferraro FJ, Livingston DH, Odom J, Swan KG, McCormack M, Rush BF. The role of sigmoidoscopy in the management of gunshot wounds to the buttocks. *Am Surg* 1993;**59**:350–2.

    A large retrospective study of 70 patients, 26 of whom required celiotomy (37.1%). All patients with gross blood in the urine or on digital rectal examination had major injuries. Microscopic hematuria was found in 17 patients, none of whom had genitourinary injuries. Biplanar X-rays were obtained to determine trajectory. In contradistinction to previous authors who advocated mandatory rigid proctosigmoidoscopy in all patients who have sustained gluteal gunshot wounds, they advocate selected use of rigid proctosigmoidoscopy in patients with a transpelvic trajectory without blood present on digital rectal examination.

5. Grossman MD, May AK, Schwab CW *et al.* Determining anatomic injury with computed tomography in selected torso gunshot wounds. *J Trauma* 1998;**45**:446–56.

    Large retrospective study which demonstrates the utility and accuracy of CT scan for trajectory determination in hemodynamically stable victims of gunshot wounds.

6.   Ivatury RR, Rao PM, Nallathambi M, Gaudino J, Stahl WM. Penetrating gluteal injuries. *J Trauma* 1982;**22**: 706–9.

Retrospective review from a busy urban trauma center. Twelve of the 45 patients who sustained gluteal gunshot wounds (26.7%) and four of the 15 patients who sustained gluteal stab wounds (26.7%) required operative intervention. The work-up included physical examination, urinalysis, rigid sigmoidoscopy, biplanar plain film chest, and abdominopelvic X-rays. Gross or microscopic hematuria resulted in a cystogram with or without a retrograde urethrogram. Diagnostic peritoneal lavage was liberally used for equivocal physical examinations. All patients were admitted for observation and serial examinations. There were no missed injuries and one non-therapeutic laparotomy.

7.   Levine H, Simon RJ, Smith TR, Ivatury R, Stahl W. Guaiac testing in the diagnosis of rectal trauma: what is its value? *J Trauma* 1992;**32**:210–12.

What is its value? None.

8.   Mangiante EC, Graham AD, Fabian TC. Rectal gunshot wounds: management of civilian injuries. *Am Surg* 1986;**52**:37–40.

Forty-three patients retrospectively identified as having sustained rectal injuries from handguns or shotguns were reviewed. Gross blood was present at digital rectal examination in 80% and rigid proctoscopy identified the injury in 91% of patients. While this study demonstrates the utility of these studies when positive, it is not possible to comment on the accuracy of negative studies.

9.   Maull KI, Snoddy JW, Haynes BW. Penetrating wounds of the buttock. *Surg Gynecol Obstet* 1979; **149**:855–7.

This retrospective review of 15 patients is the earliest paper to formally discuss penetrating gluteal injuries, although sporadic case reports can be traced back to 1902 (Fenner ED. Report of six cases of penetrating wounds of the abdomen submitted to abdominal section. *Ann Surg* 1902;**35**:15–24). The paradigm for assessment proposed by the authors, physical examination, plain film X-ray studies, trajectory determination, and further diagnostic work-up of the areas at risk, has remained fundamentally unchanged. It is interesting to note that this review had no references.

10.   Mercer DW, Buckman RF, Sood R, Kerr TM, Gelman J. Anatomic considerations in penetrating gluteal wounds. *Arch Surg* 1992;**127**:407–10.

In an interesting approach to triaging patients into high-risk and low-risk categories for major injuries, the authors assessed the entrance wound site in relationship to the intertrochanteric line. They demonstrated that 35.1% of gunshot wounds and 23.5% of stab wounds above the intertrochanteric line were associated with major injuries, as compared with one of 27 wounds below that line. They assumed that all patients were injured while standing and therefore had an inferior trajectory direction.

11.   Nagy, KK, Krosner SM, Joseph KT, Roberts RR, Smith RF, Barrett J. A method of determining peritoneal penetration in gunshot wounds to the abdomen. *J Trauma* 1997;**43**:242–6.

Large study of 429 consecutive patients with abdominal gunshot wounds evaluated with diagnostic peritoneal lavage. Using a threshold of 10 000 $RBC/mm^3$, they demonstrated an accuracy of 98% for identifying the presence or absence of intra-abdominal injury. Unfortunately, this technique cannot rule out significant injuries of the extraperitoneal organs.

12.   Phillips T, Sclafani SJA, Goldstein A, Scalea T, Panetta T, Shaftan G. Use of the contrast-enhanced CT enema in the management of penetrating trauma to the flank and back. *J Truma* 1986;**26**:593–601.

Prospective study which demonstrated the added efficacy of contrast enema-enhanced CT scans in assessing the abdomen, pelvis, and retroperitoneum. The subsequent rapid adoption of the technique by trauma centers confirms its utility.

13.   (a) Vo NM, Russell JC, Becker DR. Gunshot wounds to the buttocks. *Am Surg* 1983;**49**:579–81.

(b) Vo NM, Russell JC, Becker DR. Gunshot wounds to the buttocks. *Connecticut Med* 1983;**47**:685–6.

Retrospective reviews of two Connecticut institutions' experience. Twenty-five per cent had intra-abdominal injuries and underwent laparotomy. The initial work-up included physical examination, biplanar abdominal X-rays, and trajectory determination as extraperitoneal or intraperitoneal. All of the latter group underwent laparotomy, only one of which was non-therapeutic.

## Class III references

14.   (a) Gilroy D, Saadia R, Hide G, Demetriades D. Penetrating injury to the gluteal region. *J Trauma* 1992; **32**:294–7.

(b) Demetriades D, Rabinowitz B, Sofianos C. Gluteal artery aneurysms. *Br J Surg* 1988;**75**:494.

Eight cases of gluteal region pseudoaneurysms are described, six secondary to gluteal stab wounds and two from gluteal gunshot wounds, presenting between one hour and three months postinjury. Four were incorrectly diagnosed as abscesses and incised under local anesthesia.

15.   Holland AJA, Ibach EG. False aneurysm of the inferior gluteal artery following penetrating buttock trauma:

case report and review of the literature. *Cardiovasc Surg* 1996;**4**:841–3.

An interesting case report of sciatic nerve palsy and dysesthesia with an inferior gluteal artery false aneurysm three months after a gluteal stab wound. A good, concise discussion of the topic.

16. Williams W, Jackson GF, Greene C. Superior gluteal artery aneurysm. *J Trauma* 1977;**17**:477–9.

A case report of a superior gluteal artery pseudo-aneurysm secondary to a gluteal gunshot wound which presented 22 months after injury.

**Gluteal gunshot wounds**

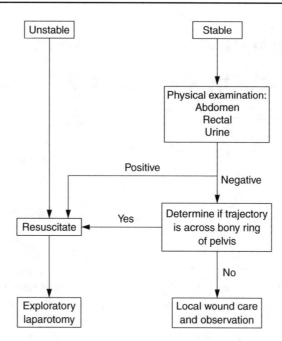

# 15 Evaluation of vascular proximity in penetrating extremity trauma

*Michael D Grossman*

## Hemodynamic status

Patients sustaining proximity penetrating extremity trauma (PPET) are at risk for limb loss and death. Limb loss in urban civilian series is less than 5% and in recent military conflicts less than 10%. Mortality rates attributable to peripheral vascular injury are under 1% for both groups.[1–8]

Patients may be initially segregated based on hemodynamic status. The vast majority of hemodynamically unstable patients require immediate operative therapy. If hypotension is due to associated injury, evaluation of PPET can occur in the operating room via a combination of ankle-brachial indices and intraoperative arteriography if needed.

## Vascular injury

Hemodynamically stable patients are differentiated based on the presence or absence of "hard" vascular signs. These include pulsatile bleeding, expanding hematoma, palpable thrill or audible bruit, and evidence of distal ischemia: pallor, paresthesia, paralysis, pain, pulselessness, and poikilothermia. When operating for any single hard sign, vascular injury will be encountered in 50–90% of cases.[3,5–10] When operating for a combination of hard signs, vascular injuries will be encountered in 90–100% of cases.[3,11] Pulses may be present in 35% of patients with vascular injury but another physical sign will usually be present.

The majority of hemodynamically stable patients with PPET have either no signs or "soft" signs of injury.[9,12–16] Soft signs include a history of hemorrhage at the scene, stable hematoma, injury to anatomically related nerve or bone, diminished but palpable pulse. It may be difficult to distinguish soft signs from signs of distal ischemia, particularly in patients with pre-existing vascular disease. The ability of soft signs to predict vascular injury depends upon the confirmatory study used.[8] While arteriographic abnormalities may be present in 2–20%[9,10,12–19] of these patients the number of injuries requiring repair may be in the range of 2–4%.[9,10,12–16] Soft signs are non-specific and may be due to injuries to associated structures. Nonetheless, they may be indicative of a trajectory in close proximity to the neurovascular bundle. Thus all patients with PPET and soft signs should undergo API.

Many patients with PPET have only a penetrating wound in proximity to a major vessel. The definition of proximity is variable and complicated by imprecise knowledge of trajectory in most series of PPET. The yield of operative exploration or angiography using proximity as the only criterion for these interventions is low, ranging between 2% and 20%.[9,10,12–16] The lowest figures are encountered when patients with any clinical abnormality are excluded (true absence of soft signs) and all extremity wounds are included. When there is overlap with patients having soft vascular signs, and wounds which are clearly distant from the neurovascular bundle are excluded, the incidence of vascular injury is higher. We recommend API for the evaluation of patients with PPET and no signs of vascular injury because it is an easy test to perform and interpret and because trajectory may be difficult to determine in all but the most obvious cases.

## Arteriography

Arteriography may be warranted in some patients with hard vascular signs. These include patients who have multiple potential levels of injury such as shotgun wounds or multiple gunshot wounds, patients with preexisting vascular disease and wounds in which choice of surgical approach would be influenced by precise localization of the site of injury. The latter include wounds of the thoracic outlet. In every case the delay involved in departmental multiplanar arteriography must be weighed against time elapsed since injury and degree of ischemia. When there is significant ischemia, a long period of time since injury or another indication for immediate surgery (associated injury), intraoperative angiography should be used.

## Arterial pressure index

The arterial pressure index (API) is highly specific for major arterial injury of the extremities.[20,21] When a threshold API of 0.9 is used as an indication for arteriography, specificity is 100%. Sensitivity of API for all types of arterial injury is approximately 70% but is higher than this when injuries that did not subsequently undergo repair are excluded from consideration. API functions well to detect any lesion that reduces flow in major axial arteries. Lesions of the profunda femoris and brachii will not be detected. For patients with API > 0.9, further evaluation may be desirable depending on clinical suspicion of non-flow limiting lesions.

Color-flow duplex (CFD) examination has excellent specificity for non-flow limiting lesions of major arteries when compared with arteriography.[22] Sensitivity is 50%, with most missed injuries involving small branch vessels. CFD might be used in some patients with API < 0.9 but in most circumstances arteriography would be required to further characterize any abnormality.

Utilizing the strategy of API measurement, arteriography for API < 0.9, and selective CFD for API < 0.9, the rate of occult or missed arterial injuries should approximate the rate of false-negative arteriography. This approach is much more cost effective than routine exclusion arteriography in PPET.

## Arterial injury

Major arterial injuries are those resulting in ischemia or bleeding. Thrombosis, laceration, large AV fistulas, and large pseudoaneurysms should be repaired at the time of diagnosis. Minor arterial injuries include intimal irregularities or flaps, focal narrowing, and small false aneurysms or AV fistulas. There have been several studies providing Class II data[17,23,24] that support the contention that minor injuries may be observed. From 75% to 90% will not require repair. Intimal irregularities and focal narrowing are most likely to resolve. All

studies addressing this issue assert that very careful follow-up is needed to detect worsening injuries (mostly pseudoaneurysms and AVFs) which require repair.

## Observation

The concept of observation for minor arterial injury requires a follow-up protocol. Injuries will have been identified by arteriography; it is unclear whether follow-up arteriography or duplex examination is preferred to reimage abnormalities. The most recent long-term follow-up of this type used duplex examination in 43% of cases.[17c] Development of new signs or symptoms requires immediate reevaluation.[17,23-25] The optimal interval and duration of follow-up are not known.

## Stenting

Stenting of arterial injuries has been reported in small studies containing class III data.[26] Utility in treatment of false aneurysm and AVF in areas that would require extensive surgical dissection has been promoted. It is likely that the role for these devices will expand for the treatment of subclavian/proximal axillary arterial injury.

## Notes on the references

It should be noted that evaluation of ideal strategies for PPET involves analysis of literature concerning diagnostic testing. The ideal study of diagnostic testing includes two cohorts of patients, one subjected to the "test" diagnostic procedure and one to the "gold standard" diagnostic procedure, with each diagnostic procedure interpreted by an individual blinded to the patients' disease and results of other diagnostic studies. This would permit unbiased evaluation of the test diagnostic procedure. Determination of sensitivity, specificity, positive, and negative predictive value follows from such an evaluation. Randomized prospective clinical trials have no relevance to this methodology. With respect to evaluation of tests designed to detect vascular injury following PPET, the gold standard studies include operative exploration and arteriography. We would rate studies that meet the aforementioned criteria as Class I insofar as interpretation of testing strategies is concerned. Class II studies are defined as prospective studies, which compare the test procedure with a gold standard such as arteriography but without blinded interpretation. Included as Class II references for the purposes of this chapter are studies that examine epidemiological factors and contain more than 100 cases. Class III studies are those with fewer than 100 cases, no standard of comparison for test studies, and clinical reviews.

## Class II references

1. Tonkovic I, Petrovic M, Fiolic Z *et al*. War injuries of the arteries. *Lijecnicki Vjesnik* 1997;**119**:316.

   Translated from Czech. A large contemporary review of extremity vascular wounds from the Slovenian war. Examines associated injuries and outcomes. One hundred and ninety-seven patients with 231 injuries. Over 50% were lower extremity, orthopaedic injuries were observed in 34%, venous injuries in 47%. The amputation rate was 8% for this series. The study is of interest because it reflects a favorable success rate in a group of patients with very high-energy wounds. The amputation rate is higher than that reported in contemporary civilian series.

2. Sheriff AA. Vascular injuries: experience during the Afghan war. *Int Surg* 1997;**77**:114.

   This is a large study in which data were gathered prospectively but no apparent selection or exclusion criteria were employed. The study examines 224 patients with 78 "major" and 146 "minor" vascular injuries. Mine explosions were the most common cause of injury in this series. As with the study referenced above, orthopaedic injuries (26%) and venous injuries (41%) were commonly associated. The amputation rate was 4%. Again, the series is of interest in that it provides relatively contemporary data on a "worst case" scenario with respect to PPET. Wounding energy is higher than seen in civilian series with favorable limb salvage rates.

3. Martin LC, McKenney MG, Sosa JL *et al*. Management of lower extremity arterial trauma. *J Trauma* 1994;**37**:591.

   This is a large retrospective review of civilian penetrating trauma. The series covers a five-year time span from 1987 to 1992. The methods section describes that patients with hard signs of vascular injury were taken to surgery and patients with soft signs underwent arteriograms. Patients with no clinical evidence of vascular injury were observed. Thus the approach to vascular injury described for this review is contemporary. The paper reviews 188 consecutive patients, 88% with penetrating injury. The majority (73%) presented with hard signs. Results are described based on individual arterial injury: iliac, femoral, popliteal, and tibial. Associated injuries, surgical therapy, and treatment failures are described. The rate of amputation for penetrating injury in this large civilian series

is 0%, all amputations occurring secondary to blunt injury. This is a good retrospective study with lots of interesting data presented in an organized fashion. The large number of patients presenting with hard signs supports contemporaneous studies examining the validity of physical examination as a sensitive and specific test for patients with PPET.

9. Frykberg ER, Dennis JW, Bishop K, Laneve L, Alexander RH. The reliability of physical examination in penetrating extremity trauma for vascular injury: results at one year. *J Trauma* 1991;**31**:502.

   This is another excellent study from Dr Frykberg's group, which examined the utility of physical examination in evaluating patients with PPET. Based upon the results of the study given in reference (12) these authors created a protocol for the management of PPET that used physical examination alone as the initial management tool for patients with PPET but no hard signs. Of 21 patients with hard signs, all had vascular injury requiring repair (positive predictive value 100%). Of 286 proximity wounds, two had negative physical examination but required surgery for thrombosis or bleeding of major vessels within 36 hours of injury ("immediate" negative predictive value = 99.3%). This study also generated heated discussion following its presentation in 1990. The most significant criticism was lack of long-term follow-up which would have allowed the determination of *true* negative predictive value for physical exam. Dr Frykberg, in his response to this criticism, noted that lack of long-term follow-up has not precluded acceptance of the conclusions of many studies, including those supporting exclusion angiography.

10. Weaver FA, Yellin AE, Bauer M *et al*. Is arterial proximity a valid indication for arteriography in penetrating extremity trauma? A prospective analysis. *Arch Surg* 1990;**125**:1256.

    This widely quoted prospective study examined two groups of patients with PPET: those with clinical findings and those with proximity alone. All patients underwent arteriography. There were 373 patients studied; 216 had one or more signs which included a combination of hard and soft signs. There were 157 patients with proximity alone. In the first group there were 65 (30%) "injuries" (arteriographic abnormalities), of which 19 (8.7%) were repaired. In the second group there were 17 (10%) "injuries" of which one (0.6%) was repaired. The authors conclude that arteriography in the absence of clinical signs should be abandoned and their data seem to support this conclusion. The study nicely defines inclusion criteria for clinical abnormality but does include some signs which might have mandated exploration without arteriography in other studies. Thus the rate of positive, clinically significant, arteriograms in the first group is higher than might have been observed if only soft signs were used as inclusion criteria.

11. Sirinek KR, Levine BA, Gaskhill HV III, Root HD. Reassessment of the role of routine exploration in vascular trauma. *J Trauma* 1981;**21**:339.

This large retrospective review of 390 patients is one of the last to document routine operative exploration in every patient with PPET. The patients are not selected and many patients with PPET and trajectory remote from vessels may have been excluded before the fact. Many of the injuries reported were to arteries in the neck. There were 139 (36%) vascular injuries; 102 (26%) of these were arterial, the remainder venous. Nonetheless, the study is of interest in the evolution of contemporary diagnostic algorithms in that it led the authors to adopt a policy "...similar to their colleagues in Dallas...of exclusion arteriography...". References 12 and 13, both from Dallas, reveal the outcome of that policy almost a decade after publication of this paper.

12. Frykberg ER, Crump J, Vines FS *et al*. A reassessment of the role of arteriography in penetrating extremity trauma: a prospective study. *J Trauma* 1989;**29**:1041.

This study is a prospective, randomized study of the timing and efficacy of arteriography in PPET. At the time of its presentation in 1988, it elicited great controversy. It is very well done with explicitly stated inclusion and exclusion criteria, randomization scheme, informed consent for "delayed" arteriography, and observation of "minor" injuries. There were 27 abnormal arteriograms in 152 PPET wounds; 126 wounds associated with proximity alone, 26 with soft signs. Eleven abnormalities were to non-critical branch vessels; of the remaining 16 abnormalities, only one (an AV fistula) was immediately repaired. One of the 15 observed injuries (pseudoanuerysm) was repaired 10 weeks later. The remainder were watched and resolved on follow-up arteriogram (11) or clinical exam (3). The greatest strength of the study is the careful definition of abnormalities associated with "positive" arteriograms in PPET and the scheme for observational management of these injuries. The data provide strong support for the conclusion that the incidence of significant vascular injury in patients with minimal or no clinical findings is very low. The suggested approach to "minimal" arterial injury was unique at the time and supported only by short-term follow-up of a small cohort.

13. Francis H III, Thal ER, Weigelt JA, Redman HC. Vascular proximity: is it a valid indication for arteriography in asymptomatic patients? *J Trauma* 1991;**31**:512.

This study examines the yield of angiography in asymptomatic patients with PPET. A prospective series evaluating 146 patients over two years. The accuracy of arteriography was measured relative to findings at surgery. Patients with negative arteriograms were not explored but follow-up was conducted in 64% of patients over an average of nearly eight weeks. Proximity is defined as "within 1 cm of a major vessel". Exclusion criteria included hard signs and these were defined as pulse deficit, bruit, thrill, history of arterial hemorrhage, expanding hematoma, nerve deficit, fracture, and massive soft tissue deficit. It should be noted that these exclusion criteria include several soft signs and so the study more truly examines the "asymptomatic" population with PPET. Eighty-nine per cent of arteriograms were negative. Of the 17 positive arteriograms, only seven (4.4%) were "true positive" at exploration. The majority of repaired injuries were intimal injuries. The authors conclude that this prospective study of a well-defined group of patients demonstrates that arteriography is unnecessary in asymptomatic patients with PPET. This is a well-done study that addresses the definition of asymptomatic patients by prospectively excluding those with soft signs and distant, tangential injuries.

14. Reid JD, Weigelt JD, Thal ER, Francis H III. Assessment of proximity wounds to major vascular structures as an indication for arteriography. *Arch Surg* 1988;**123**:942.

A large retrospective study that served as the precursor to the study referenced above. This study reviewed 507 unselected patients undergoing arteriography following PPET. There were 36 (6.7%) positive arteriograms of which 19 (3.7%) were "true positive" at exploration. The value of this study is the large number of patients reviewed. The authors concluded that arteriography based on proximity alone may not be worthwhile.

15. Anderson RJ, Hobson RW, Lee BC *et al*. Reduced dependency on arteriography for penetrating extremity trauma: influence of wound location and non-invasive vascular studies. *J Trauma* 1990;**30**:1063.

This is a large retrospective study that examined the utility of arteriography in an unselected group of 454 patients. Of 412 arteriograms in patients with minimal or no physical signs, 44 (11%) were positive. The number of positive arteriograms, which were "true positive" at exploration, is not given so comparison with the incidence figures from the previously referenced studies is difficult. The authors note that wounds of specific anatomic location such as the lateral arm and thigh did not result in any positive arteriograms while wounds of the antecubital fossa and posteromedial thigh resulted in positive arteriograms in 14% and 8% of cases respectively. The study also reports a preliminary experience with B-mode ultrasound in 23 of these patients all of whom underwent confirmatory arteriograms. Sensitivity is reported as 83%, specificity 100%.

16. Henderson V, Nambsian R, Smith ME, Yim KK, Organ C. Angiographic yield in penetrating extremity trauma. *West J Med* 1991;**155**:252.

A large retrospective review that excludes patients with hard signs and examines the yield of arteriography in PPET. There were 284 arteriograms in 268 patients. The overall yield for positive arteriograms was 57/284 (20%). For patients with "abnormal clinical findings" (soft signs) the angiographic yield was 51%; for patients with proximity as the sole indication, yield was 11/194 (6%). When these 11 cases are analyzed, only three (1.5%) patients had significant injuries, one of which was venous. The authors conclude that arteriography for proximity *is* justified in patients with PPET caused by gunshot wounds but not in stab wounds. This is a useful study because it presents data nearly identical to contemporaneous studies but reaches opposite conclusions. The authors recommend a maximally conservative approach and suggest that physical examination is insensitive in detecting vascular injuries in patients with PPET.

17. Validation of non-operative management of occult vascular injuries: prospective cohort evaluation.
    (a) Frykberg ER, Vines FS, Alexander RH. The natural history of clinically occult arterial injuries: a prospective evaluation. *J Trauma* 1988;**29**:577.

    A small prospective study which independently qualifies as class III data due to its small size and limited follow-up. Because it is the inception study for the cohort described in the following two studies it is most reasonable to include it here. Twenty clinically occult injuries demonstrated on arteriogram were followed by arteriogram in 15/20 cases and one enlarging pseudoaneurysm was detected and repaired (see reference 12 above). Clinical follow-up of 19/20 injuries was for periods ranging between three days and 19 months. No complications were encountered. The authors conclude that non-operative management of clinically occult vascular injuries is safe provided follow-up and careful instructions are provided.
    (b) Frykberg EF, Crump JM, Dennis JW, Vines FS, Alexander RH. Nonoperative observation of clinically occult arterial injuries: a prospective evaluation. *Surgery* 1991;**109**:85.

    The cohort mentioned above is followed. Additional cases are added. There are 47 patients with 50 clinically occult vascular injuries. All injuries identified by arteriogram. Forty of the injuries were due to penetrating trauma; note the addition of some blunt trauma patients to the study at this point. Concentrating on the 40 PPET cases, three (7.5%) underwent surgery following identification, one of the explorations revealed a normal artery (true false negative for physical exam = 5%). Of the 50 occult injuries, arteriographic follow-up was achieved in 39. Clinical follow-up was achieved in all patients via physical exam and API over a mean period of 3.1 months (three days to 27 months).
    (c) Dennis JW, Frykberg ER, Velndez HC, Huffman S, Menawat SS. Validation of nonoperative management of occult vascular injuries and accuracy

of physical examination alone in penetrating extremity trauma: a 5–10 year follow-up. *J Trauma* 1998;**44**:243.

This study reports 5–10 year follow-up for two patient cohorts. The first is the original group of patients who had confirmatory arteriography (n = 43), the second group consists of 287 patients with PPET who underwent observation without confirmatory angiography. Mean follow-up for the first cohort was 9.1 years, for the second 5.4 years. In the first group, four (9%) patients had clinical deterioration of known injuries within the first month and required surgery; 23/39 (58%) patients were contacted in follow-up; 17 (43%) underwent duplex examination. There were no late complications in this group. In the second group, four (1.3%) patients required delayed surgery within the first week and 78 (29%) patients with 90 injuries were seen in follow-up or contacted by phone and had no problems. The authors conclude that the data provide support for the safety of physical examination as a reliable predictor of significant vascular injuries. Discussion following presentation of the paper again focused on the limited number of patients seen in follow-up. It would seem that even 29 and 58% follow-up for a trauma cohort constitutes an excellent result.

18. Ordog GJ, Balasubramanium S, Wasserberger J *et al.* Extremity gunshot wounds: Part one – identification and treatment of patients at high risk of vascular injury. *J Trauma* 1994;**36**:358.

    This is a massive review, the largest I am aware of, from a single institution. The review covers 14 years, from 1978 to 1992, and reports on 16 316 patients with 18 349 extremity injuries. The study examines two time periods, one in which exclusion arteriography was used and the second in which exclusion arteriography was replaced by duplex Doppler ultrasonography (Ddu). Although the results section of this paper is poorly organized and difficult to read, the paper satisfies criteria for classification as level II evidence. The summarized data support conclusions that Ddu replaced exclusion arteriography in evaluating asymptomatic or minimally symptomatic patients with PPET. Significant cost savings are suggested. Though a difficult read, the study is recommended because of the large volume of patient data.

20. Johansen JH, Lynch K, Paun M, Copass M. Non-invasive vascular tests reliably exclude occult arterial trauma in injured extremities. *J Trauma* 1990;**31**:515.

    This paper was presented at the same meeting as reference 9 above. It too generated significant controversy. The study is prospective. Patients with hard signs were excluded. Patients with PPET and soft signs or no signs had API determination. Patients with API < 0.9 underwent arteriography. Patients with API > 0.9 were managed "expectantly" with serial API and/or (in 64 cases) duplex sonography (du). Patients with positive du or new clinical signs underwent immediate arteriography. There were 100 extremities, 96 patients, 82 penetrating injuries. There were 17 limbs with normal clinical exam and API > 0.9 and 16 of these had abnormal arteriograms, of which seven underwent "repair" (two fasciotomies for diffuse spasm). For 79 limbs with API > 0.9, 64 underwent subsequent du. There were 5 minor lesions discovered in this group within two weeks of injury; one was repaired during the following year. This study does not segregate based upon presence of soft signs but does provide data supporting the conclusion that API can detect injuries in clinically "normal" (no hard signs) extremities. In fact, only one anatomically flow-limiting lesion (brachial artery) had a normal physical exam in this series. Again, the decision regarding which lesions "required" repair remains subjective, as with all of these studies.

21. Nassoura ZE, Ivatury RR, Simon RJ *et al.* A reassessment of Doppler pressure indices in the detection of arterial lesions in proximity penetrating injuries of the extremities: a prospective study. *Am J Emerg Med* 1996;**14**:151.

This study is the largest I know of examining the utility of API. It compares API to arteriography in each of 258 patients with 323 extremity wounds allowing calculation of sensitivity and specificity. Using API < 0.9 as a threshold "abnormal" value, the study was true negative in 283 (88%), false negative in 11 (3.4%), true positive in 29 (8.9%), and false positive in 0 cases. Sensitivity for API compared with arteriography was 72.5%, specificity 100%, positive predictive value 100%, and negative predictive value 96%. The false-negative rate is consistent with that reported for physical examination alone; injuries identified in this small subgroup required repair in 5/11 (1.5%) cases, yielding a very low clinically significant false-negative rate and commensurately higher sensitivity. The data support the conclusion that API is a useful test for screening for vascular injury in PPET. It is of interest to note that approximately 100 negative arteriograms would be required to detect an occult injury requiring repair. Again, the definition of which injuries required repair is subjective and not subject to blinding.

## Class III references

4. Fainzilber G, Roy-Shapira A, Wall M, Mattox KL. Predictors of amputation for popliteal artery injuries. *Am J Surg* 1995;**170**:568.

This review of 80 consecutive patients with 81 popliteal artery injuries reports an amputation rate of 6.2% for the 76 patients with penetrating mechanism. This is consistent with historic data citing higher amputation rates for popliteal injury. Associated injuries are described and an association between amputation and fractures is reported with an odds ratio of +2.7. Fasciotomy based upon clinical criteria is recommended to reduce the potential of limb loss. The diagnosis of popliteal artery injury in this series was based upon emergency center arteriography in 57%, departmental arteriography in 22%, and clinical grounds alone (presumably hard signs) in 21%. The study is of interest because of the concentrated experience with popliteal injury. The reader should note that the study by Martin described in reference 3 contained 40 popliteal injuries.

5. Frykberg ER. Advances in the diagnosis and treatment of extremity vascular trauma. *Surg Clin North Am* 1995;**75**:207.

An excellent review with 111 references. Concise and clearly written. Provides the framework for the evolution of diagnostic strategies away from routine exclusion arteriography. Table 4 is particularly worthwhile as it documents the incidence of occult injury in PPET and the concomitant number of those injuries which required operative repair. An algorithm is presented for evaluation of PPET. The section on treatment focuses on Frykberg's own work describing non-operative management of occult injuries. There is minimal information on selection of conduit, prioritization of repair in blunt injury, management of concomitant venous injury, and factors affecting limb salvage.

6. Austin OMB, Redmond HP, Burke PE, Grace PA, Bouchier-Hayes DB. Vascular trauma: a review. *J Am Coll Surg* 1995;**181**:91.

This is a very large review, which is broad based and covers the entire field of vascular trauma. It has 222 references, which may be its most redeeming feature. The topics covered are not dealt with in sufficient detail to be particularly useful.

7. Edwards JM, Moneta GL. Peripheral venous injury. *Adv Trauma Crit Care* 1993;**8**:217.

This is a well-written review with 37 references. It is easy to read. It very nicely reviews modern series and includes a concise discussion of repair techniques.

8. Shackford SR, Rich NM. Peripheral vascular injury. In: Feliciano DV, Moore EE, Mattox KL, eds. *Trauma*, 3rd edn. Stamford, Connecticut: Appleton and Lange, 1996.

This is a superb review which should be the starting point for any inquiry into the subject. The chapter deals with all phases of peripheral vascular injury but supplies enough detail to be of practical value. The data displayed in Table 43.6 are particularly relevant to the diagnostic approach to patients with PPET. The algorithm shown in Figure 43.12 has many similarities to the approach suggested herein. There are 151 references.

19. Gomez GA, Kreis DJ, Ratner L *et al*. Suspected vascular trauma of the extremities: the role of arteriography in proximity injuries. *J Trauma* 1986;**26**:1005.

  Although smaller than other referenced studies, this is one of the earliest to suggest a diminishing role for exclusion arteriography. It reviews 72 patients who had no symptoms following PPET and underwent arteriography strictly for exclusion of vascular injury. Fifty-five (76%) studies were normal, 17 (23.7%) were abnormal but none of these 17 were operated upon. These include injuries to branch vessels and minor arteries. The study may have included patients with remote wounds that would have had a very low potential for vascular injury.

22. Bergstein JM, Blair JF, Edwards J *et al*. Pitfalls in the use of color flow duplex ultrasound for screening of suspected arterial injuries in penetrated extremities. *J Trauma* 1992;**33**:395.

  A smaller study which compares color flow duplex (CFD) to arteriography. It reports on 67 patients with 75 injured extremities. All patients underwent confirmatory arteriography. Based upon the definition that any arteriographic abnormality in the presence of normal CFD represents a false negative, CFD sensitivity and specificity were determined. CFD was 99% specific, 50% sensitive with positive predictive value of 66% and negative predictive value of 97%. Two small psuedoaneurysms were missed and one geniculate pseudoaneurysm was misread as a popliteal injury. The authors conclude that CFD may be useful to screen for vascular injury in PPET provided any abnormality on CFD is studied with arteriogram.

23. Stain SC, Yellin AE, Weaver FA, Pentecost MJ. Selective management of non-occlusive arterial injuries. *Arch Surg* 1989;**124**:1136.

  This study represents class III evidence because of the number of patients presented. Nonetheless, it is a larger experience than that reported by Frykberg in his initial study. Fifty patients with 61 non-occlusive injuries were reviewed following prospective data collection. There were 19 intimal defects, four flaps, 26 pseudoaneurysms, two stenoses, and 10 AV fistulas. Between one and 12 weeks, 30 were reimaged with arteriograms; 21 of 24 (87%) injuries to major arteries were improved. This study does not have the follow-up period of the Frykberg series and lumps minor and major arterial injury together. Resolution of 87% of minor injuries to named arteries supports the contention that such injuries will heal spontaneously, particularly intimal defects and stenoses.

24. Hoffer EK, Sclafani SJ, Herskowitz MM, Scalea TM. Natural history of arterial injuries diagnosed with arteriography. *J Vasc Int Rad* 1997;**8**:43.

  This is a review of 86 patients with 105 injuries, all classified based on arteriography. The injuries include 13 occlusions that may have presented with hard signs mandating repair in other studies. The remainder of injuries includes narrowing (33), intimal irregularity (23), pseudoaneurysms (12), AV fistulas (13), extravasation (5), and dilatation (2). There were 25 of these injuries which worsened or were repaired (presumably all occlusions). This study does not include data on clinical presentation. It focuses on the fate of minor arterial injuries (some of which seem major) and concludes that many will heal on their own.

25. Tufaro A, Arnold T, Rummel M, Matsumoto T, Kerstein M. Adverse outcome of nonoperative management of intimal injuries caused by penetrating trauma. *J Vasc Surg* 1994;**20**:656.

  A five-year retrospective review of 118 patients who initially presented with soft signs of injury following PPET. There were 23 angiographic abnormalities, seven were intimal injuries treated by observation alone. The 16 other minor injuries were characterized as "significant" intimal injuries and were explored upon presentation. Within 6–39 months, 6/7 observed patients returned with pulse deficits and underwent operative repair. There was no limb loss. The study concludes that the yield of arteriography in patients with soft signs is higher than for patients with proximity alone and that observation of intimal injuries may be associated with adverse outcomes. Although retrospective this study is interesting. The reader may interpret the results somewhat differently from the authors.

26. Ohki T, Veith FJ, Marin ML, Cynamon J, Sanchez LA. Endovascular approaches for traumatic arterial lesions. *Semin Vasc Surg* 1997;**10**:272.

  This is a good review that references a number of small series introducing the concept of endovascular surgery in trauma. The authors describe its utility for central or difficult-to-access injuries including subclavian/axillary artery pseudoaneurysms. Advantages and pitfalls are described. There are 24 references. The authors have since published another review (1999) reporting added experience in the use of covered stents for upper extremity vascular injury.

**Vascular proximity in penetrating extremity trauma**

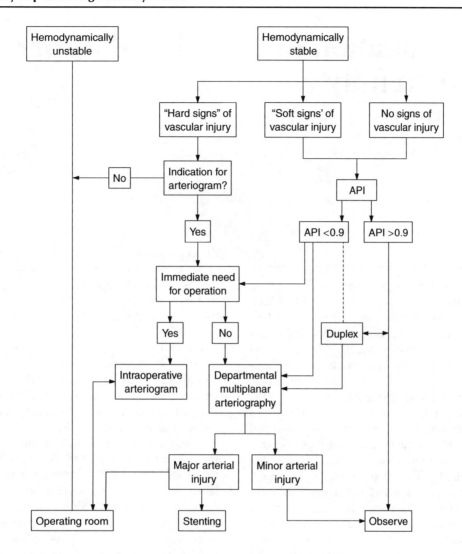

# 16 Evaluation of the injured upper extremity

*Steven L Frick, Michael A Gibbs*

## Introduction

Upper extremity trauma is common, accounting for one-third of all injuries. It is estimated that 16 million upper extremity injuries sufficiently severe to restrict activity occur annually in the United States. The upper extremity functions to position the hand in space and allow prehensile activity. The preservation of this function is the goal of treatment of upper extremity injuries. Principles of trauma care dictate, however, that the specific care of upper extremity injuries should proceed only after life-threatening injuries are identified and treated. Severe limb-threatening injuries must not distract the trauma care provider from basic trauma life support protocols. Upper extremity injuries are rarely life threatening, although associated injuries may be. Upper extremity injuries that may pose an immediate threat to life are those associated with massive ongoing hemorrhage, usually associated with a proximal level complete or incomplete traumatic amputation.[1]

Proper initial management of upper extremity injuries can facilitate patient transport, reduce the risk of future morbidity and decreased function, decrease blood loss, and reduce the risk of infection. Emergency department evaluation is directed first at identifying those injuries requiring emergent therapy. Limb-threatening injuries to the upper extremity include vascular injuries with loss of distal perfusion, compartment syndromes, crush injuries, open fractures, and complex soft tissue wounds. Isolated closed fractures or dislocations in the upper extremity are rarely limb threatening.

## Initial evaluation: primary survey and resuscitation, splinting

During the primary survey, ongoing hemorrhage from upper extremity wounds should be controlled by direct pressure. Clamping of vessels is strongly discouraged, as the risk of damage to associated neural and vascular structures is high. Following the initial evaluation and resuscitation, skeletal integrity is assessed by evaluation for swelling, deformity, abnormal motion, crepitance or tenderness. In the setting of marked deformity or instability of the upper extremity because of fractures or dislocations, splinting will aid in decreasing blood loss by stabilizing the skeleton and encouraging vascular tamponade and clot formation. It will also decrease the pain associated with the injury and facilitate safe patient transport and transfer.

By conferring some stability to the limb with a splint, the risk of further injury to the neurovascular and soft tissue structures of the extremity will also be diminished. Initial splinting should be in the position at which the extremity is found, unless there is compromise of the distal circulation or marked deformity. In these cases the limb should be splinted after applying longitudinal traction to realign the limb. Splints should be applied so that they do not constrict the extremity and compromise distal perfusion. In general, injuries to the shoulder girdle can be immobilized by securing the arm at the side of the torso. Arm, elbow, and forearm injuries may be immobilized with splints to hold the limb in an anatomically neutral position. Extremes of elbow flexion should be avoided as this may cause increased pressure on the brachial artery as it courses anterior to the elbow, further compromising distal perfusion.

## Secondary survey: systematic evaluation

In evaluating extremity injuries, a systematic approach is helpful. Injuries to multiple elements or systems are associated with higher energy trauma and an increased risk of morbidity. The systems of the extremity to assess are:

- vascular
- neurologic
- skeletal
- soft tissue and skin.

Severe injury to three or more systems may lead to consideration of primary amputation, although there are currently no established or validated criteria for primary amputation in upper extremity injuries.

## Vascular system

A diligent search for arterial injury is mandatory. Failure to diagnose vascular injury may result in significant morbidity, threatening limb viability and function. Capillary refill, skin color and temperature, and the strength of distal pulses should be noted and compared with the contralateral extremity. Because of the rich collateral network in the upper extremities, pulses may remain normal distal to the site of significant arterial injuries. A careful neurologic examination is also essential. The presence of a neurologic deficit can be an important marker of occult arterial injury, as these injuries coexist in as many as 50% of cases. In addition, the absence of neurologic function or a deterioration in neurologic function may be an important sign of an evolving compartment syndrome.[2,3]

When perfusion is compromised distal to a fracture or dislocation that is not reduced, a qualified physician should perform a reduction maneuver and splint the extremity and the vascular status should then be reassessed. In cases where splints have been applied prior to arrival in the emergency department and the patient presents with distal ischemia, the splints may be constricting the extremity and contributing to the poor perfusion. The splints should be removed to facilitate a complete examination of the extremity, which is then resplinted in an appropriate position. A reassessment of distal perfusion should then be performed.

Physical "hard signs" and "soft signs" of vascular injury have been described to assist the clinician during the evaluation of the patient at risk for vascular trauma. It should be recognized that the vascular physical examination can be compromised in the hypotensive patient. Clinical signs of vascular injury may remain absent or equivocal until the intravascular volume has been normalized and tissue perfusion has been restored.

Most clinically significant extremity vascular lesions manifest unequivocal physical findings or "hard signs". These include pulse deficits, distal ischemia, active hemorrhage, an expanding or pulsatile hematoma or the presence of a bruit or thrill. One or more

hard signs reliably predict the presence of arterial injury. "Soft signs" represent more equivocal physical findings which should alert the physician to the potential for vascular injury. These include: small, stable hematomas; injury to an anatomically related nerve; unexplained hypotension; and a history of hemorrhage that is no longer present. "Proximity" is an additional soft sign, defined as a wound in which the path of a penetrating agent could potentially cross the normal anatomic position of a major artery.

The presence of hard signs of vascular injury is diagnostic of arterial trauma and in the vast majority of cases, their presence is an indication for immediate surgery without further time-consuming evaluation. The benefit of performing arteriography in this setting is outweighed by the risk of increased ischemia time and/or ongoing hemorrhage. In rare circumstances, arteriography in the patient with hard signs of vascular injury is a useful endeavor. These include:

- injuries with multiple possible sites of vascular disruption (e.g. shotgun wounds)
- injuries associated with extensive bony or soft tissue destruction
- injuries in patients with preexisting vascular disease.

In these situations a limited intraoperative arteriogram may serve as a reasonable, less time-consuming alternative to formal multiplanar studies in the radiology suite.

Traditionally, the presence of soft signs of vascular injury was considered an appropriate indication for screening arteriography. More recent studies have questioned the utility of these findings, suggesting that they do not accurately predict the presence or absence of vascular injury. The presence of soft signs merits further evaluation with non-invasive testing (e.g. arterial pressure index and/or duplex Doppler ultrasonography). The assessment of penetrating extremity trauma in "proximity" to major vessels, but without clinical signs of vascular injury, remains an area of controversy. Routine screening arteriography for proximity alone is expensive, of limited clinical benefit, and associated with non-trivial complications. More recently, several authors have suggested that clinically important arterial injuries can be effectively ruled out by other means.

Measurement of the arterial pressure index (API) is an integral part of the physical examination and should be performed in all patients with proximity injury or other soft signs who lack absolute indications for immediate surgery. The API is determined by obtaining Doppler pressures in the distal vessels of the injured extremity (radial/ulnar) and dividing this number by the brachial Doppler pressure of an uninjured arm. A value of <0.90 is considered abnormal.

Several studies have assessed the accuracy of the API in patients with penetrating extremity trauma.[4,5]

Duplex Doppler ultrasonography has been used as a diagnostic modality in vascular surgery for many years. It is non-invasive, safe, and allows for serial patient evaluations. Duplex imaging gives real-time assessments of flow velocities and waveform characteristics, allowing the physician to understand the hemodynamic changes of an arterial injury. In addition to detecting the presence of vascular disruption, duplex Doppler can also characterize different injury patterns. Several studies have addressed the use of duplex scanning in proximity injury and have found it to be both sensitive and specific. The limitations of duplex scanning are that state-of-the-art equipment is expensive and not widely available and it requires skill in operation and interpretation. A learning curve will be required for clinicians to become proficient in its use.[6,7]

Hard signs of vascular trauma, or soft signs corroborated by further studies, should prompt the trauma care provider to obtain immediate consultation from a vascular surgeon for definitive care.

## Neurologic system

Peripheral nerve injuries in the upper extremities can result in marked loss of function. The status of the nerves supplying the upper extremity (axillary, median, radial, ulnar) should be assessed and documented. When possible, this should be done before any deformity reduction, as the initial exam may have significant bearing on later treatment decisions. Patients with neurologic deficits associated with fractures or dislocations that are not reduced should have a reduction performed by a qualified physician, followed by reassessment of neurologic function. When a neurologic deficit is noted prior to reduction and persists following reduction, then observation is the most likely course. If the patient does not have a neurologic deficit prior to a reduction but develops one after reduction, then nerve entrapment in the fracture site or joint is possible and operative exploration should be considered.

Patients with neurologic deficits and stable skeletons are divided into two categories: sharp penetrating trauma or blunt trauma. Open injuries with a sharp mechanism of injury (laceration, stabbing) and a neurologic deficit consistent with the zone of injury should undergo operative exploration and nerve repair. Open injuries caused by blunt trauma and closed blunt injuries with distal neurologic deficits should generally not undergo operative exploration, unless there is an associated vascular injury which is being addressed operatively. If a neurologic injury is identified intra-

operatively, the nerve should be tagged with a suture and plans made for delayed repair with possible nerve grafting, as the extent of nerve damage (zone of injury) is difficult to define acutely following blunt trauma. Nerve deficits related to gunshot wounds are placed into the blunt trauma category, as studies of nerve injuries after ballistic trauma have shown that most injuries are secondary to the blast effect and not anatomic division of the peripheral nerve. Patients who develop significant swelling and compression causing a nerve deficit should undergo early operative exploration of the nerve. The nerve is explored, decompressed, and then observed for recovery of function.

The results of nerve repair in the upper extremity are dependent on the mechanism of injury, age of the patient, and distance from the site of the nerve injury to the motor endplate or sensory organ. Those injuries that can undergo primary repair without tension in a clean, vascular wound bed have the best chance for success. The results of nerve repairs in the upper extremity are better than those in the lower extremity and aggressive attempts at repair or reconstruction are recommended.[1]

## Skeletal system

Physical examination for skeletal stability should be performed, with any areas of deformity, crepitus, abnormal motion or tenderness noted. Any lacerations or wounds in proximity to a fracture or dislocation indicate an open injury. Areas with gross deformity, crepitus, severe swelling or ecchymosis, bone tenderness or significant wounds should be evaluated with radiographs. At least two orthogonal views of the injured area should be taken. The views should be taken by moving or rotating the X-ray machine and not the patient's extremity. Moving the extremity to obtain the second view (orthogonal to the first) may result in motion only through a fracture or dislocation, causing unnecessary pain and potential further injury, while often not obtaining an orthogonal view of the proximal fragment. When fractures are identified, the joints above and below the fracture should be carefully analyzed radiographically to identify any associated intraarticular components of the injury.

Upper extremity open fractures are managed with the same treatment goals and principles as open fractures elsewhere.[8] The goals are to preserve limb viability, prevent infection, and preserve/restore function. Proper assessment of open fractures includes obtaining and evaluating the following information:

- history or mechanism of the injury
- vascular and neurologic status

- skin condition and size of the wound
- presence of muscle crush or loss
- extent of periosteal stripping or bone necrosis
- fracture pattern
- contamination of the wound
- recognition of any associated compartment syndrome.

Open fracture treatment includes tetanus prophylaxis, immediate antibiotic therapy, emergent wound evaluation, irrigation and debridement, skeletal stabilization, soft tissue coverage and wound closure. These are high-energy injuries, commonly associated with other injuries, and compartment syndrome is more likely.[9–11]

The initial management of the extremity includes placement of a sterile dressing over the wound and splinting. Tetanus prophylaxis should be administered in the emergency department and intravenous antibiotics started. As soon as the patient's overall condition allows, the wound should be explored under sterile conditions in the operating room. Intraoperative assessment and debridement are critical in the successful management of severe open fractures. The zone of injury concept (entire expanse of extremity affected by the injury) is key for proper debridement. This concept includes extension of wounds to allow exposure and evaluation of all tissues (superficial and deep) which might be contaminated or contain non-viable tissues. The purpose of the wound evaluation and debridement is to remove all contaminants and excise all non-viable tissues, converting the wound to a clean environment with excellent perfusion, thus maximizing wound healing and prevention of infection.

In severely contaminated or devitalized wounds, multiple "second-look" debridements may be required to convert the wound to a clean and well-perfused environment. The wound is typically left open with second-look debridements scheduled at 48–72 hour intervals until the following criteria are met:

- wound clean without residual contamination
- viable soft tissue envelope present
- closure without undue tension possible.

If coverage is not possible secondary to a lack of a viable soft tissue envelope or wound tension, consideration should be given to coverage using local or free tissue transfers and skin grafting. Early free flap coverage (within 3–5 days) of severe wounds has been shown to decrease infection rates.

The eventual function of the extremity is usually not determined by the bony injury but rather by the extent of the soft tissue, vascular, and neurologic injuries. Thus, treatment of open fractures should attempt to maximize preservation of a healthy soft tissue envelope

(skin, subcutaneous tissues, fascia, muscles and tendons, periosteum).[12] Orthopedic consultation should be obtained immediately after identification of an open fracture, as there is some evidence that delay in initial operative management (>6 hours) of these injuries may increase the morbidity associated with the injury.

Closed fractures should be managed by initial splinting, appropriate radiographs to allow proper identification of the fracture pattern and extent, and orthopaedic consultation for definitive management. These injuries are rarely life or limb threatening. An exception to this is a closed scapulothoracic dissociation. This is a complete disruption of the attachments of the scapula and upper extremity to the thorax and can be life threatening because of associated injuries to the vascular structures in the thoracic outlet.[13,14]

Definitive treatment of closed upper extremity fractures should be undertaken once the patient has been stabilized medically. Fractures typically managed non-operatively include clavicle, scapular body, and humeral shaft fractures.[15,16] Operative treatment is generally preferred for fractures with intraarticular extension and displacement, such as glenoid fractures, distal humerus fractures, olecranon and radial head fractures, and distal radius fractures.[17] Operative management of displaced proximal humerus fractures and displaced fractures of the radius and ulna is also frequently employed as improved functional outcomes are obtained after surgical stabilization of these injuries.[18,19] Most closed upper extremity fractures undergoing surgical repair are managed with open reduction and internal fixation with plate and screw constructs, although intramedullary nailing has proponents for certain fractures and patient groups.[20–22] Closed dislocations of the shoulder and elbow are managed by closed reduction and a period of immobilization, followed by protected range of motion and rehabilitative therapy.[23] Recurrent dislocations are an indication for operative treatment. Upper extremity dislocations with associated fractures are managed by operative stabilization of the fractures and reduction of the joint, followed by early motion and rehabilitation.

### Skin and soft tissues

Open injuries should be evaluated for any underlying bone, tendon, nerve or artery injury. Clean, sharp wounds should be irrigated and debrided and undergo repair of underlying injured structures. Antibiotics may be given but are of unproven benefit in patients with clean upper extremity soft tissue injuries. Contaminated sharp wounds and wounds from blunt trauma should undergo irrigation, debridement, and delayed repair and closure in most circumstances. Tetanus prophylaxis should be given and antibiotics administered based on clinical assessment of the level of contamination and soft tissue injury.[24,25]

Closed soft tissue injuries should be examined for signs of a crush injury or compartment syndrome. Patients with massive crush injuries should undergo hydration to protect against renal dysfunction. All patients with significant soft tissue injuries should be evaluated to rule out compartment syndrome. Compartment syndrome is a condition in which the circulation and function of tissues within a closed space are compromised by increased pressure within that space. The osseofascial boundaries of the anatomic compartments of the arm and forearm enclose muscles, nerves, arteries, and veins, thus making these structures susceptible to injury by compartment syndromes. They occur more frequently in the forearm and can occur following any condition resulting in elevated tissue pressure within the compartment. Tissue pressure is elevated by two mechanisms: increasing volume within a compartment, usually as a result of hemorrhage or edema, or decreasing volume available within a compartment, commonly caused by excessive external compression by a bandage, cast, splint or tight fascial closure. Frequently occurring traumatic conditions resulting in compartment syndrome are fractures, burns, crush injuries, prolonged limb compression, blunt and penetrating trauma, and postischemic swelling.[2,3]

The predominant symptom of compartment syndrome is pain, specifically pain out of proportion to that expected given the patient's injury. The earliest sign is tenseness and swelling throughout the boundaries of a compartment. Other signs include pain with passive stretch of the muscles of the involved compartment, hypoesthesia/paresthesias in the distribution of nerves that traverse the compartment, and/or weakness of the muscles of the compartment. Tissue pressure measurements are often a useful adjunct in the diagnosis of compartment syndrome. Controversy exists regarding the critical compartment pressure threshold for fasciotomy. Most authors believe that the threshold varies depending on the patient's blood pressure as well as the physiologic state of the tissues of the compartment. The treatment of compartment syndrome is emergent fasciotomy to decompress the involved compartment and restore tissue perfusion.[2,3,26]

## Conclusion

The upper extremity differs significantly from the lower extremity in a few areas that influence treatment decisions in severe injuries. First, the collateral circulation of the upper extremity is rich, allowing more aggressive, definitive early management of fractures with a lower infection rate than in the lower extremities. Second, nerve repairs in the upper extremity are generally more successful than in the lower extremity. Last, the currently available prosthetic replacements for the upper extremity are not as functional as those for the lower extremity. Each of these differences leads to more aggressive attempts at salvage of severe injuries in the upper extremity.[27] The sequential goals of preserving life, limb, and function should be remembered during treatment decision making. Injuries requiring emergent diagnosis and treatment should be specifically sought during the initial phase of management and include vascular injuries with distal ischemia, compartment syndromes and crush injuries, open fractures or dislocations, and complex soft tissue wounds.

## Class I references

10. Dellinger EP, Caplan ES, Weaver LD *et al*. Duration of preventive antibiotic administration for open extremity fractures. *Arch Surg* 1988;**123**:333–9.

    A prospective randomized trial of one-day versus five-day administration of intravenous antibiotics for open extremity fractures did not show a benefit for longer duration of antibiotic therapy.

15. Andersen K, Jensen PO, Lauritzen J. Treatment of clavicle fractures: figure of eight bandage versus a simple sling. *Acta Orthop Scand* 1987;**58**:71–4.

    This prospective study found no advantage to the use of figure of eight bandages as compared to simple sling immobilization for clavicle fractures.

23. Josefsson PO, Gentz CF, Johnell O. Surgical versus nonsurgical treatment of ligamentous injuries following dislocation of the elbow joint: a prospective, randomized study. *J Bone Joint Surg (Am)* 1987;**69**:605–8.

    Thirty consecutive patients with an elbow dislocation without fracture were randomly assigned to either surgical or non-surgical treatment of the ligamentous elbow injury. There was no evidence that surgical repair of the ligaments was better than nonoperative treatment.

## Class II references

1. Manord JD, Garrard CL, Kline DG, Sternbergh WC, Money SR. Management of severe proximal vascular and neural injury of the upper extremity. *J Vasc Surg* 1998;**27**:43–7.

    A retrospective study of 46 patients with severe neural and vascular injuries of the proximal upper extremity, all of whom had aggressive attempts at limb salvage with revascularization and delayed nerve reconstruction. The majority of patients improved with aggressive intervention and the authors suggest that early amputation should be carried out only in cases of massive tissue loss or when an attempt at limb salvage may endanger the patient's life. The initial clinical presentation was a poor predictor of final outcome.

2. Gelberman RH, Garfin SR, Hergenroeder PT. Compartment syndromes of the forearm: diagnosis and treatment. *Clin Orthop* 1981;**161**:252–60.

Reviews the methods of evaluation and treatment of forearm compartment syndrome in 26 patients. The most reliable physical findings of compartment syndrome were marked pain on passive digital extension and decreased sensibility or paresthesias in the hand. Fasciotomy techniques for the volar, dorsal, and mobile wad compartments of the forearm are described.

4. Lynch K, Johansen K. Can Doppler pressure measurement replace "exclusion" arteriography in the diagnosis of occult extremity trauma? *Ann Surg* 1991;**214**:737.

Ninety-three consecutive patients underwent calculation of the API and 21 arterial injuries were identified. An API of <0.90 had a sensitivity of 95% and a specificity of 97%.

5. Johansen K, Lynch K, Paun M. Non-invasive vascular tests reliably exclude occult arterial trauma in injured extremities. *J Trauma* 1991;**31**:515.

Evaluation of 100 traumatized limbs in 96 consecutive patients found the negative predictive value of an API >0.90 to be 99%.

6. Bynoe RP, Miles WAS, Bell RM. Noninvasive diagnosis of vascular trauma by duplex ultrasonography. *J Vasc Surg* 1991;**14**:43–6.

One hundred and ninety-eight consecutive patients with penetrating extremity trauma underwent duplex scanning followed by arteriography, surgical exploration or clinical follow-up. Duplex scanning had a sensitivity of 95% and a specificity of 99% for arterial injury.

7. Fry WR, Smith RS, Sayers DV. The success of duplex ultrasound arterial scanning in diagnosis of extremity vascular trauma. *Arch Surg* 1993;**128**:1368.

In a study of 175 patients with 20 documented arterial injuries, duplex scanning was 100% specific, 97% sensitive, and 97% accurate.

11. Patzakis MJ, Wilkins J, Moore T. Use of antibiotics in open tibial fractures. *Clin Orthop* 1983;**178**:31–5.

Data from 363 open tibial fractures demonstrated that antibiotic therapy is effective in reducing the infection rate in open tibial fractures. A 24% infection rate was noted in patients receiving no antibiotics, while patients receiving a cephalosporin and an aminoglycoside had only a 4.5% incidence of infection.

16. Zagorski JB, Latta LL, Zych GA. Diaphyseal fractures of the humerus: treatment with a prefabricated brace. *J Bone Joint Surg* (Am) 1988;**70**:607–10.

Excellent results can be obtained in isolated humerus fractures with the use of prefabricated braces. Of 170 patients treated with this method, 167 had an excellent or good result.

17. Knirk JL, Jupiter JB. Intra-articular fracture of the distal end of the radius in young adults. *J Bone Joint Surg* (Am) 1986;**68A**(5):647–59.

A retrospective study of 40 young adults with 43 intraarticular distal radius fractures at six-year follow-up demonstrated a higher incidence of radiographic arthritis in those patients whose fractures healed with articular incongruity.

18. Anderson LD, Sisk TD, Tooms RE, Park WI III. Compression-plate fixation in acute diaphyseal fractures of the radius and ulna. *J Bone Joint Surg* (Am) 1975;**57**(3):287–97.

Two hundred and forty-four patients with 330 diaphyseal forearm fractures were treated with compression plate fixation with a greater than 96% union rate and good restoration of forearm function in 85%.

19. Chapman MW, Gordon JE, Zissimos AG. Compression-plate fixation of acute fractures of the diaphysis of the radius and ulna. *J Bone Joint Surg* (Am) 1989;**71**:159–69.

Eighty-seven patients with 129 diaphyseal fractures of the forearm were treated with compression plate fixation, with a 98% union rate and a 92% excellent or satisfactory functional result. Refracture after plate removal only occurred after use of 4.5 mm plates and therefore 3.5 mm plates are recommended.

20. Bell MJ, Beauchamp CG, Kellam JF. The results of plating humeral shaft fractures in patients with multiple injuries: the Sunnybrook experience. *J Bone Joint Surg* (Br) 1985;**67**:293–6.

Thirty-eight patients with multiple injuries and 39 humeral shaft fractures underwent plating of the humerus. Excellent results were achieved and nursing care and management of other injuries was facilitated by rigid fixation of the humerus fractures. Complications were infrequent (one non-union, one infection, one fixation failure).

21. Bleeker WA, Nijsten MW, ten Duis H-J. Treatment of humeral shaft fractures related to associated injuries: a retrospective study of 237 patients. *Acta Orthop Scand* 1991;**62**:148–53.

The authors demonstrated that treatment of humeral shaft fractures is best dictated by associated injuries. Isolated humeral shaft fractures were best treated with bracing and multiply injured patients had better results with operative stabilization.

22. Brumback RJ, Bosse MJ, Poka A. Intramedullary stabilization of humeral shaft fractures in patients with multiple trauma. *J Bone Joint Surg* (Am) 1986;**68**:960–70.

Intramedullary fixation of humeral shaft fractures in 61 multiply injured patients was employed utilizing Ender nails or Rush rods and a closed insertion technique. Union was obtained in 94% of patients and 62% had excellent clinical results.

24. Ordog GJ, Sheppard GF, Wasserbaerger JS. Infection of minor gunshot wounds. *J Trauma* 1993;**34**:358.

 In over 3000 patients with low-energy gunshot wounds and no skeletal injury, the rate of infection without antibiotic therapy was only 1.8%.

25. Cassell OC, Ion L. Are antibiotics necessary in the surgical management of upper limb lacerations? *Br J Plast Surg* 1997;**50**:523–9.

 A prospective controlled trial of 250 patients with soft tissue lacerations of the upper extremity (nerve, tendon, and muscle lacerations included), comparing one group (113 patients) who received co-amoxiclav with a group that did not (137 patients). There was no difference in the rate of infection between the groups. The authors conclude that antibiotic administration after surgical management of sharp upper extremity lacerations is unnecessary.

26. Heppenstall BR, Sapega AA, Izant T *et al*. Compartment syndrome: a quantitative study of high energy phosphorus compounds using 31P-magnetic resonance spectroscopy. *J Trauma* 1989;**29**:1113–19.

 A basic science report of the pathogenesis of compartment syndrome and its effects on cellular metabolism. Traumatized muscle has a lower threshold for injury by compartment syndromes. The critical threshold for irreversible muscle damage was dependent on both the mean arterial blood pressure and the intracompartmental pressure.

## Class III references

3. Mubarak SJ. A practical approach to compartment syndromes. *AAOS Instr Course Lect* 1983;**32**:92–102.

 Reviews the presenting symptoms and signs of compartment syndromes and recommends compartmental pressure monitoring and a threshold of 30 mmHg (critical closing pressure of normal capillary beds) for decompression of suspected compartment syndromes.

8. Patzakis MJ. Management of open fracture wounds. *AAOS Instr Course Lect* 1987;**36**:367–9.

 Review of open fracture treatment principles, in particular the author's extensive experience with the use of empiric antibiotics to decrease the incidence of infectious complications.

9. Brumback RJ. Open tibial fractures: current orthopaedic management. *AAOS Instr Course Lect* 1992;**41**:101–17.

 An excellent review of the principles of open fracture care management, applicable to the management of these injuries in all anatomic locations.

12. Norris BL, Kellam JF. Soft tissue injuries associated with high energy extremity trauma: principles of management. *J Am Acad Orthop Surg* 1997;**5**:37–46.

 The principles of soft tissue injury management include early initial evaluation, skeletal stabilization, serial examinations and debridements if necessary, and early soft tissue coverage, followed by appropriate rehabilitation.

13. Oreck SL, Burgess A, Levine A. Traumatic lateral displacement of the scapula: a radiographic sign of neurovascular disruption. *J Bone Joint Surg (Am)* 1984;**66**:758–63.

 This article describes the clinical entity of scapulothoracic dissociation, a potentially life- and limb-threatening complication of massive upper extremity trauma. It is recognized by lateral displacement of the scapula and acromioclavicular dislocation or fracture and is associated with distal neurologic and vascular deficits. Arteriography is recommended to identify the level of arterial disruption.

14. Sturm JT, Perry JFJ. Brachial plexus injuries in blunt trauma: a harbinger of vascular and thoracic trauma. *Ann Emerg Med* 1987;**16**:404–6.

 Injury to the brachial plexus may be associated with major injuries to the thorax and the vascular supply to the upper extremity.

27. Dirschl DR, Dahners LE. The mangled extremity: when should it be amputated? *J Am Acad Orthop Surg* 1996;**4**:182–90.

 A review of the various rating scales designed to aid the clinician in determining if a lower limb should be amputated primarily or if attempts at salvage are warranted. None of the currently available scales are designed for the upper extremity, but the major decision factors are similar for the upper and lower extremities.

## Initial assessment

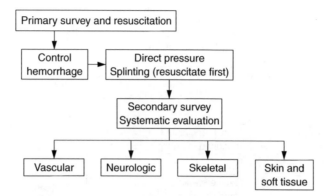

## Vascular system

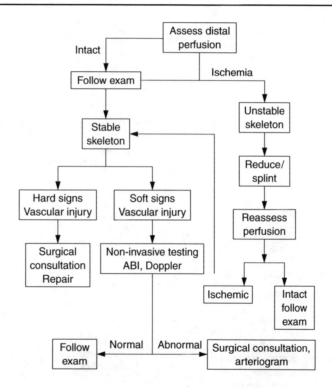

## Neurologic system

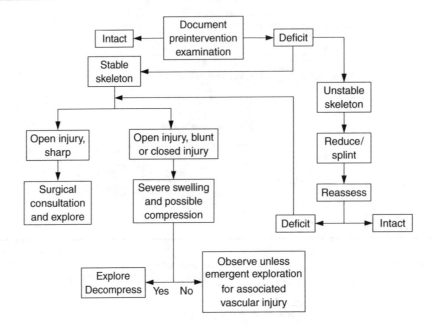

## Skeletal system

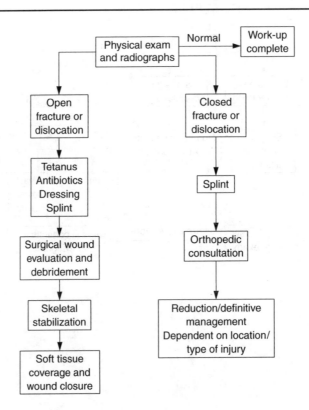

## Skin and soft tissues

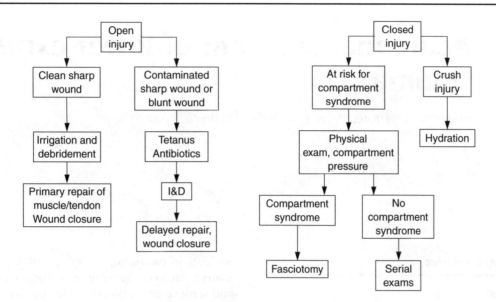

# 17 Acute management of lower extremity trauma

*Roger N Passmore, Peter J Nowotarski, Brent L Norris*

## Proximal femur injuries

### Introduction

Fractures and/or dislocations of the proximal femur occur frequently in the elderly from relatively low-energy mechanisms such as same-level falls. However, proximal femur injuries in the younger patient require higher energy mechanisms, the most common being motor vehicle accidents. The energy required to injure the proximal femur commonly causes associated injuries both local (abdominal injury) and distant (head injury). Proximal femur injuries can be divided into four distinct and separate injuries based on the location of the fracture:

- femoral head fractures (FHFx)
- femoral neck fracture (FNFx)
- intertrochanteric fracture (ITFx)
- subtrochanteric fracture (STFx)

### History and physical

Evaluation of the patient with a suspected proximal femur injury requires a thorough history and physical examination. Mechanism and position of the extremity at the time of injury are a very important part of the history. Awake and alert patients universally complain of groin and/or hip pain. Initial inspection of the involved extremity often reveals a shortened, externally rotated limb. Pain on palpation of the groin and trochanteric region is common. Attempts at moving the extremity are met with extreme spasm and pain and should be avoided. Crepitance should not be sought. Although vascular injury occurs infrequently, examination should include palpation of the femoral, popliteal, dorsalis pedis, and posterior tibial pulses. Penetrating or open injuries to the proximal femur should alert the

evaluating physician to the possibility of vascular injury. Neurologic examination should include motor and sensory evaluation of the knee and foot.

### Radiographs and classification

Radiographic assessment of the suspected proximal femur injury should include an AP pelvis, AP and lateral of the hip, and AP and lateral of the femur. The diagnosis of a proximal femur fracture and/or dislocation is confirmed with these radiographs.

Femoral head fractures are uncommon and are often associated with a dislocation of the hip and/or an acetabular fracture. The classification scheme for femoral head fractures is based on location of the fracture, associated femoral neck fracture, and associated acetabular fracture.

Femoral neck fractures occur commonly in the elderly from rather trivial mechanisms.[1] However, an isolated displaced femoral neck fracture in a young patient is rare. Most occur from high-energy mechanisms and frequently have associated injuries (multiply injured patient). *A femoral neck fracture in a patient less than 50 years old is an orthopaedic emergency.* Classification is again based on location of the fracture and degree of displacement.

Intertrochanteric fractures are the most common proximal femur fracture in the elderly. They are relatively uncommon in the younger patient and can be difficult to treat. The number of fragments and their associated displacement are related to the significant muscle forces acting on this region of the femur. Classification is based on the number of fracture fragments present on the radiographs.

Subtrochanteric fractures usually result from significant axial loading. Strong bending moments and torsional loads can also propagate fractures in this region of the femur. The anatomy and physiology of this region of the femur also make it difficult to treat. Tremendous loads are routinely placed through the subtrochanteric region of the femur. Classification of these injuries is important and based on whether the fracture extends to the intertrochanteric region.

## Additional studies

Fractures of the proximal femur are usually clinically apparent and routine plain films of the region are usually adequate to diagnose the injury. Additional studies are usually unnecessary but occasionally the occult femoral neck fracture may elude diagnosis on plain radiographs. Occasionally a MRI is needed to determine definitively the occult injury to the proximal femur.[2] Bone scan can be helpful but is not as good at detecting occult injury in the early evaluation period. CT scan of the proximal femur with bone windows will give excellent detail of the fracture and the degree of comminution but is usually not necessary.

## Early treatment

Initial treatment should consist of obtaining appropriate diagnosis of the injury and associated injuries. During acquisition of the diagnosis, ongoing resuscitation should be performed because it is not uncommon for the fractured proximal femur to bleed 500–1000 ml. Splinting of the extremity with longitudinal traction can be effective in diminishing the blood loss and associated pain at the fracture site. Once hemodynamically stable, early surgical management is the most effective means of managing these injuries.[3] If surgical intervention is to be significantly delayed (longer than 48 hours), skeletal traction with a distal femoral transfixion pin is appropriate. Otherwise longitudinal traction through skin or Bucks traction is adequate.

The importance of recognizing a femoral neck fracture in the young adult (less than 50 years old) cannot be overemphasized. Early diagnosis and appropriate surgical treatment (less than eight hours following injury) have been shown to be critical factors in obtaining a good clinical outcome.

## Late treatment

Surgical treatment of proximal femur injuries has yielded excellent results and should be considered the standard of care for these injuries.[4–10] Non-operative treatment of proximal femur injuries remains an option but only with patients who cannot tolerate surgical intervention.

## Complications

Patients with proximal femur fractures can develop complications related to the injury as well as the treatment. Bleeding and infection are two early complications associated with this injury. Late complications are numerous and depend on the specific fracture but include avascular necrosis of the femoral head, nonunion of the fracture, loss of fixation, loss of hip motion, prosthetic dislocation, deep venous thrombosis, and pulmonary embolus.[11]

# Femoral shaft fractures

## Introduction

Fractures of the femoral shaft are usually a result of high-energy injuries. Prior to the advent of modern treatment techniques, fractures of the femur were extremely disabling and often fatal injuries. The morbidity and mortality associated with this injury have been significantly lowered over the last several decades.

## History and physical

Diagnosis of an acute traumatic injury to the femoral shaft is generally quite apparent. Shortening of the limb, swelling, severe pain, and spasm are present. Clinical evaluation of the distal portion of the injured extremity should include a thorough neurologic and vascular examination. Physical examination of the knee for effusion and ligamentous injury is necessary as 10–20% of femoral shaft fractures have an associated major knee ligament injury. Penetrating injuries and open femoral shaft fractures should heighten the clinician's concern for vascular injury, intimal or other. Although rare, compartment syndrome of the thigh should be sought early on during the evaluation of the patient and manifests as tense swelling in the thigh with associated sensory changes and paresthesias. Both compartment syndrome and/or a vascular injury require emergent limb-saving fasciotomy and revascularization respectively. Again, aggressive resuscitation should be performed early in the management of femoral shaft fracture because these fractures have accounted for 1–21 blood loss in multiply injured patients. Recent literature reports that the mortality of bilateral femoral shaft fractures approaches 30%. Whether this is related to associated injuries or hemorrhage is unknown.

## Radiographs and classification

Initial AP and lateral radiographs of the femur should include the hip and knee joint. An AP pelvis can be helpful in determining whether an associated femoral neck fracture has occurred with the femoral shaft fracture. Also associated hip dislocations and/or acetabular fractures can be evaluated with an AP pelvis radiograph. These images are often adequate for the diagnosis of the femoral shaft fracture.

Classification of femoral shaft fractures is based on location and degree of comminution of the fracture. The utility of classification of femoral shaft fractures lies mainly with dialog and research and less with prognosis and treatment.

## Additional studies

Additional studies are usually unnecessary in securing the diagnosis of a femoral shaft fracture. Penetrating and/or open fractures occasionally necessitate radiographic evaluation of the vascular system.

## Early treatment

Initial management of femoral shaft fractures should be aggressive resuscitation. Splinting of the extremity and longitudinal traction are helpful in controlling hemorrhage, pain, and spasm associated with femoral shaft fractures.

## Late treatment

When patients are stable, early surgical management of the femoral shaft fracture, usually with an intramedullary nail, has improved patient outcomes.[12–15] Femoral shaft fractures have a high union rate and a relatively low complication rate with surgical management.[16] Non-operative treatment of femoral shaft fractures has little to no role in Western medicine.

## Complications

Treatment of diaphyseal fractures of the femur has relatively few complications. Infection and hemorrhage are rare following surgery. Deep venous thrombosis and fat emboli syndrome, although relatively uncommon, can be life threatening. Non-union, although rare, can be difficult to treat. Malunion when it does occur is usually rotation and often requires corrective procedures.

## Distal femur fractures

### Introduction

Fractures of the distal femur occur in two populations of patients: the elderly, after low-energy trauma, and the young adult following high-energy trauma. The mechanism of injury in the young population is most often direct impact on a flexed knee (dashboard strike) whereas the mechanism of injury in the elderly population is usually from axial load combined with bending or rotational forces. Distal femur fractures account for almost a third of all femur fractures.

## History and physical

Patients with a suspected distal femur fracture often have associated injuries. The initial evaluation should be directed toward life-threatening injuries. A secondary survey should include a thorough examination of the entire lower extremity. Patients will complain of pain in the knee region. Swelling and/or effusion are extremely common. Tenderness to palpation of the entire knee region and deformity are clinical signs of a distal femur fracture. Abrasions over the patella anteriorly are common and should be differentiated from open fractures. Open fractures (relatively common) occur with the proximal fragment piercing the anterior lateral thigh (quadricep muscle) most of the time. Distal femur fractures require a thorough vascular examination because of associated vascular injuries to the popliteal artery. Neurologic examination should include evaluation of the motor and sensory portions of the posterior tibial nerve, superficial peroneal nerve, and deep peroneal nerve. If pulses are diminished or absent, longitudinal traction to realign the limb should be performed followed by repeat vascular examination (Doppler pulse recordings may be necessary). Sustained absence of pulse despite longitudinal traction warrants radiographic evaluation of the vascular system. Compartment syndrome of the leg should be suspected if the limb has been dysvascular for greater than six hours.

## Radiographs and classification

Initial radiographic evaluation should include an AP and lateral of the knee. Distal femur fractures should be considered intraarticular unless proven otherwise by radiographs. Oblique radiographs of the knee can aid in accurately diagnosing distal femur fractures. Additionally, an AP and lateral of the femur to rule in or out contiguous injuries and comparison knee radiographs are helpful.

Classification schemes are based on the degree of intraarticular involvement and comminution of the metaphyseal fracture. They have been quite useful in predicting knee function and outcome following various treatment methods.

## Additional studies

Arguably the most useful but least obtained plain radiographs for suspected distal femur fractures are traction AP and lateral radiographs of the knee. These easily obtained radiographs can provide a tremendous amount of information regarding the degree of injury to the distal femur. An additional imaging study frequently obtained and invaluable when evaluating comminuted intraarticular fractures of the distal femur is the CT scan. Axial and sagittal images of the distal femur are extremely important for preoperative planning of the surgical reconstruction of the distal femur.

## Early treatment

Initial management of distal femur fractures should include thorough evaluation of associated injuries with particular attention to vascular injuries of the affected extremity. Splinting with a knee immobilizer or posterior plaster slab is an excellent early intervention. It aligns the limb to better protect the vasculature, decrease the pain and spasm, and protect the soft tissues from further injury. Definitive surgical management of distal femur fractures has evolved significantly and is now the treatment of choice. Only a few indications for non-surgical management of distal femur fractures now exist.

## Late treatment

Displaced intraarticular fractures of the distal femur are best managed with open reduction and internal fixation. Three indications exist for emergent surgical intervention: open fractures, fractures associated with vascular compromise, and fractures associated with compartment syndrome. Surgical management of intraarticular distal femur fractures is demanding and requires adherence to several recently defined surgical principles.[17–19] Good to excellent outcomes can still be obtained in the appropriate surgeon's hands.

## Complications

Complications are numerous and arise when one deviates from the previously mentioned surgical principles. Early complications include infection and wound dehiscence. Knee stiffness will occur if range of motion exercise is not started in the early postoperative period. Non-union occurs relatively frequently, as does malunion and loss of fixation. Traumatic arthritis can develop if anatomic reduction of the joint surface is not obtained.

## Extensor mechanism injuries

### Introduction

The intact knee extensor mechanism requires a combination of intact muscle, tendon, retinaculum, and bone to function appropriately. Patella fractures, quadriceps rupture, and patella tendon rupture will disrupt the function of the knee extensor mechanism. These are relatively common injuries that occur from a variety of mechanisms: direct blows, falls, dashboard impacts, and eccentric muscle contraction under a heavy load.

### History and physical

Patients with suspected extensor mechanism injury complain of anterior knee pain and swelling. The second most common complaint is inability to actively extend or straighten the leg. Patients with partial extensor mechanism disruption can often extend the leg but will complain of pain, weakness and/or the leg giving way on them with activity.

Careful physical exam should cover the entire lower extremity. Extensor mechanism injuries are usually isolated injuries but can occur in the multiply injured patient. Evaluation of the skin around the knee should be performed, looking for open injuries. Lacerations must be proven not to communicate with an extensor mechanism injury or the knee joint. An effusion is common but depends on an intact capsule. If the capsule is disrupted, then diffuse periarticular swelling is noted. Tenderness to palpation of the quadriceps, patella, patellar ligament and/or tibial tubercle is common. Additionally, palpation of the anterior knee region often identifies a defect in the extensor mechanism either at the quadriceps insertion, patella fracture or patellar ligament origin.

Occasionally, swelling is so massive that a defect cannot be palpated. In patients without neurologic injury, the inability to extend or straighten the leg (especially against gravity) is pathognomic for extensor mechanism injury. A thorough evaluation of the major knee ligaments is needed but occasionally must be postponed until definitive treatment of the extensor mechanism injury has been performed. Although nerve and vascular injury is uncommon, a thorough evaluation will strengthen the diagnosis of extensor mechanism injury.

### Radiographs and classification

Radiographic evaluation of the knee is important to confirm/diagnose the level of extensor mechanism injury. AP, lateral, and "sunrise" radiographs should be obtained. The AP image will reveal most patella fractures. The lateral image should be evaluated for patella fracture displacement and patellar position relative to the tibial tubercle. The sunrise image will show vertical fractures and joint displacement. A common radiographic abnormality, bipartite patella (superior lateral growth center which never unites with the patella), should not be mistaken for a patella fracture.

Classification of extensor mechanism injuries is divided into partial and complete. Patella fractures are classified based on direction of fracture lines and displacement. Displaced fractures are defined as fracture separation greater than 3 mm and articular step-off of greater than 2 mm.

## Additional studies

Additional studies should be considered if plain radiographs do not reveal the injury and the diagnosis remains in question. MRI is the most useful test after plain radiographs. Injuries to the quadriceps tendon and patellar ligament are easily identified, even the partial injuries which can be clinically elusive.

## Early treatment

Initial management consists of placing and maintaining the knee in an extended position. A knee immobilizer is quite effective in reaching this end. Measures should be taken to control pain and swelling in the region of injury.

## Late treatment

Definitive management of extensor mechanism injuries depends on numerous factors including but not limited to whether the injury is open or closed, the level of injury, the completeness of the injury (partial versus complete), the displacement of the patella fracture, and the overall health of the patient.[20] Some extensor mechanism injuries can be treated with casting (partial quadriceps tendon rupture, non-displaced patella fractures) while others require surgical intervention (complete tendon/ligament ruptures, displaced patella fractures).[21,22] Complications associated with extensor mechanism injuries include misdiagnosis, late diagnosis, extensor lag, weakness of the knee extensors, patellofemoral arthritis, knee stiffness, infection, and loss of fixation, to name a few. Outcomes are generally good but early appropriate diagnosis, attention to detail in operatively treated injuries, and appropriate use of physical therapy to rehabilitate the extensor mechanism of the knee are important factors.

## Complications

Loss of knee extension power, loss of knee motion, and knee pain are relatively infrequent but a few of the complications related to extensor mechanism injury. Traumatic arthritis of the patellofemoral joint can follow comminuted patella fractures.

## Knee dislocations

### Introduction

Traumatic knee dislocation is an uncommon injury occurring with an incidence of one in 10 000 orthopaedic injuries and may result in poor functional outcomes, including amputation. Therefore, proper initial and definitive management is essential. Low-velocity sports injuries and high-velocity knee dislocations secondary to motor vehicle collisions and falls are the usual mechanisms of injury. Suspicion of injury is high in all multitrauma patients with swollen, ecchymotic, and deformed lower extremities.[23]

Treatment principles and prognosis of knee injuries with three or four ligaments disrupted without dislocation on presentation (presumed knee dislocations spontaneously reduced) are identical to complete dislocations.

### History and physical

Knee dislocation is suspected with deformity, swelling, open wounds, and ecchymosis but spontaneously reduced dislocations may appear normal on inspection. Prior to any reduction, the screening exam is performed, consisting of palpation of distal pulses, assessment of motor function by toe and ankle dorsiflexion and plantarflexion and sensory function of dorsal and plantar light touch, in addition to evaluating potential tight swelling of the foot, leg, and calf compartments. Open wounds are noted and sterilely dressed.

Anatomic considerations are pertinent to pathoanatomy and associated injuries. The anterior and posterior cruciate ligaments are the primary restraints to anterior and posterior tibial femoral subluxation respectively. The medial and lateral collateral ligaments are termed secondary restraints and prevent valgus and varus instability of the knee. The popliteal artery and vein are vulnerable because of tethering proximally by the adductor hiatus and distally by the soleus fascia at the posterior knee. The peroneal nerve is tightly restrained at the fibular neck and is susceptible to stretch injury during varus displacement. Associated injuries include major vascular disruptions (30%), peroneal nerve palsy (25%), open injuries (5–20%), associated knee joint and ipsilateral limb fractures in 30–60% of cases.

## Radiographs and classification

Anteroposterior and lateral knee radiographs are quickly evaluated for direction of dislocation and associated fractures when treatment is not delayed. Reduction of the dislocated knee is performed under sedation in the emergency room as soon as screening exam and radiographs are complete and always before transfer to another facility. Postreduction detailed neurovascular examination and repeat anteroposterior, lateral, and oblique radiographs are reviewed to confirm reduction and neurovascular status.

The most common classification of knee dislocation is based on direction of displacement of the tibia with respect to the femur: anterior, posterior, medial, lateral, and posterolateral (often irreducible).

## Additional studies

MRI is a helpful preoperative tool for evaluating the status of the major knee ligaments, articular cartilage, and meniscus. The policy of routine lower extremity angiogram to evaluate occult vascular injury in all patients regardless of clinical vascular status has been replaced by a more selective approach based on the arterial pressure index (API) measurement using a Doppler probe and standard blood pressure cuff. An API is obtained by a Doppler arterial pressure measurement in the injured extremity distal to the injury divided by a pressure measurement in an uninjured limb. When the API is less than 0.9 arteriogram is indicated.[24] If angiogram demonstrates a vascular lesion, immediate vascular consultation for vascular bypass grafting is obtained.[25] Formal angiography can also be obtained early (less than four hours) in the injury if frank ischemia is present. If postreduction examination demonstrates absent pulses and a long period of ischemia exceeding 4–6 hours then immediate vascular surgery exploration with "on the table" arteriogram is indicated to minimize further ischemia time involved with a formal angiography. When the API is greater than 0.9 close clinical examination without arteriography is employed.

## Early treatment

Reduction and immobilization of the dislocated knee are paramount in the early stages of management. Thorough evaluation of the leg for neurologic and vascular status as well as compartment syndrome is necessary. In-line traction and manual pressure on the tibia opposite the direction of tibial displacement is the principal reduction maneuver followed by splinting. Elevation,

ice, and pain management are also helpful adjuncts. Often the dislocated knee will require surgical reconstruction but the avoidance of missed diagnosis and preventable complications will improve the outcome. The goal of revascularization within six hours of injury is important to avoid infection and late amputation. Fasciotomies are indicated to prevent post-reperfusion compartment syndrome sequelae, especially when ischemia time exceeds 4–6 hours.

## Late treatment

Emergent surgical treatment is indicated in cases of "irreducible" dislocation and open knee dislocations for irrigation and debridement and stabilization, usually with external fixation. Definitive treatment options have evolved over the past two decades from the standard six weeks of plaster casting to surgical repair or reconstruction of all torn ligaments for most patients.[26] Though no prospective randomized comparative studies exist, surgery is recommended for most patients within the first three weeks of injury.[27]

Preoperative duplex arterial scanning or angiography is mandatory if an intraoperative tourniquet is to be used, as inflation of tourniquet weeks after a knee dislocation can cause acute arterial occlusion from an intimal flap tear. Open surgery is favored over arthroscopic techniques if surgery is done early because arthroscopic fluid extravasation from the acutely injured knee can precipitate compartment syndrome. Surgical exploration does not seem to affect the rate and degree of recovery of peroneal nerve injuries in less than half the cases. Exceptions include elderly, sedentary, and critically ill multiply injured patients. Postoperative rehabilitation may require up to 12 months to complete with most patients achieving good but not normal knee function and motion.

## Complications

Major complications can arise from knee dislocations and their treatment. Early complications include compartment syndrome, dysvascular extremity, amputation, and neurologic injury. Late complications include amputation, infection, knee stiffness, knee instability, and traumatic arthritis. Most of these complications can be avoided with prompt diagnosis and early surgical management of these injuries by an experienced surgeon.

## Proximal tibia fractures (tibial plateau fractures)

### Introduction

The proximal tibia is composed of medial and lateral

articular surfaces supporting their respective femoral condyles, separated by the tibial eminence. Fractures of the proximal tibia may be extraarticular or involve one or both of the articular surfaces. The peak incidence of these fractures is seen in males around the fourth decade due to high-energy trauma, whereas the peak incidence for women is the seventh decade and involves osteopenic fractures.

## Mechanism of injury

Fractures of the tibial plateau occur either as a result of high-energy trauma (MVC, fall from height) or from low-energy mechanisms such as falls from standing height in elderly patients with osteoporotic bone. Tibial plateau fractures may also be the result of a sports-related injury. Fractures of the medial tibial plateau are often the result of axial loading with a varus (medial) stress, while fractures of the lateral tibial plateau result from axial load with a valgus (lateral) stress.

## History and physical

Physical examination often reveals a painful, swollen extremity with a pronounced knee effusion (hemarthrosis). The affected limb may be shortened or have an obvious varus or valgus deformity. Swelling may extend distally into the lower leg and can cause compartment syndrome in extreme cases. The history of trauma is usually readily available from the patient or from the paramedics in the case of multiple injury. A complete physical examination should be performed to assess the neurovascular status of the limb. Pulses should be documented as palpable, Dopplerable or absent. Sensibility of the leg and motor examination should also be recorded.

## Radiographs

Plain radiographs are the first imaging modality to be obtained to evaluate a patient with a tibial plateau fracture. Standard views are AP and lateral and 45° obliques are usually adequate for initial evaluation. For those injuries with significant deformity, traction views taken while longitudinal traction is being performed are valuable to further define fracture pattern. CT is a valuable adjunct that gives greater detail to the bony anatomy and the overall joint alignment. MRI is also helpful for any associated ligamentous injury but is not as informative for bony detail as a CT scan.

## Classification

### Schatzker classification

Lateral condyle

- Type I – split fracture
- Type II – split depression
- Type III – compression

Medial condyle

- Type IV (A) – high-energy fracture
- Type IV (B) – osteoporotic fracture

Bicondylar

- Type V – medial and lateral condyles
- Type VI – metaphysis separated from diaphysis

### AO classification

- A – extraarticular
- B – partial articular
- C – intraarticular

Each further subdivided into 1, 2 or 3 based on the degree of comminution (1 = least, 3 = most).

## Associated injuries

Associated injuries are common with fractures of the tibial plateau. It has been reported that up to 50% of tibial plateau fractures have a meniscus injury and 25% have a ligamentous injury (collateral or cruciate). Collateral ligament injury is also frequent involving the opposite collateral ligament from the tibial plateau fracture.[28] Injuries of the anterior cruciate ligament are also common, particularly with split depression or bicondylar fractures. Fractures of the medial tibial plateau are often associated with varus deformity and associated injury to the peroneal nerve with resultant foot drop. Fractures involving the ipsilateral lower extremity are also common and the entire limb from pelvis to foot must be examined with radiographs when indicated.

## Emergent management

The initial management of the patient with a tibial plateau fracture should follow basic trauma protocols. The vascular supply to the limb must be documented with pulses being palpable, Dopplerable or absent. Capillary refill to the toes may still be present even in the absence of pulses due to collateral circulation. If the pulses are diminished in a limb with significant deformity, then longitudinal traction with varus or valgus stress to correct the deformity will often improve distal blood supply. A thorough evaluation of the proximal tibia should be performed to rule out any open injury in communication with the fracture site. The compartments of the leg should also be palpated to check for possible compartment syndrome. The cardinal signs of compartment syndrome are pain with passive range of motion, pallor, pulselessness, and paresthesias; however, the most specific is pain with passive extension of the toes.

Finally, a thorough assessment of the remainder of the limb is performed looking for other areas of tenderness, swelling or crepitance. The leg is then splinted with a long leg posterior splint or a knee immobilizer.

## Definitive treatment

A variety of treatment options are available for tibial plateau fractures. Non-displaced or minimally displaced fractures often can be adequately treated with closed reduction and casting with non-weight bearing for 8–12 weeks. The majority of displaced articular fractures are best treated with open reduction and internal fixation.[29] Open injuries with soft tissue compromise or contamination are often initially managed with either external fixation until the soft tissue envelope will tolerate a surgical incision or definitive treatment in an external fixator. Some minimally displaced fractures can be treated with arthroscopic-assisted reduction with percutaneous screw fixation.[30]

## Complications

Early complications following tibial plateau fractures are primarily related to the degree of soft tissue injury and the association of an open injury.[31] Compartment syndrome is infrequent but is important to recognize early. Infection can follow an open fracture but can also follow surgical treatment of these injuries and requires debridement with long-term intravenous antibiotics. Wound dehiscence or skin slough is also problematic in those fractures with significant associated soft tissue injury and may require rotational muscle flap coverage or free tissue coverage.[32] Late complications include malunion and non-union which both necessitate further surgery. Posttraumatic arthrosis is also fairly common due to articular injury at the time of fracture. Instability from unrecognized or untreated ligament injury is another reported complication.

## Tibial shaft fractures

### Introduction

Tibial shaft fractures are the most common long bone fractures with almost 500 000 occurring each year in the United States. There is a large spectrum of injury ranging from stress fractures due to repetitive microtrauma to low-energy fractures (falls from standing height, sports injuries) to high-energy injuries (MVC, falls from heights). Due to the relatively thin soft tissue envelope over the distal half of the tibia, treatment options are sometimes dictated not by the fracture itself but rather by the status of the surrounding soft tissue.

## Mechanism of injury

Fractures of the tibia may be the result of either low-energy or high-energy trauma. Examples of low-energy trauma include sports-related injuries and falls from standing height. High-energy mechanisms include MVC and falls from heights. Low-energy fractures are usually torsional stresses about a fixed foot leading to a spiral fracture. Bending forces produce short oblique or transverse fractures. High-energy mechanisms are associated with comminution at the fracture site or segmental fractures. Pedestrian versus automobile accidents frequently result in tibial fractures due to the height of the car bumper.

## History and physical

The deformity associated with a fracture of the tibia is often readily apparent due to the subcutaneous nature of the bone. Patients will complain of severe pain localized to the area of the fracture associated with pronounced soft tissue swelling. The neurovascular status of the limb should be assessed with documented pulses, sensory, and motor examinations. Gross deformity should be corrected with traction if decreased pulses are noted. The compartments should be assessed for possible compartment syndrome. Any break in the skin should be assessed for possible continuity with the fracture site.

## Radiographs

The initial radiographic assessment of a patient with a possible tibial shaft fracture should include AP and lateral views of the entire length of the tibia from knee to ankle. If significant deformity is present, then traction views of the tibia are helpful. Ancillary studies such as CT and MRI are usually not indicated.

## Classification

There is no universally accepted classification system.

### Descriptive classification system

- Level of injury – proximal diaphyseal, middle diaphyseal, distal diaphyseal
- Open versus closed injury (see classification for open fractures below)
- Associated fibula fracture (at same or different level from tibia fracture)
- Degree of comminution
- Fracture pattern (transverse, oblique, spiral, segmental)

### Gustilo-Anderson classification for open fractures

- Grade I     Clean laceration <1 cm, typically inside-out wound, no fracture comminution
- Grade II     Laceration >1 cm in length with soft tissue stripping/muscle injury, some degree of comminution
- Grade III     Laceration >10 cm in length with extreme soft tissue stripping including skin, muscle, neurovascular structures; high degree of comminution
  - IIIA     Adequate soft tissue coverage of bone present, gunshot wound
  - IIIB     Periosteal stripping and exposed bone requiring soft tissue procedure (muscle flap, free flap) for coverage
  - IIIC     Vascular injury requiring repair

## Associated injuries

Ligamentous injuries to the knee occur in a reported 22% of tibial shaft fractures. Associated fractures of the ipsilateral lower extremity (femur, knee, ankle, foot) are not uncommon.

## Emergent management

The initial management of a patient with a suspected tibial shaft fracture should include basic trauma protocols. After this is established, the neurovascular status of the limb should be assessed. Pulses should be assessed and classified as palpable, Dopplerable or absent. If significant deformity is present, then longitudinal traction is helpful in improving distal blood flow. Sensibility and motor function to the foot should be assessed at this time. The soft tissue envelope should then be evaluated for possible open injury or compartment syndrome. Finally, the leg should be placed in a long leg posterior splint or a short leg posterior splint with a knee immobilizer. Any open wounds should be covered with moist sterile gauze. Open fractures also require administration of tetanus prophylaxis and intravenous antibiotics with a cephalosporin such as cefazolin.

## Definitive treatment

Stable fractures with minimal displacement and shortening which are closed may be treated with closed manipulation and casting.[33] Unstable fractures and those open fractures with minimal soft tissue contamination are most commonly treated with intramedullary nailing.[34–36] Those fractures with severe contamination, soft tissue stripping or vascular injury are best treated with irrigation and debridement followed by external fixation. Once the wounds have stabilized, the external fixator may be converted to an intramedullary nail or the external fixator can be used as definitive treatment.

## Complications

Early complications following tibial shaft fractures are most frequently the sequelae of injury to the surrounding soft tissue. Compartment syndrome requires emergent fasciotomy and, if unrecognized or untreated, can lead to loss of the limb. Infection following open fracture or internal fixation of closed fracture is also an early complication. Skin slough is another serious complication that may require soft tissue coverage either by local flap or free tissue transfer. The combination of infection with skin slough often leads to definitive treatment by amputation as a salvage procedure. Late complications are often related to the healing of the fracture. Non-union is a particular concern in tibial shaft fractures because of the marginal blood supply to the diaphysis, especially distally. Malunion is another frequent complication which may follow any form of treatment, but is more commonly seen after closed manipulation and casting.

## Distal tibia fractures (tibial plafond fractures)

### Introduction

Fractures of the tibial plafond are relatively infrequent, involving 1% of lower extremity fractures and 5–10% of tibia fractures. They are also referred to as pilon (hammer) fractures as the talus is driven into the distal tibial articular surface by axial loading. These fractures are differentiated from the much more common ankle fractures by the involvement of the distal tibial articular surface, which is undisturbed in the majority of simple ankle fractures. Plafond fractures have an associated fracture of the tibia in approximately 25% of cases.

### Mechanism of injury

Tibial plafond fractures are primarily the result of axial compression with the talus being driven up into the distal tibial articular surface. Varying degrees of rotational forces may give the fracture a spiral configuration. Low-energy injuries are frequent and can follow falls from standing height or sports-related injuries (ski boot fractures). High-energy injuries typically result from falls from heights or MVC. The more plantarflexed the foot at impact, the more posterior involvement of the plafond. Conversely, with more dorsiflexion of the foot, more anterior involvement of the plafond will be noted.

## History and physical

Examination typically reveals a painful, swollen distal tibia with the inability to bear weight. The history usually involves forced rotation or axial compression. A thorough neurovascular examination is vital to determine any associated limb-threatening injuries. Gross deformity should be corrected with gentle longitudinal traction. The surrounding soft tissue envelope should be assessed for injury, contamination, and the possibility of compartment syndrome. Finally, the entire lower extremity from pelvis to foot should be examined to rule out ipsilateral fractures.

## Radiographs

Initial radiographs should include AP and lateral views of the entire length of the tibia from knee to ankle. If deformity is present, traction views with gentle longitudinal traction are very helpful. CT is a valuable imaging modality to better visualize the tibial articular surface and fracture pattern. CT has essentially replaced trispiral tomograms. Comparison views are also helpful for comminuted fractures as a "template" for future fracture reduction.

## Classification

### Ruedi and Allgower

- Type I – simple fracture pattern with no articular displacement
- Type II – simple fracture pattern with >2 mm displacement
- Type III – comminuted distal tibia with several articular fragments

### AO classification

- A – extraarticular
- B – partial articular
- C – intraarticular

1 no comminution
2 some comminution
3 extremely comminuted

## Associated injuries

Injuries accompanying tibial plafond fractures include fractures of the ipsilateral lower extremity and disruption of the pelvic ring. In addition, lumbar spine compression/burst fractures are also not uncommon, particularly after high-energy trauma. In the evaluation of any patient with a high-energy fracture of the tibial plafond, the entire lower extremity and lumbar spine should be examined clinically for associated injury.

## Emergent management

The entire lower limb and spine should be evaluated for possible injury. Gross deformity should be corrected with manual traction. Appropriate radiographs need to be obtained after gross alignment has been restored. A thorough neurovascular examination is mandatory to rule out associated vascular injury with ischemia of the foot and to assess sensibility and motor function. The soft tissue envelope should then be assessed to rule out open fracture and compartment syndrome. Open injuries should then be covered with a sterile dressing. Finally, the limb should be splinted in a short leg posterior splint. At this time, ancillary studies (CT) may be obtained.

## Definitive treatment

Closed treatment with casting is acceptable for non-displaced fractures. The majority of tibial plafond fractures have significant articular displacement and require anatomic restoration of the joint which is achieved only through open reduction and internal fixation.[37–40] Open fractures require emergent irrigation and debridement. Gross contamination and fractures with a marginal soft tissue envelope should be provisionally or definitively treated with external fixation.

## Complications

Early complications are often related to the degree of injury to the soft tissue. There is a very high infection risk with open, comminuted fractures (approaching 25–30%). In addition to infection, another complication is lack of soft tissue coverage due to wound breakdown. This can lead to the need for free tissue transfers and possible osteomyelitis and in some instances requires amputation as definitive treatment. Late complications involve bony healing, with malunion being frequently reported without rigid internal fixation or with severely comminuted fractures. Non-union is common, particularly following open fractures with some degree of bone loss. This typically will respond to bone-grafting procedures once the soft tissue envelope heals. Posttraumatic arthrosis can result from cartilage injury suffered at the time of fracture or from imperfect reconstruction of the distal tibial articular surface. The treatment for painful, debilitating arthrosis of the tibiotalar joint is ankle fusion.

## Ankle fractures

### Introduction

Fractures of the ankle are very common with 23 000 fractures or sprains occurring daily in the United States. These fractures are commonly seen as a twisting injury during sports activities from "rolling over" of the ankle. Ankle fractures may be associated with subluxation or frank dislocation of the talus from the ankle mortise. Rupture of the syndesmotic ligaments is also often associated with ankle fractures. These fractures are differentiated from tibial plafond fractures by the lack of involvement of the articular surface of the distal tibia.

### Mechanism of injury

The most common mechanism of injury leading to ankle fracture involves the twisting of the tibia on a planted foot. The position of the foot at the time of impact and the direction of the deforming force determine the fracture pattern. Forces can be transmitted through the interosseous membrane and exit the fibula proximally as high as the fibular neck. These "high" fibula fractures are referred to as Maisonneuve fractures.

### History and physical

The patient with an ankle fracture will usually report some type of twisting injury immediately prior to the fracture. The ankle typically will be very swollen and tender with inability to bear weight. It is important to document areas of tenderness and swelling particularly on the medial side of the ankle because injuries to the deltoid ligament may be present even when there is no apparent fracture on the radiograph. Tibiotalar subluxation/dislocation is not uncommon and should be corrected with longitudinal traction and plantarflexion

of the ankle followed by dorsiflexion to maintain reduction. The soft tissue envelope should also be assessed for open injury or any neurovascular compromise.

### Radiographs

The standard radiographic series of the ankle includes the AP, mortise (oblique), and lateral views. If gross deformity is present, this should be corrected prior to the radiographs if possible. Ideally, the entire length of the fibula should be visualized to rule out a high fibula fracture. Additional stress radiographs are also beneficial in certain circumstances to assess for ligamentous injury.

### Classification

#### *Denis-Weber system*

Determined by the level of the fibula fracture.

- Type A – fibula fracture distal to the level of the tibiotalar joint
- Type B – fibula fracture at the level of the tibiotalar joint
- Type C – fibula fracture proximal to the level of the tibiotalar joint

#### *Lauge-Hansen system*

Based on the position of the foot and direction of force.

*Supination-adduction*
Typically transverse distal fibula fracture with vertical fracture of medial malleolus.

*Supination-external rotation*
Most frequent ankle fracture.

- Stage I – strain of anterior inferior tibiofibular ligament (AITF)
- Stage II – AITF strain with fibula fracture
- Stage III – AITF strain, fibula fracture, and PITF strain
- Stage IV – AITF strain, fibula fracture, PITF strain, and medial malleolus fracture or deltoid ligament strain/rupture

*Pronation-external rotation*
- Stage I – medial malleolus fracture or deltoid rupture
- Stage II – medial malleolus or deltoid injury with AITF
- Stage III – medial malleolus or deltoid injury, AITF, and lateral malleolus
- Stage IV – medial malleolus or deltoid injury, AITF, lateral malleolus, and PITF strain

*Pronation-abduction*
Horizontal fractures of both medial and lateral malleoli.

## Associated injuries

There are a variety of subtle injuries which can accompany fractures of the ankle. Ligamentous injury may occur either laterally or medially. Osteochondral fractures involving the talus sometimes are present, particularly following ankle fracture/dislocation. In addition, lateral process talus fractures may accompany ankle fracture and can complicate treatment. Injury to the peroneal tendons may lead to persistent lateral ankle pain or frank dislocation.

## Emergent management

The ankle and foot should be examined thoroughly for any neurovascular compromise. If gross deformity is present, it should be corrected with longitudinal traction. The soft tissue envelope then requires evaluation to rule out open fracture. An adequate assessment includes palpation of the entire foot and the entire length of the fibula to rule out associated ligamentous injuries or a high fibula fracture. Finally, the injured extremity should be immobilized in a short leg posterior splint.

## Definitive treatment

Some minimally displaced fractures can be adequately treated with cast immobilization for 6–8 weeks. The majority of ankle fractures, including all fracture/dislocations, require open reduction with internal fixation.[41,42] Some open fractures with significant bone loss or contamination necessitate multiple irrigation and debridements with external fixation.[43]

## Complications

Early complications following ankle fracture are related to the soft tissue envelope. Open fractures have a higher incidence of infection, which requires irrigation and debridement with long-term intravenous antibiotics. Wound breakdown following soft tissue injury can necessitate free flap coverage. Late complications include non-union, malunion, and posttraumatic arthrosis. Each of these requires additional surgery for bone grafting or corrective osteotomy. Painful arthrosis may ultimately require ankle fusion for adequate pain relief.

## Foot fractures (hindfoot, midfoot, and forefoot)

Foot fractures may involve the hindfoot (calcaneus, talus), midfoot (navicular, cuboid, cuneiforms, tarsometatarsal joints) or forefoot (metatarsals, toes) or any combination of these structures. While traditionally overlooked in the management of multitrauma patients, these injuries and their treatment play a primary role in the long-term function of the patient. Correct diagnosis and early appropriate treatment are paramount in the end result of a painless, plantigrade foot for ambulation and weightbearing.

## Hindfoot

### Osteochondral injuries to the talus

#### Introduction

These injuries are relatively uncommon and frequently misdiagnosed as injuries to the lateral ligament complex of the ankle. While they can accompany lateral ligament injuries and ankle fractures, they can also be seen as isolated injuries. The typical mechanism of injury is one of an inversion strain applied to a planted foot. The patient reports the typical pain seen with lateral ligament injuries. Swelling and tenderness are often reported as well. If misdiagnosed as ligament injuries and left untreated, these injuries can lead to chronic symptoms of persistent pain, stiffness, recurrent ankle effusion, and occasional locking of the ankle.

#### History and physical

The patient with an osteochondral injury to the talus will typically report an inversion injury to the ankle with resultant pain. The patient may or may not be able to bear weight on the injured foot. Examination reveals painful swelling most pronounced along the lateral side of the ankle. The patient may also report a painful "catching" sensation. The range of motion of the injured ankle is typically much less than the contralateral side.

#### Radiographs

Standard AP and lateral radiographs are usually adequate to make the diagnosis in 70–100% of cases. An area of lucency is generally seen in the area of the talar dome. If the osteochondral fragment has a large amount of bone present, then it can be seen in a displaced position on radiographs. If the diagnosis is equivocal, then bone scan is a useful adjunct. Magnetic resonance imaging is the most sensitive study and is very good at demonstrating both the size and stability of the fragment.

### Emergent management

Because these injuries are typically the result of low-energy mechanisms and present as isolated injuries, a thorough physical examination coupled with the appropriate radiographs is usually adequate to make the diagnosis. If the diagnosis is equivocal, then the use of MRI is very helpful to further document the size and stability of the fragment. The patient should then be splinted in a short leg posterior splint.

### Definitive treatment

The treatment of osteochondral fractures of the talus depends on two factors: size and stability of the osteochondral fragment. For a stable, non-displaced fragment, the preferred treatment is cast immobilization until healing has occurred. The treatment for unstable fragments with overlying cartilage is controversial. These injuries usually require surgical intervention with arthroscopic or open debridement of the bed of the fragment and drilling of the subchondral bone to stimulate healing of the fragment. Unstable fragments require debridement of the fragment bed and either removal or internal fixation of the fragment, depending on its size and location.

### Complications

The main complication following ostechondral injuries of the talus is degenerative arthrosis. There is a reported 75% incidence of arthrosis regardless of treatment. Smaller fragments that are stable have the best prognosis. Large, unstable fragments and those that have gone untreated have a more unfavorable prognosis.

### Talar neck fractures

### Introduction

Fractures of the talar neck are fairly common fractures. The typical mechanism is axial loading with forced dorsiflexion of the foot. Some degree of medial or lateral stress may also be present. Due to the tenuous nature of the blood supply to the talus, *displaced* fractures involving this bone must be treated as a *surgical emergency*.

### History and physical

The patient with a fracture of the talar neck will usually complain of pain over the ankle region. The ankle is usually very swollen and range of motion is very limited. The mechanism of injury is usually high energy such as MVC or fall from height. The entire foot and leg must be examined for associated injury and possible compartment syndrome. A thorough neurovascular examination is also mandatory.

### Classification

Hawkins' classification for talar neck fractures is most commonly used.

- Type I – non-displaced vertical fracture
- Type II – displaced fracture with subluxation of subtalar joint
- Type III – displaced fracture with subtalar and tibio-talar subluxation/dislocation
- Type IV – type III fracture with subluxation of talus from talonavicular joint

### Radiographs

Standard AP and lateral radiographs are typically adequate for diagnosis of talar neck fracture. With some fractures of the talus, CT is an important adjunct to better characterize displacement and fracture pattern.

### Emergent management

Displaced fractures of the talar neck are a *surgical emergency* and require rapid diagnosis and treatment. The blood supply to the body of the talus is tenuous and the longer a displaced fracture of the talar neck is left unreduced, the higher the risk of resultant avascular necrosis. After complete examination of the injured extremity, appropriate radiographs may be taken. If a displaced talar neck fracture is seen, a single attempt at closed reduction should be performed under sedation. If the fracture reduces, a short leg posterior splint should be applied, followed by urgent definitive surgical treatment. If the talus remains dislocated, emergent ORIF should be performed.

### Definitive treatment

Non-displaced (type I) fractures can be adequately treated with closed means and non-weight bearing until bony union occurs. Displaced fractures of the talar neck require emergent anatomic reduction with secure internal fixation.[44] Open fractures of the talar neck require emergent irrigation and debridement followed by internal fixation.

### Complications

The most frequent complication following talar neck fracture is avascular necrosis due to disruption of the blood supply to the talus. The incidence of avascular necrosis varies with displacement and type of fracture as follows: type I 0–13%; type II 42–50%; type III 84–91%; type IV ~100%. Posttraumatic arthrosis of subtalar or tibiotalar joints is also reported due to either cartilage injury at the time of injury or collapse of the articular surface with resultant degenerative arthrosis. Malunion and non-union are also infrequent complications requiring corrective osteotomy, bone grafting or hindfoot fusion.

## Calcaneus fracture

### Introduction

Fractures of the calcaneus are relatively infrequent injuries. They are the result of axial loading on the hindfoot. The most frequent mechanisms of injury are MVC and falls from heights. These fractures may be either intra-articular or extraarticular. Associated injuries are common with up to 30% of patients suffering concomitant lumbar spine compression/burst fractures. Injuries to the ipsilateral lower extremity and the pelvis are also fairly frequent with calcaneus fracture.

### History and physical

The patient with a calcaneus fracture will typically report significant heel pain. Swelling is usually dramatic and compartment syndrome of the foot is a reported sequela of calcaneus fracture. The neurovascular status of the foot should be assessed as well as the soft tissue envelope. The foot should be elevated and iced. Open fractures should be covered with a moist sterile dressing. The foot should then be splinted with a short leg posterior splint. The entire lower extremity and lumbar spine should be examined clinically to assess for associated injury.

### Radiographs

Standard radiographs for initial evaluation include lateral and axial views. Oblique views (Broden's view) are also helpful to evaluate the subtalar joint. CT is very important as an adjunctive modality in order to assess the fracture pattern, joint surfaces, and degree of displacement. Occasionally, comparison views are beneficial to serve as a "template" or to assess degree of joint depression and loss of heel height.

### Classification

*Sanders*
Most common, based on CT scan, I–IV based on number of fracture lines and posterior facet fragments.

*Crosby and Fitzgibbons*
Three types based on posterior facet comminution on CT.

- Type I – posterior facet fragments non-displaced
- Type II – posterior facet fragments displaced but not comminuted
- Type III – posterior facet comminution

### Emergent management

After initial neurovascular examination of the foot, the degree of soft tissue injury should be assessed. The foot should be closely examined to rule out open fracture. The degree of swelling must also be determined to rule out possible compartment syndrome. The entire ipsilateral lower extremity and spine should then be assessed for associated injuries, in particular fractures of the lumbar spine. Once appropriate radiographs have been obtained, the foot should be splinted in a short leg posterior splint and appropriate ancillary studies (CT) ordered.

### Definitive treatment

Closed treatment with casting is usually adequate for non-displaced fractures or some displaced extraarticular fractures. Displaced intraarticular fractures require anatomic restoration of the joint surfaces and heel height/width in order to maximize a successful outcome.[45] Grossly contaminated fractures require irrigation and debridement with or without the use of an external fixator. Some severely comminuted fractures are unreconstructable at the time of surgery; salvage is by primary subtalar fusion.

### Complications

Early complications following calcaneus fracture are usually related to associated soft tissue injury. Infection can follow ORIF and is particularly problematic after open fracture of the calcaneus. Wound problems are frequent after attempted ORIF with skin slough occasionally requiring soft tissue coverage with free tissue transfer. Late complications are the result of cartilage injury, imperfect reduction or inadequate restoration of heel morphology. Posttraumatic arthrosis can present up to two years after fracture and may eventually require subtalar fusion. Peroneal tendon impingement can also result from increased heel width and lead to chronic lateral ankle pain. Chronic heel pain can result from injury to the heel pad at the time of fracture. Difficulty with shoe wear is particularly problematic and for some patients is the chief complaint following even adequately treated calcaneus fractures.

## Midfoot

### Navicular fracture

Fracture of the navicular bone is relatively uncommon. Three types of fracture are described: stress fracture, acute fracture, and avulsion fracture. Displaced intra-articular fractures have been classified by Sangeorzan as follows:

- type I – coronal fracture
- type II – coronal fracture with medial displacement of forefoot
- type III – comminuted with lateral angulation.

Diagnosis is relatively straightforward with an adequate radiographic series of the foot. AP, lateral, and oblique views of the foot are considered standard. Treatment is non-operative for non-displaced fractures. Displaced fractures with intraarticular incongruity necessitate open reduction with internal fixation.[46]

### Tarsometatarsal joint complex (Lisfranc) injuries

#### *Introduction*

Injuries to the tarsometatarsal joints are complex and notoriously difficult to diagnose and treat. The mechanism of injury is typically that of axial loading with forced plantarflexion of the midfoot. Historically, the injury was that of a horse rider being thrown or forcefully dismounting with a twisting mechanism to a foot hung in the stirrup. The Lisfranc joint is named after a surgeon in Napoleon's army who performed amputations at the tarsometatarsal level for frostbite. Most injuries are high energy such as MVC and falls from heights.

#### *History and physical*

Physical examination reveals a swollen midfoot with tenderness, inability to bear weight, and swelling. The patient usually gives a history of axial loading and twisting with immediate pain. The deformity may be mild or significant. The foot should be thoroughly examined for open injuries and the soft tissue assessed for possible compartment syndrome. After appropriate radiographs have been obtained, the foot should be immobilized in a short leg posterior splint.

#### *Radiographs*

The standard radiographic series for evaluation of the foot contains three views: AP, lateral, and oblique. These three views are usually adequate for the diagnosis, demonstrating subluxation or frank dislocation of one or several metatarsals. Occasionally only subtle findings will be present and stress views are helpful to demonstrate ligamentous instability. CT is of limited use in the event of concomitant fracture.

#### *Classification*

The classification system described by Hardcastle is most commonly used.

- Type A – total incongruity involving all five metatarsals
- Type B – partial incongruity; typically only one or two metatarsals involved
- Type C – divergent with either total or partial incongruity

#### *Emergent management*

The patient should first be resuscitated according to the principles of basic trauma protocol. The foot and entire lower extremity should be thoroughly assessed for any concomitant injury. The soft tissue envelope should also be thoroughly assessed for possible open injury and compartment syndrome. After appropriate radiographs have been obtained, the foot should be splinted in a short leg posterior splint.

#### *Definitive treatment*

Sprains of the Lisfranc joint may be adequately treated with cast immobilization. Any displacement or instability noted on stress radiograph mandates treatment with open reduction and internal fixation.[47] Open fractures require immediate irrigation and debridement prior to fixation.

#### *Complications*

The most frequent complications involve the soft tissue of the foot. Infection following open or closed injury treated with open reduction is significant, requiring irrigation and debridement with long-term intravenous antibiotics. Wound problems and skin slough are also problematic with the sometimes severe swelling of soft tissue following these injuries. Posttraumatic arthrosis is also a complication seen as a result of either cartilage damage at the time of injury or inadequate reduction.

## Forefoot

### Base of fifth metatarsal fracture

Fractures of the base of the fifth metatarsal are common. There are two specific types of fracture frequently encountered: proximal avulsion fractures (ballerina fracture) or proximal diaphyseal fractures (Jones fracture). Fractures of the base of the fifth metatarsal may be either acute or a stress fracture. Physical examination reveals pain localized to the lateral midfoot with associated swelling. The patient may or may not be able to bear weight and sometimes cannot recall one specific traumatic event preceding the fracture. Appropriate radiographs include AP, lateral, and oblique foot views.

Treatment is usually conservative with closed treatment with short leg cast. Screw fixation is sometimes necessary for high-performance athletes or non-united fractures.[48] The most frequent complication is non-union, especially following Jones fractures, which requires ORIF and bone grafting.

## Metatarsophalangeal joint injuries

Injuries to metatarsophalangeal joints range from mild sprain to complete rupture of capsuloligamentous structures. These injuries represent hyperextension injury to the toe, often referred to as turf toe. Physical examination reveals painful swelling to the first metatarsophalangeal joint with decreased range of motion. Ecchymosis may be present and represents more severe injury. Foot radiographs (AP, lateral, and oblique) are usually adequate to reveal the diagnosis in the case of dislocation of the MTP joints. Ancillary studies such as bone scan or MRI are sometimes helpful in the case of ligamentous or capsular disruption. MTP joint injuries are typically treated with taping or brief periods of splinting with the use of NSAIDS for pain. Severe cases sometimes require surgical repair and exploration for possible osteochondral injuries. MTP dislocation of the first MTP joint is an unusual injury but one which should not be taken lightly. Closed reduction of the MTP joint is mandatory as soon as the diagnosis is made. Some dislocations of the first MTP joint are irreducible and require open reduction for correction of deformity. Cases of rupture of the capsuloligamentous structures are best treated with early surgical repair followed by immobilization.

## Class I references

4. Brien WW, Wiss DA, Becker V Jr *et al.* Subtrochanteric femur fractures: a comparison of the Zickel nail, 95 degrees blade plate, and interlocking nail. *J Orthop Trauma* 1991;**2**:458–64.

A prospective, randomized study evaluating the results of three different types of fixation for subtrochanteric fracture of the femur. The operative time was longest for the 95-degree blade plate, and shortest for the interlocking nail. The average blood loss was also significantly greater for those patients treated with the 95-degree blade plate in comparison to the other two groups. There were also more malunions in the group treated with the 95-degree blade plate, but this was not statistically significant. There was no difference between any group in regards to infection or non-union. The authors conclude that the treatment of choice for nonpathologic subtrochanteric fracture of the femur is interlocking nailing.

5. Desjardins AL, Roy A, Paiement G *et al.* Unstable intertrochanteric fracture of the femur: a prospective randomized study comparing anatomical reduction and medial displacement osteotomy. *J Bone Joint Surg* 1993;**75B**:445–7.

A prospective, randomized study of unstable intertrochanteric femur fracture fixation. The study found no difference in walking ability, social status, or failure of fixation but did notice increased operative time and blood loss in the group treated with medial displacement osteotomy. The authors concluded that the use of the modern sliding hip screw made the medial displacement osteotomy rarely indicated for these fractures.

6. Goldhagen PR, O'Conner DR, Schwarze E. A prospective comparative study of the compression hip screw and the gamma nail. *J Orthop Trauma* 1994;**5**:367–72.

A prospective, randomized study of compression hip screw fixation compared to the gamma nail in 75 patients with peritrochanteric fracture of the femur. No difference in perioperative and intraoperative parameters was noted. The gamma nail allowed earlier weight bearing but this was not statistically significant. Overall, the gamma nail had equivalent results but the authors found that the insertion was technically more demanding with a steeper learning curve.

37. Wyrsch B, McFerran MA, McAndrew MA *et al.* A randomized, prospective study evaluating the surgical management of pilon fractures. *Orthop Trans* 1994; **18**:720.

The authors present the only prospective, randomized study of open plating with external fixation and minimal internal fixation. Major complications occurred in 55% of the open reduction group and in only 18% of the external fixation/minimal internal fixation group. The authors concluded that external fixation and limited internal fixation resulted in significantly less soft tissue complications than traditional open reduction with internal fixation.

41. Phillips WA, Schwartz HS, Keller CS *et al.* A prospective randomized study of the management of severe ankle fractures. *J Bone Joint Surg* 1985;**67A**:67–78.

This prospective, randomized study evaluates 134 patients with closed SE-IV or PE-IV ankle fractures. The patients were randomized to closed treatment after satisfactory reduction versus open reduction with internal fixation. Forty-two patients with an unsatisfactory closed reduction were then randomized to open reduction internal fixation with either medial fixation only versus medial and lateral fixation. The study is weakened by a follow-up of only 51% of the enrolled patients at 3.5 years. Significantly higher scores were seen for patients treated with standard open reduction internal fixation. The numbers were too small to draw a conclusion of fixation methods. Open reduction with internal fixation is recommended for all SE-IV and PE-IV ankle fractures.

## Class II references

2.  Quinn SF, McCarthy JL. Prospective evaluation of patients with suspected hip fracture and indeterminate radiographs: use of T1-weighted MR images. *Radiology* 1993;**187**:469–71.

    A prospective, consecutive evaluation of 20 patients presenting with a suspected fracture of the femoral neck. The patients were evaluated with MRI scans, which were found to be 100% predictive for femoral neck fracture. In addition, the cost of the MRI scan was less expensive than computerized tomography or a bone scan.

7.  Haentjens P, Casteleyn P, DeBoeck H *et al*. Treatment of unstable intertrochanteric and subtrochanteric fractures in elderly patients. *J Bone Joint Surg* 1989;**71A**: 1214–25.

    A consecutive series of 37 patients greater than 75 years of age treated with primary bipolar hemiarthroplasty. Seventy-five per cent good to excellent results were reported based on functional results. These results were then retrospectively compared to results achieved after open reduction and internal fixation of the same type of fracture. The patients treated with hemiarthroplasty had faster and easier rehabilitation, and also had decreased incidence of atelectasis, pneumonia, and pressure sores. Early weight bearing after hemiarthroplasty was felt to be the major advantage.

8.  Wiss DA, Brien WW. Subtrochanteric fractures of the femur: results of treatment by interlocking nailing. *Clin Orthop* 1992;**283**:231–6.

    A prospective, consecutive study of 95 subtrochanteric fractures of the femur treated with intramedullary nailing. The average time to healing was 25 weeks. There were three delayed unions, one nonunion, and six malunions. The authors conclude that closed, interlocked, intramedullary nailing is the preferred treatment for this type of fracture regardless of fracture pattern or degree of comminution.

12. Brumback RJ, Uwagie-Ero S, Lakatos RP *et al*. Intramedullary nailing of femoral shaft fractures. Part II.

Fracture-healing with static interlocking fixation. *J Bone Joint Surg* 1988; **70A**:1453–62.

A prospective, consecutive study of 97 patients with 100 fractures of the femoral shaft treated with statistically locked intramedullary nailing. A healing rate of 98% was reported. Two patients required dynamization procedures for delayed union. The authors concluded that routine dynamization of intramedullary nails is unnecessary following femoral shaft fracture, unless there is evidence of delayed union.

16. Brumback RJ, Toal TR Jr, Murphy-Zane MS, Novak VP, Belkoff SM. Immediate weight-bearing after treatment of a comminuted fraction of the femoral shaft with a statically locked intramedullary nail. *J Bone Joint Surg* 1999;**81A**:1538–44.

    An excellent two-part study evaluating the effect of immediate weight bearing after comminuted femoral shaft fractures. The first part is a biomechanical study evaluating different makes and diameter nails for fractures of the femur with no cortical contact. The second phase of the study utilized a 12-mm diameter intramedullary nail in a consecutive series of 28 patients. The patients were allowed immediate weight bearing after surgery. All fractures united and there were no broken screws or nails. The authors conclude that early weight bearing is not detrimental and may actually be beneficial in a multiply injured patient by allowing earlier mobilization.

28. Bennett WF, Browner B. Tibial plateau fractures: a study of associated soft tissue injuries. *J Orthop Trauma* 1994;**8**:183–8.

    This prospective, consecutive study evaluates 36 patients with tibial plateau fractures for injuries to other associated structures. Associated injuries included medial collateral ligament (20%), lateral collateral ligament (3%), peroneal nerve (3%), meniscus (20%), and anterior cruciate ligament (10%). Schatzker type II and IV injuries were associated with the highest frequency of soft tissue injury. The study recommended diagnostic arthroscopy for nondisplaced type I fractures and pre- and post-fixation stress testing for all tibial plateau fractures.

42. Boden SD, Labropoulos PA, McCowin P *et al*. Mechanical considerations for the syndesmosis screw: a cadaver study. *J Bone Joint Surg* 1989;**71A**: 1548–55.

    A cadaveric study in which the syndesmotic ligaments were divided and the interosseus membranes were sectioned to different levels. Rigid fixation of both the medial and lateral sides of the ankle results in minimal widening of the mortise even if the interosseus membrane has been sectioned as high as 15 cm proximal to the ankle. When the medial side could not be stabilized (as in a deltoid ligament injury), the syndesmosis showed significant instability once the interosseus membrane had been divided part 4.5 cm proximal to the ankle.

## Class III references

1.  Hinton RY, Smith GS. The association of age, race, and sex with the location of proximal femoral fractures in the elderly. *J Bone Joint Surg* 1993;**75A**:752–9.

    Retrospective review of the medical records of 27 370 patients with a diagnosis of femoral neck fracture. The ratio of intertrochanteric fractures to femoral neck fractures increased with age in women but remained stable in men. The authors also found fracture occurrence highest in white women, followed by white men, black women, and black men, respectively.

3.  Parker MJ, Myles JW, Anand JK *et al.* Cost–benefit analysis of hip fracture treatment. *J Bone Joint Surg* 1992;**74B**:261–4.

    A consecutive series of 1400 patients with femoral neck fractures. The benefit analysis of different types of treatment was assessed. Quality adjusted life-years were evaluated and higher scores were noted for non-displaced femoral neck fractures treated surgically than those treated conservatively. High morbidity and mortality was noted for displaced femoral neck fractures treated conservatively. The authors concluded that surgical treatment of non-displaced and displaced femoral neck fractures yielded better long-term results from a quality of life standpoint than conservative treatment.

9.  Baumgaertner MR, Curtin SL, Lindskog DM, Keggi JM. The value of the tip–apex distance in predicting failure of fixation of peritrochanteric fractures of the hip. *J Bone Joint Surg* 1995;**77A**:1058–64.

    A retrospective study of 198 fractures of the hip treated with the fixed-angle sliding hip-screw. The authors used a new measurement termed the tip–apex distance, which measured from the tip of the screw to the articular surface of the femoral head on both the A/P and lateral projection. The authors found that a tip–apex distance of >25 mm had a much higher incidence of screw cutout. Other factors associated with failure of fixation were increasing age of the patient, an unstable fracture, a poor reduction, and use of a high-angle side-plate.

10. Lu-Yao GL, Keller RB, Littenberg B *et al.* Outcomes after displaced fractures of the femoral neck: a meta-analysis of one hundred and six published reports. *J Bone Joint Surg* 1994;**76A**:15–25.

    A meta-analysis of studies, which revealed a non-union rate of 33% and an avascular necrosis rate of 16%. The rate of reoperation within two years was 20–36%. An increase in mortality was noted at 30 days after injury treated with a primary hemiarthroplasty but the absolute difference between mortality after hemiarthroplasty and open reduction and internal fixation was not significant.

11. Pagnani MJ, Lyden JP. Post-operative femoral fracture after intramedullary fixation with a gamma nail: a

case report and review of the literature. *J Trauma* 1994;**37**:133–7.

    A review of the use of the gamma nail for peri-trochanteric fracture of the femur revealed that this treatment has been successful but specific complications have arisen. The most devastating of these is the development of a femur fracture below the tip of the nail. This requires reoperation and fixation options should be considered at the time of original nail insertion.

13. Butler MS, Brumback RJ, Ellison TS *et al.* Interlocking intramedullary nailing for ipsilateral fractures of the femoral shaft and distal part of the femur. *J Bone Joint Surg* 1991;**73A**:1492–502.

    A review of 23 patients with ipsilateral femoral shaft and distal femur fractures. The supracondylar/ intercondylar portion was fixed first, followed by intramedullary nailing. Range of motion averaged greater than 115° at the knee, and all fractures united at an average of 19 weeks. Three patients, however, needed additional surgery because of missed coronal fractures of the femoral condyle, and the authors concluded that the presence of a coronal fracture of the femoral condyle is a relative contraindication to this procedure.

14. Lhowe DW, Hansen ST Jr. Immediate nailing of open fractures of the femoral shaft. *J Bone Joint Surg* 1988;**70A**:812–20.

    Reamed intramedullary nailing was performed immediately after irrigation and debridement of 67 open femoral shaft fractures. Complications included infection (two patients, one superficial and one deep), loss of fixation in four patients, and seroma in two patients. Late complications included malunion in three patients, leg length discrepancy in three patients, and sciatic nerve palsy in one patient. The authors concluded that immediate reamed nailing after irrigation and debridement for open femoral shaft fractures can be performed with an acceptable rate of complications.

15. Winquist RA, Hansen ST Jr, Clawson DK. Closed intramedullary nailing of femoral fractures: a report of five hundred and twenty cases. *J Bone Joint Surg* 1984;**66A**:529–39.

    The authors retrospectively reviewed 520 femur fractures in 500 patients. The rate of union after intramedullary nailing was 99.1%. Complications included infection (0.9%), shortening (2.0%), and malrotation (2.3%). Knee range of motion averaged 130°. Also discussed in the article is a classification system. The authors recommend static locking in all but the most simple fracture patterns.

17. Iannocone WM, Bennett FS, DeLong WG *et al.* Initial experience with the treatment of supracondylar femoral fractures using the supracondylar intramedullary nail: a preliminary report. *J Orthop Trauma* 1994;**8**:322–7.

A study of 41 fractures stabilized using the supra-condylar/intercondylar intramedullary nail. Thirty-two fractures healed uneventfully, but there were five delayed unions and four non-unions. The delayed unions required either revision of fixation or dynamization. The non-unions required revision of fixation and bone grafting. Thirty-five knees achieved at least 90° of flexion.

18. Ostermann PA, Neumann K, Ekkernkamp A *et al.* Long-term results of unicondylar fractures of the femur. *J Orthop Trauma* 1994;**8**:142–6.

    This study involved 24 fractures of the distal femur treated with open reduction and lag screw fixation. After a mean of 62 months' follow-up, 20 patients had an excellent result, three had a satisfactory result, and one had an unsatisfactory result. The patients who did not have an excellent result had accompanying injuries. The authors concluded that open reduction with internal fixation of these fractures provides excellent long-term results.

19. Zehntner MK, Marchesi DG, Burch H *et al.* Alignment of supracondylar/intercondylar fractures of the femur after internal fixation by AO/ASIF technique. *J Orthop Trauma* 1992;**6**:318–26.

    A study of 59 supracondylar/intercondylar fractures of the femur evaluated at a mean follow-up of 67 months. A comparison and skeletal alignment was made with the uninjured limb. Differences in varus/valgus of up to 5° were noted in 74%, ante/recurvatum in 78%, and rotation in 83% of patients. The authors concluded that restoration of the distal femoral angle is more difficult than restoration of saggital plane and rotation. A satisfactory functional result was compatible with angulation differences up to 5° in any plane.

20. Weber MJ, Janecki CJ, McLeod P *et al.* Efficacy of various forms of fixation of transverse fractures of the patella. *J Bone Joint Surg* 1980;**62A**:215–20.

    The classic article on the modified tension band. This paper compares the stability of four forms of patella fixation: cerclage, Magnusson technique, classic tension band, and modified tension band. The authors determined that the Magnusson and the modified tension band were better but almost equal and that the retinacular repair contributes to the stability of the fracture fixation.

21. Haas SB, Callaway H. Disruptions of the extensor mechanism. *Orthop Clin North Am* 1992;**23**:687–95.

    This study presents an extensive review both of quadriceps and patellar tendon disruptions. Different methods of repair are discussed. A description of each method is also included. In addition, some of the newer repairs are compared with the classic repairs.

22. Saltzman CL, Goulet JA, McClellan RT. Results of treatment of displaced patellar fractures by partial patellectomy. *J Bone Joint Surg* 1990;**72A**:1279–85.

    This is a retrospective review of 40 patients with displaced patellar fractures. Follow-up averaged 8.4 years. The average range of motion was 94% compared to the uninjured side. Average quadriceps strength measured 85% of the uninjured side. The series reported 78% good to excellent results and 22% fair and poor results. A transverse fracture pattern was associated with significantly better results than a comminuted fracture. Partial patellectomy can be a good alternative for specific indications.

23. Schenck RC Jr, Hunter RE, Ostrum RF, Perry CR. Knee dislocations. *Instr Course Lect Series – AAOS* 1999;**48**: 515–22.

    A comprehensive review of knee dislocations including specific sections on physical examination, radiographic evaluation, and treatment (including surgical management). Also includes sections on timing of repair of ligamentous disruptions and vascular injuries. Early anatomic repair/reconstruction is the recommended approach.

24. Bandyk D. Vascular injury associated with extremity trauma. *Clin Orthop* 1995;**318**:117–24.

    This article reviews common orthopaedic injuries associated with vascular injury and indications for arteriogram. Early amputation is related to prolonged ischemia, and soft tissue injury that precludes a viable, functional extremity. Traumatic knee dislocation is associated with a relatively high incidence (16–40%) of injury to the popliteal artery. The author also concludes that orthopedic stabilization should precede vascular repair when the bony skeleton is unstable, joints are dislocated, or subsequent bone manipulation may disrupt the arterial reconstruction.

25. Green NE, Allen BL. Vascular injuries associated with dislocation of the knee. *J Bone Joint Surg* 1977;**59A**: 236–9.

    A retrospective review of 245 knee dislocations. A 32% incidence of vascular injuries is reported. The study found vascular repair should be completed by six to eight hours from injury in order to give the best chance for limb survivability. An amputation rate of 86% was reported when vascular repair was not performed within the first eight hours after injury. The presence of a warm but pulseless foot mandates exploration of the popliteal artery.

26. Fanelli GC, Giannotti BF, Edson CJ. Arthroscopically assisted combined anterior and posterior cruciate ligament reconstruction. *Arthroscopy* 1996;**12**:5–14.

    This article reviews the results of 21 arthroscopically assisted posterior cruciate and posterior lateral corner reconstructions. The PCL was reconstructed with allograft Achilles tendon, or autograft patellar tendon. Posterior lateral instability was treated with long head of biceps femoris tendon tenodesis. A significant improvement in knee functional scores was noted following ligament reconstruction.

27. Meyers MH, Harvey JP Jr. Traumatic dislocation of the knee joint: a study of eighteen cases. *J Bone Joint Surg* 1971;**53A**:16–29.

A retrospective review of 15 patients with knee dislocation after low- and high-energy trauma. Three patients had destruction of the vascular supply to the leg (two after posterior dislocation, and one after anterior dislocation). Six patients had peroneal nerve injury and none recovered nerve function. Authors recommend immediate closed reduction, early repair of ligaments, careful monitoring of the vascular status of the limb (arteriogram if necessary), and immobilization in a plaster cast for six weeks followed by protected weight bearing for six weeks.

29. Honkonen SE. Indications for surgical treatment of tibial condyle fractures. *Clin Orthop* 1994;**302**:199–205.

A retrospective review of 131 tibial plateau fractures utilizing radiographic parameters related to clinical results. Medial tilt of the plateau was poorly tolerated but lateral tilt up to 5° had no detrimental effect. Articular step-off less than or equal to 3 mm was also associated with a good result. The authors conclude that tibial plateau fractures that meet the above criteria should be operatively fixed and any associated instability should also be addressed.

30. Guanche CA, Markman AW. Arthroscopic management of tibial plateau fractures. *Arthroscopy* 1993;**9**:467–71.

This study reports the initial experience of arthroscopic treatment of tibial plateau fractures. Five patients with a tibial plateau fracture (Schatzker type I (2), II (1), III (2)) were included. No complications were reported in the series, and all fractures united uneventfully. The authors reported the advantages of better joint visualization, less dissection, and thorough irrigation of the joint. Arthroscopic assisted fixation of tibial plateau fractures is a viable alternative for a select subgroup of these injuries.

31. Moore TM, Patzakis MJ, Harvey JP. Tibial plateau fractures: definition, demographics, treatment rationale, and long-term results of closed traction management or operative reduction. *J Orthop Trauma* 1987;**1**: 97–119.

A retrospective review of 10 years' experience with 988 fractures of the tibial plateau. Forty-four percent of these fractures were treated surgically and 56% were treated by traction and early motion. The authors concluded that anatomic reduction and early motion were major factors in a successful outcome. The surgical complication rate was 19%, with the most common complication being infection. The complication rate of traction was 8%.

32. Young MJ, Barrack RL. Complications of internal fixation of tibial plateau fractures. *Orthop Rev* 1994;**23**:149–54.

A retrospective review of all cases of tibial plateau fractures treated by open reduction and internal fixation over a three-year period. A total of 45 patients

were included. The goals of early internal fixation followed by early motion were obtained in all patients. A very high incidence of infection and wound complications was seen following double plating for severe, bicondylar fractures. The authors felt that severe, comminuted fractures of the tibial plateau may be better treated with non-operative treatment or limited internal fixation.

33. Sarmiento A, Gersten LM, Sobol PA *et al.* Tibial shaft fractures treated with functional braces: experience with 780 fractures. *J Bone Joint Surg* 1989;**71B**:602–9.

A retrospective review of 7,809 fractures of the tibial shaft treated with case immobilization followed by conversion to a functional brace. Six per cent of patients required early conversion to operative stabilization due to failure of closed treatment. The non-union rate was 2.5%. The authors found an average healing time for isolated tibial shaft fractures 17.4 weeks and the average healing time for tibial and fibular fractures was 21.5 weeks. Sixty per cent of the patients healed with shortening averaging 7.1 mm. Twenty-five per cent of the patients healed with more than 5° of varus. Anterior and posterior angulation also occurred in approximately 20–30% of cases. The authors do not comment on malrotation.

34. Riemer BL, DiChristina DG, Cooper A *et al.* Non-reamed nailing of tibial diaphyseal fractures in blunt polytrauma patients. *J Orthop Trauma* 1995;**9**:66–75.

This study reviews the efficacy of non-reamed nailing of tibial shaft fractures. Average time to union was 32 weeks with 39% of patients needing a second procedure to complete union. The reoperation rate was higher for grade III open injuries than for grades I or II open injuries. The rate of reoperation was also higher for more comminuted or segmental fractures. The authors recommend non-reamed nailing for grade III open fractures but not for grade I or II fractures where reamed nailing is the treatment of choice.

35. Whittle AP, Russell TA, Taylor JC *et al.* Treatment of open fractures of the tibial shaft with the use of interlocking nailing without reaming. *J Bone Joint Surg* 1992;**74A**:1162–71.

This technique article presents a rationale for the use of small diameter intramedullary nails without reaming. The clinical results document no increase in infection rate. In addition, the malunion rates were much lower in comparison to the historical treatment of external fusion.

36. Wu CC, Shih CH. Complicated open fractures of the distal tibia treated by secondary interlocking nailing. *J Trauma* 1993;**34**:792–6.

The authors of this article combine the historical treatment of open tibial shaft fractures using external fixation with conversion to intramedullary nailing early in the course of treatment. The results of this study were encouraging in that there was no significant increase in the infection rate and the incidence of pin-tract infection was decreased due to the limited time in an external fixator.

38. Brumback RJ, McGarvey WC. Fractures of the tibial plafond: the pilon fracture. Evolving treatment concepts. *Orthop Clin North Am* 1995;**26**:273–85.

This article reviews the evolving changes in the treatment of the pilon fracture. It includes a discussion of the various classification systems and comparison of the results of open reduction with internal fixation with external fixation and limited internal fixation.

39. Helfet DL, Koval K, Pappas J et al. Intraarticular "pilon" fracture of the tibia. *Clin Orthop* 1994;**298**: 221–8.

A retrospective review of the treatment of 34 high-energy pilon fractures. Of the fractures in the study, 28 were treated with open reduction with internal fixation and the remaining six were treated with external fixation with limited internal fixation. Type II fractures had 65% good results and type III fractures had 50% good results. The final score was correlated to the accuracy of the articular reconstruction. The authors concluded that open reduction with internal fixation was appropriate for most of these injuries.

40. Tornetta P III, Weiner L, Bergmen M et al. Pilon fractures: treatment with combined internal and external fixation. *J Orthop Trauma* 1993;**7**:489–96.

A retrospective review of the results of external fixation with minimal internal fixation for the treatment of pilon fractures. Seventeen fractures are presented with 69% good results for type III injuries. Only one deep infection occurred in the study.

43. Bray TJ, Endicott M, Capra SE. Treatment of open ankle fractures: immediate internal fixation versus closed immobilization and delayed fixation. *Clin Orthop* 1989;**240**:47–52.

A retrospective review of 31 patients with open ankle fractures followed for an average of 11 years. Half of the patients were managed with closed reduction and delayed fixation and the other half with standard immediate open reduction internal fixation after irrigation and debridement. One patient from each group had an infection. Functional scores were the same for each group. Immediate open reduction internal fixation had faster recovery and no higher risk of infection than the conservatively treated group.

44. Szyszkowitz R, Reschauer R, Seggl W. Eighty-five talus fractures treated by ORIF with five to eight years of follow-up study of 69 patients. *Clin Orthop* 1985;**199**: 97–107.

A retrospective study of the results of surgical treatment of 69 displaced talus fractures. A significant number of patients were found radiographically to have evidence of ankle and subtalar arthrosis. However, the clinical results were much more encouraging,

with 82% of patients reporting good or excellent results. The authors conclude that open reduction with internal fixation offers significantly better results for displaced fractures than closed treatment.

45. Sanders R, Fortin P, Dipasquale T et al. Operative treatment in 120 displaced intraarticular calcaneal fractures: results using a prognostic computed tomography scan classification. *Clin Orthop* 1993;**290**:87–95.

A retrospective review of the results of 120 intraarticular fractures of the calcaneus. The article also presents an excellent classification system for calcaneal fractures based on CT findings. The classification system is based on the number of fragments of the posterior facet of the calcaneus. Both the clinical results and the ability to achieve an anatomic reduction decrease as the number of fragments increase. Severely comminuted fractures may be candidates for primary subtalar fusion. The authors also identified a significant learning curve in the treatment of these fractures.

46. Sangeorzan BJ, Benirschke SK, Mosca V et al. Displaced intra-articular fractures of the tarsal navicular. *J Bone Joint Surg* 1989;**71A**:1504–10.

A retrospective review of the surgical treatment of 21 fractures of the tarsal navicular. Three fracture types were identified: coronal, oblique in the dorsolateral to plantar–medial plane, and comminuted. The average follow-up was 44 months. A good result was achieved in 14 patients, a fair result in four, and a poor result in one. The fracture type correlated with the clinical outcome.

47. Arntz CT, Veith RG, Hansen ST Jr. Fractures and fracture-dislocations of the tarsometatarsal joints. *J Bone Joint Surg* 1988;**70A**:173–81.

A retrospective review of the treatment of 41 fracture-dislocations of the tarsometatarsal joints. The treatment was anatomic reduction with temporary internal fixation with AO screws. Follow-up averaged 3.4 years. The quality of reduction and the severity of injury were correlated with the results at final follow-up. Grade II or III open injuries had the worst results. Screws were removed at an average of 16 weeks.

48. Josefsson PO, Karlsson M, Redlund-Johnell I et al. Jones fracture: surgical versus nonsurgical treatment. *Clin Orthop* 1994;**299**:252–5.

A retrospective review of 63 patients with a fracture of the proximal diaphysis of the fifth metatarsal (Jones fracture) evaluated five years after injury. Twenty-seven of the fractures were acute and 38 were chronic or stress fractures. Almost 25% of non-surgically treated fractures required late surgery due to delayed union or refracture. Late surgery was required for 12% of acute fractures and 50% of chronic fractures. Primary surgical treatment with an intramedullary screw is recommended for higher demand patients or those with delayed union.

**Proximal femur injury**

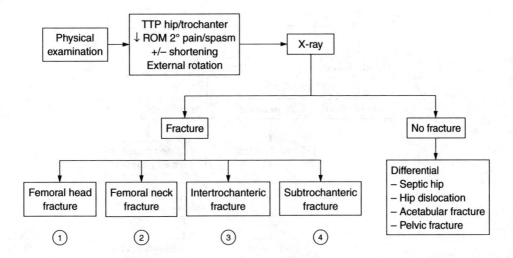

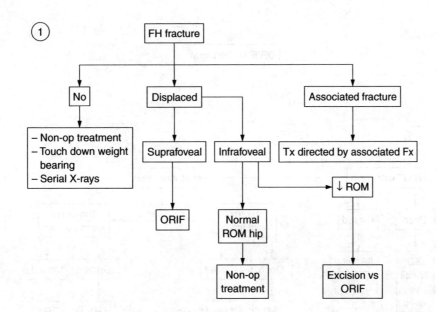

**Proximal femur injury (continued)**

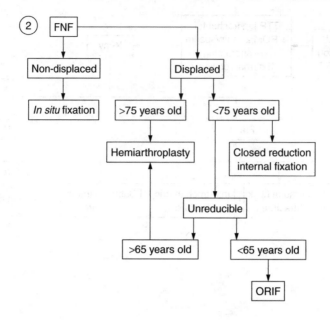

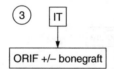

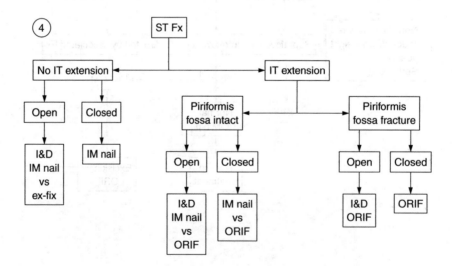

## Femoral shaft fracture

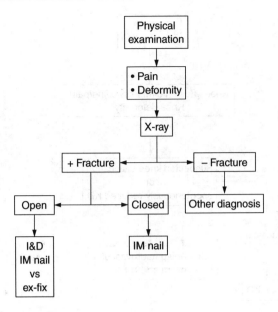

## Distal femur fractures

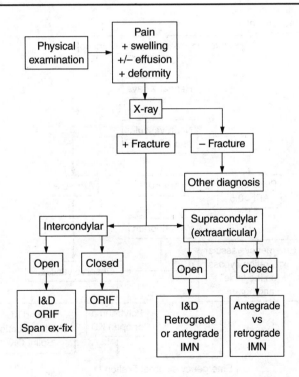

**Knee dislocation**

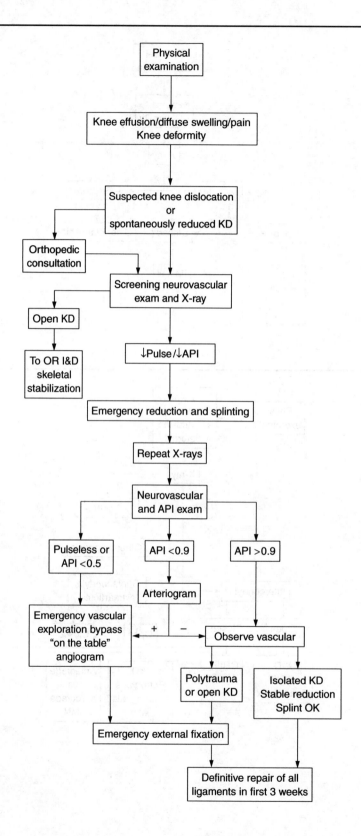

**Proximal tibia fracture**

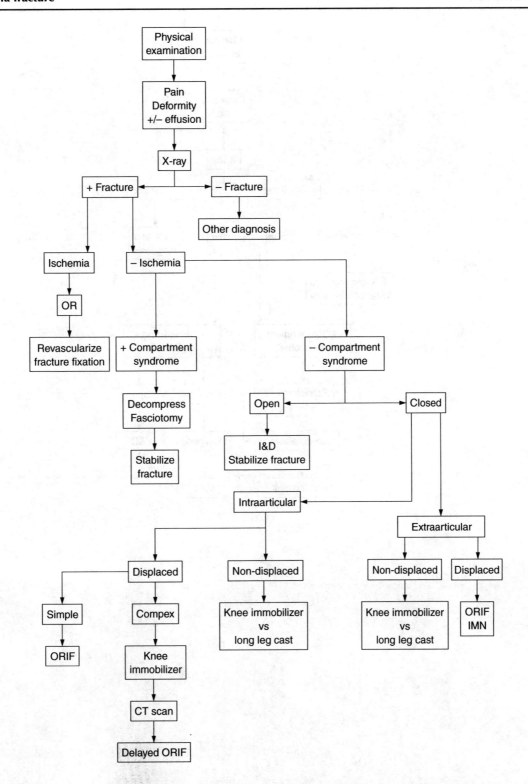

**Tibial shaft fracture**

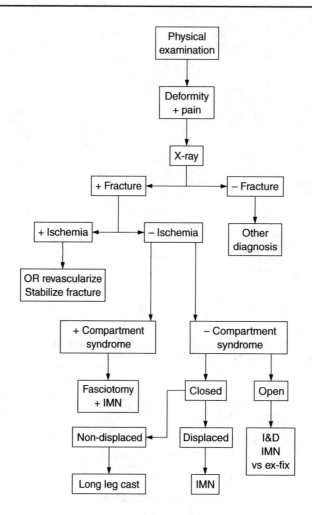

**Tibial plafond fracture**

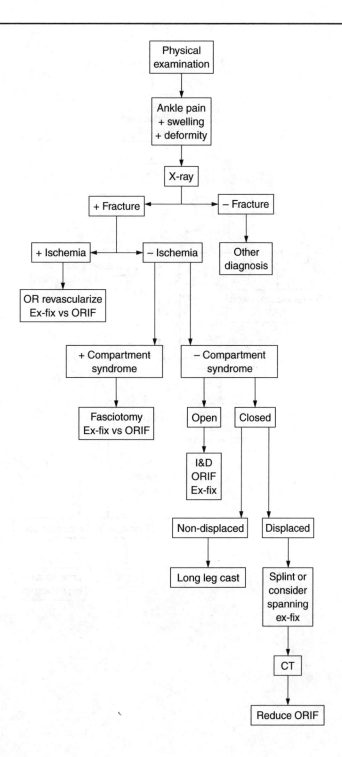

**Ankle fracture**

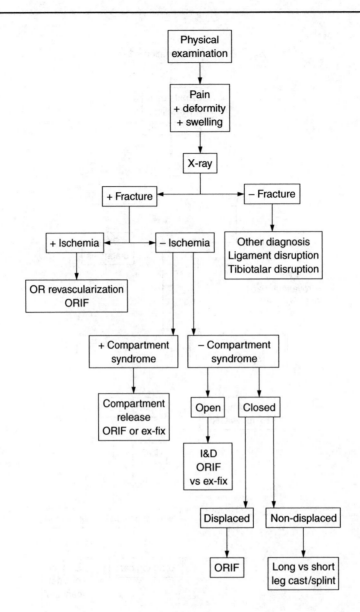

**Hindfoot fracture**

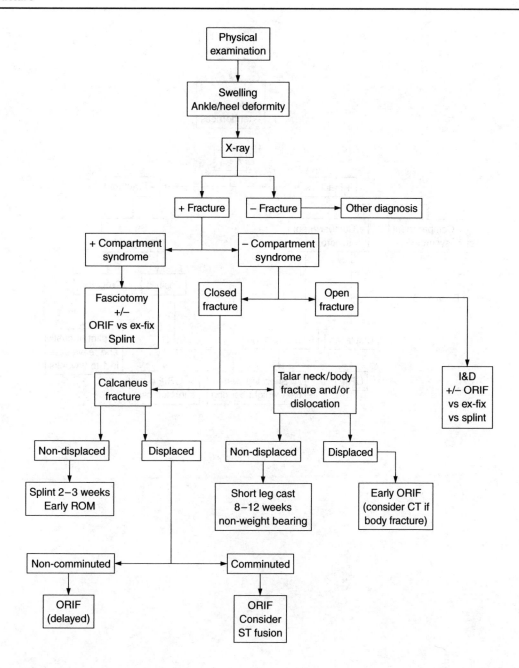

**Midfoot fracture**

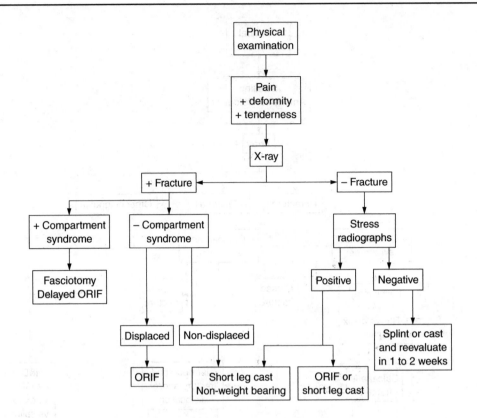

## Forefoot fracture

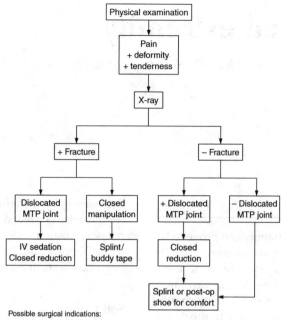

Possible surgical indications:
• open phalangeal fracture/MTP dislocation
• intraarticular fracture of great toe proximal phalynx
• irreducible dislocation of great toe MTP joint.

## Exterior mechanism injury

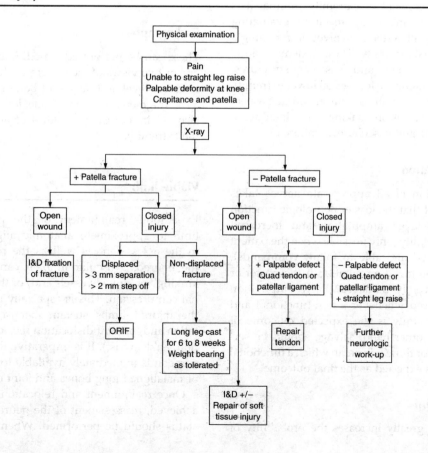

# 18 Mangled extremity

*Vicente H Gracias, Alvin Ong, Patrick M Reilly*

## Physical examination

Severe traumatic injury to the extremity can prove to be a complex problem in the care of acutely injured patients. Surgeons are faced with the critical decision of amputation versus limb salvage. An unwarranted attempt at salvage has its own associated morbidity and mortality. When evaluating a severely traumatized extremity, one must make decisions in the context of other associated injuries.

Judgment regarding limb salvage is based upon a surgeon's experience with treating multiple systemic injuries. In the assessment of extremity trauma, it is best to have an organized approach in evaluating injury sustained by all systems involved in retaining a viable and functional extremity. These systems include integument, nerve, bone, and vascular structures. Most of the current literature focuses on lower extremity trauma and this chapter will concentrate on this aspect of trauma surgical decision making. This includes a complete neurologic and vascular evaluation.

## Neurologic evaluation

Thorough evaluation of all appropriate nerves takes place. Data suggest that the loss of neurologic function correlates with delayed amputation and increased morbidity and mortality (only possible when the patient is alert and oriented and able to follow commands). Some authors recommend amputation if the posterior tibial nerve is severely damaged. Early amputation should be considered whenever a non-functional and insensate foot/extremity is the expected outcome of the injury. On the other hand, salvage should be seriously considered for those injuries in which a functional and sensate limb is expected as the final outcome.[1]

## Vascular evaluation

Vascular integrity greatly increases the probability of limb salvage. An attempt at early diagnosis of vascular compromise is needed to correlate appropriate surgical revascularization attempts. Pulses, assessments of cap refill, Doppler, and ankle brachial index (ABI) are all-important tests in assessing vascular integrity.[2]

## Soft tissue

A quick but thorough survey of the degree of contamination, muscle injury, size of skin loss, amount of devitalized tissue, and compartment pressures should be performed.

## Radiographs

These can be performed expeditiously. If time allows, one or two views of the extremity should be performed to assess level and degree of bony injury, fracture pattern, fragmentation, and bone loss. Radiographs can also aid in assessing the level of energy sustained by the extremity.

## Viable limb

Expeditious realignment of the mangled/deformed limb to approximate anatomic alignment often aids in the assessment as well as the revascularization of the injured, avascular limb. It can help in the "unkinking" of kinked vessels and/or the removal of external compression. This is especially true in cases where the injured limbs sustain extensive bony fragmentation and/or joint dislocation (i.e. knee, elbow dislocation, ankle, wrist). It is imperative that the orthopaedic surgeon is immediately available to assist in reduction of malaligned long bones and joint dislocation.

Once realignment and relocation of joints has been achieved, reassessment of the neurologic and vascular status should be performed. When this is completed, temporary stabilization with splints, packing, and redressing of wounds should be performed to prevent further soft tissue, nervous or vascular injury and contamination of wounds, respectively (it is important that wounds be examined by a limited number of qualified individuals to prevent further contamination and soft tissue injury).

Limbs with no vascular supply, long ischemia time (greater than six hours warm ischemia) and with severe neurologic and bony injury should be quickly triaged to the OR where a definitive decision on limb salvage versus amputation can be better made. All patients with type III-C fracture and complete nerve disruption of the sciatic or tibial nerve should have high consideration for amputation. No studies have shown benefit in attempted limb salvage in this group of patients compared to early amputation in the presence of significant nerve disruption. Obviously non-viable extremities require completion of amputation in the OR. Delay in amputation has been shown to result in a statistically significant increase in sepsis, disability, number of surgical procedures, mortality, and hospital costs. However, it is of paramount importance that each patient and injury should be treated on an individual case-by-case basis.[3-5]

The decision of limb salvage versus immediate amputation of any mangled extremity should be made with a team approach. Amputation should only be performed when the trauma, vascular, and orthopaedic surgeons involved all agree on the decision to amputate. The decision to amputate should never be made on the sole basis of a protocol or algorithm.[6]

## Vascular injury

Vascular compromise must be corrected as quickly as possible. Ischemia time greater than six hours has been correlated with irreversible nerve injury and loss of function. A limb with ABI < 0.9 or absent pulses must have the vascular system examined. If the patient is stable and ischemia time allows, a formal angiogram to delineate arterial injury is always useful prior to surgical exploration. If the patient is unstable or has hard signs of arterial injury such as obvious arterial bleeding or expanding hematoma, an arteriogram can be obtained in the OR. If an arterial injury is present and the patient has multiple associated injuries or is unstable, one should consider rapid vascular shunting with external fixation of bony injury. Resuscitation should then continue, with planned formal revascularization when the patient's status improves.[7,8]

## Compartment syndrome

Blunt extremity trauma without vascular injury can still be a cause of significant soft tissue damage and edema leading to compartment syndrome. In the face of associated vascular compromise, the risk of compartment syndrome escalates and empiric fasciotomy needs to be considered, especially if the ischemia time is greater than 4–6 hours. Postoperative vigilance and monitoring for compartment syndrome must still be maintained. The measurement of compartment pressures should always be performed in any patient in whom the possibility of compartment syndrome exists.

## Bony stabilization

Patient condition determines if bony stabilization should precede vascular repair. The use of temporary vascular shunts can reinstitute blood flow while limbs are brought out to length. This should be coordinated between the vascular and orthopaedic surgery teams. Bony stabilization can be intramedullary rod fixation, plate fixation, pinning or external fixation. The trauma service ultimately decides the timing and coordination of procedures (i.e. ex fix then vascular repair or temporary stent → bony stabilization then formal vascular repair or simultaneous procedure).[7]

## Limb salvage

Many attempts at objectifying the criteria for limb salvage versus amputation have been reported. Although all the data should be reviewed and studied, there is no substitute for sound clinical judgment based on experience. No one study or report has conclusively defined a guaranteed predictor for limb salvage. Scoring systems can serve as an adjunct to surgical judgment when treating a patient with severe extremity trauma. Scoring systems reported in the literature include the Predictive Salvage Index, the Mangled Extremity Severity Score (MESS), the Limb Salvage Index, and the NISSSA Scoring Index. These should only be used by the treating physician as a guideline. All eventual decisions are predominantly based on patient condition and the findings during operative exploration. Each patient should be evaluated on an individual basis.[9-12]

The ultimate decision to salvage the limb or to amputate depends not only on the injuries at hand but also the skills of the managing team. The long-term goal of limb salvage is a *functional* and not just a viable limb.

## Delayed amputation

Delayed amputation can often prove to be a difficult decision when so much effort has been expended on limb salvage. One must always bear in mind that a non-viable limb can still serve as an impetus for continued inflammatory response. ARDS and abdominal compartment syndrome have both been attributed to delayed complications associated with inappropriate attempts at limb salvage. Postoperative monitoring of fluid sequestration and hemodynamic parameters may aid in deciding whether delayed amputation should be considered in a patient who deteriorates or does not show improved hemodynamics within 24 hours of a limb salvage attempt.[2]

## Class II references

9.  Chi-Hun L, Fu-Chan W, Levin S *et al.* The functional outcome of lower-extremity fractures with vascular injury. *J Trauma* 1997;**43**(3):480–5.

    Prospective, non-randomized study. Limb salvage attempted for all lower extremity injuries with Gustilo IIIC fractures and MESS score ≤10. Excluded were below-ankle injuries and those patients treated with immediate amputation. Thirty-four patients with a total of 36 lower extremity revascularization attempts were reported. Overall, 25% secondary amputations and a 75% limb salvage rate were reported. The authors recommend that the threshold for immediate amputation be set at ≤9.

10. Johansen K, Daines M, Howey T *et al.* Objective criteria accurately predict amputation following lower extremity trauma. *J Trauma* 1990;**30**(5):568–73.

    MESS (Mangled Extremity Severity Score) is a simple rating scale for lower extremity trauma. Retrospective analysis of severe lower extremity injuries in 25 trauma victims demonstrated a significant difference between MESS values for 17 limbs ultimately salvaged and nine requiring amputation (P < 0.01). A prospective trial is included demonstrating a significant difference between MESS values in 14 salvaged and 12 doomed limbs (P < 0.01). In both the retrospective survey and prospective trial, a MESS value ≥7 predicted amputation with 100% accuracy.

## Class III references

1.  Alexander J, Piotrowski J, Graham D *et al.* Outcome of complex vascular and orthopaedic injuries of the lower extremity. *Am J Surg* 1991;**162**:111–16.

    Retrospective review of 32 patients undergoing limb salvage attempts; 56% showed persistent functional or neurologic deficit. The authors favor an aggressive approach to limb salvage attempts for type IIIC injuries. However, they recommend early amputation in the presence of significant nerve disruption. Infection was the most significant factor associated with amputation (P < 0.005) and was not avoided by the use of antibiotics.

2.  Roessler M, Wisner D, Holcroft W. The mangled extremity. When to amputate? *Arch Surg* 1991;**26**:1243–9.

    Retrospective review of 80 patients. The circulation as determined by the presence or absence of a palpable or Doppler detected pulse proved critical for successful salvage. Of six patients with no distal pulse in whom salvage was attempted and in whom 24-hour fluid balance after salvage was greater than 3 liters, five eventually required amputation.

3.  Russell W, Sailores D, Whittle T *et al.* Limb salvage versus traumatic amputation. *Ann Surg* 1991;**213**(5):473–81.

    Retrospective review of 67 patients, 70 limbs having sustained lower extremity arterial injury. Seventy-three per cent were salvaged, 27% had primary or secondary amputation (also functional loss). All patients with type IIIC fracture and amputation had complete nerve disruption of sciatic or tibial nerve (P < 0.001) None of the patients with a type IIIC in the limb salvage group had an associated nerve injury. Limb salvage was related to warm ischemia time and quantitative degree of arterial, bone, skin, and venous injury. A limb salvage index is proposed to aid in objectifying criteria for limb salvage decisions.

4.  McNamara MG, Heckman JD, Corley FG. Severe open fractures of the lower extremity: a retrospective evaluation of the Mangled Extremity Severity Score (MESS). *J Orthop Trauma* 1994;**8**(6):81–7.

    Retrospective review of 24 patients with Gustilo type IIIB and IIIC open tibia fractures. A MESS value of ≥7 was found to have a positive predictive value of 100% for amputation. Modification of nerve injury and soft tissue and skeletal injury grading was found to be more accurate while the NISSSA scoring system was more sensitive (81.8% versus 63.6%) and more specific (92.3% versus 69.2%).

5.  Bondurant FL, Cotler HB, Buckle R *et al.* The medical and economic impact of severely injured lower extremities. *J Trauma* 1988;**28**(8):1270–3.

    Retrospective review of 43 patients with major lower extremity trauma, who underwent primary or delayed amputation. Fourteen patients had primary amputation. Average hospital stay was 22.3 days with an average cost of $28 964. Twenty-nine patients had delayed amputation with an average hospitalization time of 53.4 days at an average cost of $53 462. Six patients with delayed amputation developed sepsis and died compared to none in the primary amputation group. Delay in amputation resulted in a statistically significant increase in sepsis and death, disability, number of surgical procedures, and hospital costs.

6. Bonanni F, Rhodes M, Lucke J. The futility of predictive scoring of mangled lower extremities. *J Trauma* 1993;**34**(1):99–104.

   Retrospective reviews of 58 patients with lower limb salvage attempts. Accuracy of MESI, MESS, PSI, and LSI was examined. Crossvalidation sensitivity and specificity analysis revealed no predictive utility in any of the four indices. Most failed limb salvage attempts could be identified early in the hospital course. Further efforts in the refinement of decision making concerning limb salvage are recommended.

7. Starr A, Hunt J, Rienhart C. Treatment of femur fractures with associated vascular injury. *J Trauma* 1996;**40**(1):17–21.

   Retrospective analysis of 26 patients with femoral fractures and vascular injury. Internal fixation was used safely to stabilize femoral fractures. Poor outcome was associated with a MESS score ≥6. Use of vascular shunt is discussed for prolonged ischemia time.

8. Lazarides MK, Arvanitis DP, Kopadis GC *et al*. Popliteal artery and trifurcation injuries: is it possible to predict the outcome? *Eur J Vasc Surg* 1994;**8**(2):226–30.

   Retrospective review of 18 patients with popliteal artery and/or trifurcation injuries. Amputation rate was 28%. The trifurcation group had an amputation rate of 71%. The MESI index had a higher overall predictive value of 83%. No scoring system was found to be specific enough to permit primary amputation.

11. Gregory R, Randolph G, Peclet M *et al*. The mangled extremity syndrome (MES): a severity grading system for multisystem injury of the extremity. *J Trauma* 1985;**25**(12):1147–50.

    Retrospective review of 17 trauma patients with application of a scoring system (MESI) to predict appropriate surgical management. Data suggest that a MESI score of 20 is the dividing line below which functional limb salvage can be expected and above which salvage is improbable.

12. Howe HR, Poole GV, Hansen KJ *et al*. Salvage of lower extremity following combined orthopaedic and vascular trauma. A predictive salvage index. *Am Surg* 1987;**53**(4):205–8.

    Retrospective review of 21 patients with major orthopaedic and vascular trauma to the lower extremity. Limb survival was related to the interval from injury to time of arrival in the operating room, the level of arterial injury, and the quantitative degree of muscle, bone, and skin injury. A predictive salvage index (PSI) was developed to objectify criteria. All 12 patients in the limb salvage group had PSI scores less than 8, whereas seven of nine patients in the amputated group scored 8 or greater. The study reports sensitivity for predicting amputation of 78% and specificity of 100%.

**Mangled extremity**

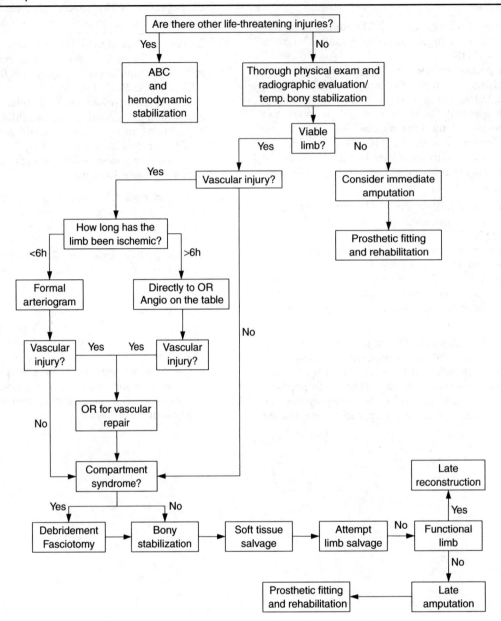

# 19 Hand injuries

*Madhav A Karunakar, James F Kellam*

## Injuries requiring urgent treatment

### History and physical examination

A complete history and physical exam should be performed. As always, life-threatening injuries are given first priority as per the ATLS protocol. The patient's age, occupation, and hand dominance may affect treatment. The mechanism of injury (laceration versus crush) will often determine the extent of tissue damage. For an open injury, the time between injury and treatment and the degree of contamination may affect operative management.

### Injuries requiring early treatment

Injuries requiring early treatment include bite wounds, flexor tendon lacerations, nerve injuries, and fracture dislocations. Less severe injuries include fingertip injuries and extensor tendons.

The management of hand compartment syndrome, a mangled hand or hand amputations is best left to an experienced hand surgeon.

### Mangled hand

Farm or industrial injuries involving hydraulic equipment, routers, milling machines or power tools are frequently heavily contaminated and often result in significant soft tissue and bone injuries. Uncontrolled hemorrhage from lacerated arterial bleeders may occur. Direct pressure is the simplest method of controlling hemorrhage. A semicompressible sterile dressing with an elastic bandage usually suffices. If heavy bleeding occurs despite direct pressure, a pneumatic arm tourniquet should be applied. If a pneumatic arm tourniquet is not available, a blood pressure cuff wrapped with cast padding to prevent unwrapping may be applied. A target pressure of 100–150 mmHg above systolic blood pressure should be maintained. An arm tourniquet will become painful after 30 minutes and should be released for five minutes every 30 minutes.[1]

The emergency management of a mangled extremity should involve copious irrigation and the application of a povidone-iodine soaked bandage. Tetanus status should be updated and prophylactic antibiotics given if indicated. A radiograph should be obtained to assist in the preoperative plan. Repeated removal of the dressings should be avoided.[2]

The role of prophylactic antibiotics in the treatment of a mangled hand is unclear. A first-generation cephalosporin will provide coverage for Gram-positive bacteria that are frequently encountered in home or factory injuries. An aminoglycoside and penicillin may be added to cover Gram-negative organisms and clostridial species in farm injuries.[3,4] The best treatment of these injuries is meticulous surgical debridement with delayed reconstruction.[3]

## Compartment syndrome

A compartment syndrome of the hand may be difficult to diagnose. A high clinical suspicion should be present if a crush injury has occurred. Often the only sign that will be present is a disproportionate amount of swelling. The pathognomic sign of compartment syndrome is pain intensified by passive stretch of involved muscles. Nerve compression may cause intense pain, paresthesias, and ultimately anesthesia. The only objective method of diagnosing a compartment syndrome is intracompartmental pressure measurements of the intrinsic compartments. The exact value of the critical pressure requiring fasciotomy is controversial. There are two methods used in the determination of this value: an absolute value >30–45 mmHg or a derived value in which the difference between the diastolic blood pressure and measured compartment pressure is <30 mmHg.[1,5] Either is considered an indication for emergent fasciotomy.

## Indications for replantation

Indications for replantation include injury to multiple digits, thumb amputation, amputation in children, and clean amputation at hand. Relative contraindications for replantation include crush or avulsion injury, single digit amputation in adults, and significant history of smoking.[6,7] Absolute contraindications include severe associated medical problems or injuries and severe multilevel injury of amputated part.[1,4]

## Emergency management

The emergency management of the amputated digit includes the following steps. A radiograph of both the injured limb and amputated part should be taken to assess bony anatomy. The wound is cleaned, irrigated with sterile normal saline, and dressed with a non-adherent gauze. An IV should be inserted for patient hydration and medications. Prophylactic antibiotics (usually a cephalosporin) and tetanus prophylaxis should be given. Clear instructions regarding NPO status for the operating room should be given to the patient. The amputated part should be cleaned, irrigated with lactated Ringer's, and then wrapped in saline-moistened gauze and placed in a sterile container. This sterile, water-tight container is placed in a large pan containing ice water. Ice should never contact the amputated part.[1]

## Fasciotomy

There are 10 compartments in the hand which can be released by four separate incisions. The interosseous muscles and adductor compartment can be released through two longitudinal incisions on the dorsum of the hand over the second and fourth metacarpals. The thenar and hypothenar compartments are opened by longitudinal incisions along the radial side of the first metacarpal and the ulnar side of the fifth metacarpal.[1]

## Replantation

Any patient who meets the criteria for replantation should be referred to a microvascular specialist as soon as possible. In many hospitals both plastic surgeons and orthopaedic surgeons with specialized certification in hand surgery will perform microvascular repairs.

## Injuries requiring early treatment

### History and physical examination

The history should include the patient's age, occupation, hand dominance, and mechanism of injury. A complete physical exam assessing tendon function, joint mobility, and range of motion should be performed. Motor strength should be tested and graded. Sensibility can be evaluated with two-point and light touch discrimination. The vascular status is assessed with color, warmth, and capillary refill. Finally, bone instability or deformity indicating fracture or dislocation is evaluated.

Major injuries include amputation of digits, a mangled hand, and compartment syndrome of the hand (see Algorithm 1).

Injuries requiring early treatment include bite wounds, flexor tendon lacerations, nerve injuries, and fractures and dislocations.

An anteroposterior and lateral radiograph of the hand should be performed to locate foreign bodies and detect fractures.

## Closed injury

Most closed hand injuries can be splinted and referred to a hand specialist. Dislocations should be reduced as soon as possible. Intraarticular fractures should be referred to a hand surgeon for treatment.

### Splinting

The hand should be splinted in the intrinsic plus or safe position. The wrist should be placed in 35° of extension. This can be estimated by aligning the long axis of the thumb with the forearm. The metacarpal phalangeal joints should be flexed in an increasing cascade from 45° to 70° starting from the index to the small finger. The interphalangeal joints should be placed in 10–15° flexion. The thumb is gently abducted away from the palm and the MCP and IP joints are placed in neutral.[1]

## Fingertip injuries

Fingertip injuries are defined as those distal to the insertion of the flexor and extensor tendons. For injuries with soft tissue loss only (no exposed bone), open treatment with healing by secondary intention is preferred. When bone is exposed, a local flap, regional flap or shortening with primary closure is preferred. The indications for each treatment are beyond the scope of this chapter.[8–11]

## Open injury

A thorough neurologic exam should be performed first. A digital block with 1% lidocaine or a wrist block should be performed. Lidocaine with epinephrine should not be used as it may result in vasospasm of the small vessels of the hand. The wound should be cleaned thoroughly. Open injuries should be irrigated with copious quantities of water and a povidone-iodine soaked dressing with elastic gauze applied. The hand should be splinted in the "safe position". Tetanus prophylaxis should be updated. If the wound is grossly contaminated, a first-generation cephalosporin or penicillinase-resistant penicillin should be given.

### Nerve injury

A primary perineural fascicular repair is possible after sharp wounds. A delay in treatment may require grafting. Early referral to a hand specialist is recommended.

### Bone injury

Open fractures should be copiously irrigated. The wounds can usually be closed primarily if early treatment is received. The indications for operative treatment are beyond the scope of this chapter.[12–16] These patients should be referred to either a plastic surgeon or orthopaedic surgeon with specialty training in hand surgery.

### Skin wound

The skin is closed with interrupted 4-0 or 5-0 monofilament in clean wounds treated less than six hours after injury. Grossly contaminated wounds may require secondary closure.[17] Secondary closure may be performed in 24–48 hours after a thorough debridement is performed. Human and animal bite wounds should never be closed primarily due to a high predisposition for infection. Antibiotic prophylaxis with a first-generation cephalosporin will effectively cover the Gram-positive organisms seen with most lacerations.

### Tendon lacerations

Tendon lacerations should be classified as either flexor or extensor. The treatment of tendon injuries is based on zones.

There are five flexor tendon zones: zone I distal to the FDS insertion; zone II metacarpal neck (fibrosseous tunnel) to FDS; zone III transverse carpal ligament to fibrosseous tunnel; zone IV transverse carpal ligament (TCL); zone V musculotendinous junction to TCL. All flexor tendons should be repaired in the operating room.[18,19]

There are five extensor tendon zones: zone I central slip insertion distal; zone II metacarpal neck to central slip; zone III extensor retinaculum to metacarpal neck; zone IV extensor retinaculum; zone V proximal to extensor retinaculum. Most extensor tendon lacerations can be safely repaired in the emergency department. In lacerations distal to the metacarpal neck, tendon retraction is usually not a problem and the tendon ends can be recovered with minimal extension of the wounds. For proximal lacerations, tendon retraction may occur, making recovery of the tendon more difficult. A 4-0 mersilene or ethibond figure of eight suture is usually sufficient for repair. The repaired tendon should be splinted in extension. Lacerations of palmaris longus do not need to be repaired.[20,21]

### Bite injury

Human bites frequently involve the organism *Eikenella corrodens*. It is sometimes difficult to determine joint penetration for fight bites. Animal bites frequently involve *Pasteurella multocida*. Mixed aerobic and anaerobic infections are common. Absolute indications for admission should include a wound >24 hours old, joint penetration, abscess, cellulitis or lymphangitis. A combination $\beta$-lactam antibiotic plus a $\beta$-lactam inhibitor are recommended.[22–24]

### Class II References

3. Fitzgerald RH Jr, Cooney WP III, Washington JA II, Van Scoy RE, Linscheid RL, Dobyns JH. Bacterial colonization of mutilating hand injuries and its treatment. *J Hand Surg* 1977;**2**:85–9.

   Meticulous surgical debridement is the best treatment of mutilating hand injuries in farm implement injuries. Antimicrobial prophylaxis with a semisynthetic penicillinase-resistant agent may be of more value in home and industrial-related injuries.

5. Matsen FA III, Winquist RA, Krugmire RB Jr. Diagnosis and management of compartmental syndrome. *J Bone Joint Surg* 1980;**62**:286–91.

   Reviews the diagnosis of compartment syndrome and the authors' preferred method of measuring compartment pressures with the infusion technique. The indications and techniques for surgical decompression are presented.

6. Urbaniak JR, Evans JP, Bright DS. Microvascular management of ring avulsion injuries. *J Hand Surg* 1981;**6**:25–30.

   Retrospective review of 24 ring avulsion injuries. Revascularization was successful with good sensibility and useful motion in nine patients. Five of seven completely amputated or avulsed digits survived but had limited motion. The recommendation for an avulsed amputated finger is generally revision amputation.

7. Urbaniak JR, Roth JH, Nunley JA, Goldner RD, Koman LA. The results of replantation after amputation of a single finger. *J Bone Joint Surg* 1985;**67**:611–19.

Retrospective review of 59 patients who underwent replantation of a single digit. Indications for single digit replantation are presented. Survival was found to be affected by the age of the patient, the number of vessels that were anastomosed, and the experience of the surgeon. Replantation distal to the flexor digitorum superficialis tendon provided a better functional result than more proximal replantation.

8. Chow SP, Ho E. Open treatment of fingertip injuries in adults. *J Hand Surg* 1982;**7**:470–6.

A prospective study discussing the role of open treatment in fingertip injuries. Healing time averaged 2–9 weeks with a low incidence of amputation neuroma, painful stump or joint stiffness. Most common complication was nail deformity.

12. McKerrell J, Bowen V, Johnston G, Zondervan J. Boxer's fractures – conservative or operative management. *J Trauma* 1987;**27**:486–90.

Retrospective review of 63 consecutive patients with isolated closed fractures of the fifth metacarpal neck. Both operative and conservative treatment resulted in good functional results and patient satisfaction. All patients regained full motion and grip strength. The residual dorsal angulation and cosmetic deformity were less in the operative group.

13. Swanson TV, Szabo RM, Anderson DD. Open hand fractures: prognosis and classification. *J Hand Surg* 1991;**16**:101–7.

A retrospective review of 200 open hand fractures. Higher infection rates occurred in the presence of wound contamination, delay in treatment greater than 24 hours, and systemic illness. Immediate wound closure is indicated for clean wounds, with an infection rate of 1.4%.

14. McLain RF, Steyers C, Stoddard M. Infections in open fractures of the hand. *J Hand Surg* 1991;**16**:108–12.

Retrospective review of 146 open fractures of the hand showed that the initial wound contamination was the factor most significantly associated with infection. There was no evidence that a delay greater than 6–8 hours in treatment increased the incidence of infection or altered outcome.

15. Pun WK, Chow SP, Lukl KD *et al.* A prospective study on 284 digital fractures of the hand. *J Hand Surg* 1989;**14A**:474–81.

Prospective study of 284 digital fractures placed in a treatment protocol based on stable and unstable injuries. Stable fractures can be treated well with early active mobilization.

16. Wehbe MA, Schneider LH. Mallet fractures. *J Bone Joint Surg* 1984;**66**:658–69.

Review of 160 mallet fractures injuries, 44 with fractures. Most mallet fractures can be treated conservatively ignoring joint subluxation and the size and amount of displacement of the bone fragment.

22. Chuinard RG, D'Ambrosia RD. Human bite infections of the hand. *J Bone Joint Surg* 1977;**59**:416–18.

A prospective protocol for the management of human bite infections of the hand. Absolute indications for admission included a bite greater than 24 hours old or the presence of cellulitis, lymphangitis, abscess, osteomyelitis or penetration of the joint capsule.

23. Talan DA, Citron DM, Abrahamian FM, Moran GJ, Goldstein EJ. Bacteriologic analysis of infected dog and cat bites. *N Engl J Med* 1999;**340**:85–92.

Prospective study of 107 cat and dog bites. *Pasturella canis* was most common in dog bites and *Pasteurella multocida* and *septica* most common in cat bites. Mixed aerobic and anaerobic infection was present in 56% of all wounds (48% dog bites and 32% cat bites). A combination B-lactam antibiotic and a B-lactamase inhibitor are recommended.

## Class III references

2. Gupta A, Wolff TW. Management of the mangled hand and forearm. *J Am Acad Orthop Surg* 1995;**3**:226–36.

Early aggressive wound excision is followed by reconstruction. Priorities in reconstruction are vascular restoration, skeletal stabilization, and soft tissue coverage.

4. Boulas HJ. Amputations of the fingers and the hand: indications for replantation. *J Am Acad Orthop Surg* 1998;**6**:100–5.

Provides guidelines for indications and contraindications to replantation.

9. Zook EG, Van Beek AL, Russell RC, Beatty ME. Anatomy and physiology of the perionychium: a review of the literature and anatomic study. *J Hand Surg* 1980;**5**:528–36.

A classic paper reviewing the anatomy and physiology of the nail. Standard terminology for the anatomy of the perionychium is proposed.

10. Stevenson TR. Fingertip and nailbed injuries. *Orthop Clin North Am* 1992;**23**:149–59.

Review of the treatment of fingertip injuries. Discusses treatment by secondary intention, primary closure, and the indication for flaps.

11. Fassler PR. Fingertip injuries: evaluation and treatment. *J Am Acad Orthop Surg* 1996;**4**:84–92.

For injuries with soft tissue loss and no exposed bone, healing by secondary intention or skin graft is the method of choice. When bone is exposed, local flaps or revision amputation should be considered.

17. Edlich RF, Rodeheaver GT, Morgan RF, Berman DE, Thacker JG. Principles of emergency wound management. *Ann Emerg Med* 1988;**17**:1284–302.

Discusses the initial assessment and treatment of wounds. Specific attention is devoted to type of sutures and tetanus prophylaxis.

18. Steinberg DR. Acute flexor tendon injuries. *Orthop Clin North Am* 1992;**23**(1):125–40.

    Review of flexor tendon anatomy, diagnosis, and five zone classification of injuries.

20. Blair WF, Steyer CM. Extensor tendon injuries. *Orthop Clin North Am* 1992;**23**(1):141–8.

    Reviews extensor tendon anatomy, zones of injury, and treatment.

21. Newport ML. Extensor injuries in the hand. *J Am Acad Orthop Surg* 1997;**5**:59–66.

    Reviews the evaluation and treatment of acute open and closed extensor tendon injuries. Contaminated wounds, open fractures, and joint capsule penetration should be treated emergently with I&D. Isolated lacerations can be repaired in the ER with 3-0 and 4-0 non-absorbable suture.

24. Fleishier GR. The management of bite wounds. *N Engl J Med* 1999;**340**:138–40.

    Review of emergency management of bite wounds. The decision to close cutaneous wounds is based on weighing the cosmetic benefits against the risk of infection. As a general rule, puncture wounds and bite wounds should be treated and left open. Closure should not be performed if the wound is older than 6–12 hours.

## Recommended reading

1. American Society for Surgery of the Hand. *The hand: examination and diagnosis*, 3rd edn. New York: Churchill Livingstone, 1990.

19. American Society for Surgery of the Hand. *The hand: primary care of common problems*, 2nd edn. New York: Churchill Livingstone, 1990.

**Management of hand injuries requiring *urgent* treatment**

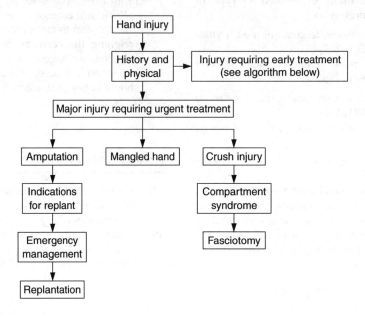

**Management of hand injuries requiring *early* treatment**

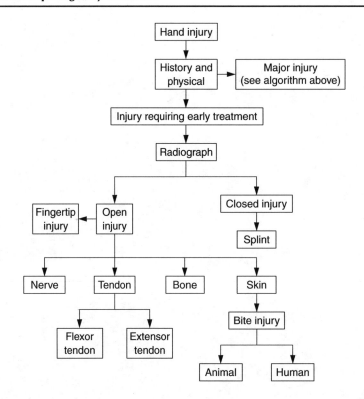

# 20 Management of the comatose patient

*Toan Huynh*

## The comatose patient

Coma represents a state of depressed consciousness unresponsive to external stimuli. A rapid, systematic management plan is crucial in the care of comatose patients after severe traumatic brain injury (TBI), defined as Glasgow Coma Scale (GCS) of 3–8. During this initial phase of care, a central premise has emerged that not all neurological damage occurs at the moment of impact but rather evolves over the ensuing hours and days. Thus, delayed insults may exert deleterious effects on the injured brain at the clinical and biochemical levels. The goal remains to maximize brain protection strategies and minimize secondary brain insults. As such, trauma patients presenting with GCS <8 should be presumed to have a head injury until proven otherwise.

## ATLS guidelines

The fundamental goals in resuscitation of head-injured patients include establishing airway control, ascertaining adequate oxygenation and ventilation, and restoring circulating volume and systemic blood pressure. The efficacy of advanced trauma life support in improving survival is generally well accepted. Since early post-injury episodes of hypotension and/or hypoxia increase morbidity and mortality from severe head injury, rapid and complete reversal of hypoperfusion constitutes the primary physiologic endpoint.

## Hypotension

Early hypotension, defined as a single observation of systolic blood pressure of less than 90 mmHg, has been prospectively evaluated and is associated with adverse outcomes.[1–3] Thus, avoidance of systemic hypotension is of paramount importance. In a multicenter study involving 717 patients, Chestnut *et al.* showed that a single episode of hypotension during the initial resuscitation (SBP <90 mmHg) increased mortality by 150%.[1] Intraoperative hypotension also adversely alters outcome, with a tripling effect on mortality.[4] If possible, mean arterial blood pressure should be maintained above 90 mmHg throughout the patient's initial course. In a subgroup *posthoc* analysis of Class I data, the evidence suggested that administration of 250 ml of hypertonic versus normal saline as the resuscitation fluid improved blood pressures and survival to discharge.[5]

## Hypoxia

Defined as $PaO_2$ <60 mmHg, hypoxia is associated with a trend toward unfavorable outcome.[1] Although experimental evidence suggests increased vulnerability of the injured brain to systemic hypoxia, no data exist to unequivocally support this contention. However, management of cerebral oxygenation, as demonstrated by cerebral extraction of oxygen via jugular bulb oxyhemoglobin saturation, may improve neurologic outcomes.[6] Furthermore, the duration of cerebral hypoxia, examined by continuous microcatheter technique, is associated with worsened neurologic recovery.[7]

## Short-duration chemical paralysis

Sedation and neuromuscular blockade provide useful adjuncts in optimizing transport of the head injury patient. Since these measures interfere with the neurological examination, a short-acting sedation agent should be used promptly to control the patient with severe agitation. Neuromuscular blockade, judiciously used when sedation alone proves inadequate, should employ short-acting agents when possible.

## Rule out hemorrhagic shock

In the unstable patient with suspected traumatic brain injury, diagnostic peritoneal lavage (or diagnostic peritoneal aspirate) or, if available, the focused assessment with sonography for trauma (FAST), constitutes the next step in the work-up. Simultaneously, chest and pelvic radiographs may identify life-threatening injuries in the respective body regions (see Chapters 9 and 11). The focus remains on determining the etiology for the shock state so that appropriate damage control measures can be initiated.

## Neurologic deterioration

When signs of transtentorial herniation, lateralization or progressive neurologic decompensation not attributable to extracranial etiologies are present, efforts should then be directed toward treatment of intracranial hypertension. Neurologic monitoring should include the following:

- serial assessment of the patient's respiratory patterns (Cheyne–Stokes, central neurogenic hyperventilation, ataxic or apneustic respiration)
- the presence of Cushing's reflex (bradycardia with hypertension)
- GCS scoring
- pupillary size and responsiveness
- movements of the upper and lower extremities and their comparative motor strengths.

Adjunctive brainstem reflexes (eyelid, corneal, oculocephalic or oculovestibular, gag) should be examined as the situation warrants and once cervical spine injury or instability has been ruled out radiographically.

In the initial resuscitative phase, methods to reduce intracranial hypertension include hyperventilation and the use of mannitol. These treatment modalities carry the potential to exacerbate intracranial ischemia or interfere with resuscitation. Ideally, invasive hemodynamic monitoring should be employed to achieve euvolemia prior to initiating osmotic therapy.

## Hyperventilation

Currently, there is no evidence to support hyperventilation as a single means of improving outcomes in comatose patients with severe head injury. Approximately 40% of patients with severe TBI develop brain swelling and elevated intracranial pressures (ICP).[8] Furthermore, uncontrolled ICP is one of the most common causes of death and neurologic disability after TBI.[9] However,

aggressive hyperventilation disproportionately reduces cerebral blood flow relative to the reduction in ICP.[10] This adverse effect of hyperventilation on brain tissue oxygenation has recently been clearly demonstrated in an animal model.[11] In a prospective, randomized trial, Muizelaar *et al.*[12] showed that chronic hyperventilation to $PaCO_2$ $25 \pm 2$ mmHg for five days resulted in adverse outcome. Therefore, chronic aggressive hyperventilation therapy should be avoided after severe TBI, particularly in the first 24 hours. Mild hyperventilation, maintaining $PaCO_2$ at levels of 30–35 mmHg, may produce a reduction in ICP. The impact of this maneuver remains to be established.

## Mannitol

The therapeutic effects of mannitol are twofold. The rheologic effects, caused by the immediate expansion of plasma in response to mannitol, lead to reduction in hematocrit and blood viscosity, and increases in cerebral blood flow and cerebral oxygen delivery.[13] Bolus administration better accomplishes this effect. The osmotic effect is delayed for 15–30 minutes and persists from 90 minutes to six or more hours. Although a common practice in the management of head-injured patients with suspected or actual raised ICP, the administration of mannitol has never been subjected to the rigor of a prospective, placebo-controlled trial. Mannitol showed superior results in controlling ICP and improving CPP and outcome in comparison with barbiturates.[14] It provides therapeutic benefits in reducing ICP in the management of head-injured patients. Serum osmolalities greater than 320 mOsm/l and hypovolemia should ideally be ruled out prior to the use of mannitol.

## Surgical lesion

In comatose patients, abnormal head CT scan consists of hematomas, contusions, edema, subarachnoid blood or compressed basal cisterns. A mass lesion (e.g. extradural, subdural, intracerebral or cerebellar hematoma) accompanied by significant midline shift (>5 mm) represents an indication for surgical removal. Early evacuation of surgical lesions appears to improve mortality and neurologic outcomes.[15,16]

## Operating room (OR)

Hemodynamically unstable, head-injured patients with hemoperitoneum should be taken directly to the operating room for exploratory celiotomy. In the presence of lateralizing signs or neurologic decompensation, intraoperative neurosurgical consultation should be obtained. If the patient responded to initial resuscitative efforts and maintained hemodynamic stability, CT scanning constitutes the next step in the diagnostic work-up. In the absence of evidence for ongoing blood loss, attention should be directed towards reversal of the shock state, immediate neurosurgical consultation if an intracranial lesion is identified on CT scan, and admission to an intensive care unit.

## ICP monitoring

Comatose patients are at high risk for intracranial hypertension.[17] Elevated ICP (>25 mmHg) is strongly associated with adverse outcome.[18] Hence, ICP monitoring is indicated in comatose patients with abnormal head CT scan on admission. In comatose patients with a normal head CT scan and two or more of the following: age over 40 years, unilateral or bilateral motor posturing and systolic blood pressure <90 mmHg, ICP monitoring should be strongly considered. Management of ICP (keeping ICP <20–25 mmHg) has been shown to improve outcomes in prospective studies.[19,20] Currently, a ventriculostomy catheter connected to an external strain gauge is recommended as the most accurate, cost-effective, and reliable method for ICP monitoring.

## Management of intracranial hypertension

Only Class II data are available to support the control of intracranial hypertension in benefiting outcome.[19,20] Currently, the upper ICP threshold of 20–25 mmHg has gained wide acceptance. The maintenance of CPP > 70 mmHg has also been demonstrated to improve mortality after severe traumatic brain injury.[21] Active management to keep CPP >70 mmHg has also resulted in improved neurologic recovery.[22,23] In practice, targeted therapy consisting of optimizing systemic oxygen delivery parameters, reducing secondary brain insults by maximizing cerebral substrate delivery (via augmented CPP), and control of intracranial hypertension may represent a physiologic approach in the care of comatose patients after traumatic brain injury.

## Class I references

11. Manley GT, Pitts LH, Morabito D *et al.* Brain tissue oxygenation during hemorrhagic shock, resuscitation, and alterations in ventilation. *J Trauma* 1999;**46**:261–7.

In a hemorrhagic shock animal model, the authors clearly showed the deleterious effects of aggressive hyperventilation (PaCO₂ 18 mmHg) on brain tissue oxygen tension, which was reduced by 40%.

12. Muizelaar JP, Marmarou A, Ward JD *et al.* Adverse effects of prolonged hyperventilation in patients with severe head injury: a randomized clinical trial. *J Neurosurg* 1991;**75**:731–9.

Prospective, randomized clinical trial consisting of 77 patients with severe TBI. This study compared clinical outcome in patients who received hyperventilation to PaCO₂ of 25 ± 2 mmHg for five days after injury with those with PaCO₂ kept at 35 ± 2 mmHg. At three and six months follow-up, patients who were not hyperventilated had more favorable outcome than their counterparts.

14. Schwartz ML, Tator CH, Rowed DW. The University of Toronto Head Injury Treatment Study: a prospective randomized comparison of pento-barbital and mannitol. *Can J Neurol Sci* 1984;**11**:434–40.

A prospective, randomized, cross-over trial which compared mannitol with barbiturates for ICP control. The mannitol group had better mortality outcome (41% versus 77%), and better CPP regulation (75 versus 45 mmHg) compared with the group receiving barbiturates.

## Class II references

1. Chestnut, RM, Marshall LF, Klauber MR *et al.* The role of secondary brain injury in determining outcome from severe head injury. *J Trauma* 1993;**34**:216–22.

A prospective multicenter study of 717 severe head injury patients demonstrating that a single episode of early hypotension (SBP <90 mmHg) increased mortality by 150%. Compared to patients whose hypotension was corrected on arrival at hospital, those who were not adequately resuscitated on arrival had worse outcome.

2. Fearnside MR, Cook RJ, McDougall P *et al.* The Westmead Head Injury Project: outcome in severe head injury. A comparative analysis of pre-hospital, clinical and CT variables. *Br J Neurosurg* 1993;**7**:267–79.

Single-center, prospective study consisting of 315 severe head injury patients showing that hypotension (SBP <90 mmHg) occurring at any time during a patient's course independently predicted poor outcome.

3. Pigula FA, Wald SL, Shackford SR *et al.* The effect of hypotension and hypoxia on children with severe head injury. *J Pediatr Surg* 1993;**28**:310–14.

This study involved 58 children with severe head injuries and revealed the detrimental effects of a single episode of hypotension, which increased mortality fourfold.

5. Vassar MJ, Fischer RP, O'Brien PE *et al*. A multicenter trial for resuscitation of injured patients with 7.5% sodium chloride. The effect of added dextran 70. The Multicenter Group for the Study of Hypertonic Saline in Trauma Patients. *Arch Surg* 1993;**128**:1003–11.

   *Post-hoc* analysis of a prospective, randomized, controlled, multicenter trial supporting the suggestion that, in patients with severe head injury, the administration of 250 cc of hypertonic saline significantly improved survival to discharge.

6. Cruz J. The first decade of continuous monitoring of jugular bulb oxyhemoglobin saturation: management strategies and clinical outcome. *Crit Care Med* 1998; **26**:344–51.

   Non-randomized study comparing jugular venous saturation-based hyperventilation with CPP-based therapy in patients with severe TBI and CT evidence of diffuse brain swelling. Patients did better with jugular venous saturation-based hyperventilation.

7. Bardt TF, Unterberg AW, Hartl R *et al*. Monitoring of brain tissue $PO_2$ in traumatic brain injury: effect of cerebral hypoxia on outcome. *Acta Neurochir* 1998; **71**:153–6.

   Prospective, uncontrolled study showing the deleterious effects of brain tissue hypoxia on mortality and poor neurologic outcome at six months follow-up in 35 patients.

8. Miller JD, Becker DP, Ward JD *et al*. Significance of intracranial hypertension in severe head injury. *J Neurosurg* 1977;**47**:503–10.

   Series of 160 patients with severe head injury who had their ICP continuously monitored. Intracranial pressure greater than 20 mmHg was associated with increased mortality and poor neurologic outcomes.

9. Narayan RK, Kishore PRS, Becker DP *et al*. Intracranial pressure: to monitor or not to monitor? *J Neurosurg* 1982;**56**:650–9.

   This study included 207 consecutive patients with severe head injury who underwent ICP monitoring. Comatose patients (GCS <8) with an abnormal CT scan had a 53–63% incidence of intracranial hypertension. Patients with elevated ICP at any stage had significantly poorer outcome (27% good, 16% moderate) compared to those with normal ICP (59% good, 18% moderate).

10. Obrist WD, Langfitt TW, Jaggi JL *et al*. Cerebral blood flow and metabolism in comatose patients with acute head injury. *J Neurosurg* 1984;**61**:241–53.

    Cohort study of 31 patients with severe TBI. Hyperventilation induced a direct effect on reduction in cerebral blood flow disproportionate to improvement in ICP.

13. Rosner MJ, Coley I. Cerebral perfusion pressure: a hemodynamic mechanism of mannitol and the pre-mannitol hemogram. *Neurosurgery* 1987;**21**:147–56.

A prospective, mechanistic study suggesting that mannitol works best when CPP <70 mmHg. Further, the rheological effect of mannitol is more profound in maximally dilated cerebral microvessels.

17. Marmarou A, Anderson RL, Ward JD *et al*. Impact of ICP instability and hypotension on outcome in patients with severe head trauma. *J Neurosurg* 1991;**75**:S59–S66.

    Analysis of data from 428 patients in the Traumatic Coma Data Bank, revealing the association of hypotension and intracranial hypertension resulting in poor outcome after severe TBI. An ICP threshold of 20 mmHg was found to correlate best with morbidity and mortality.

18. Marshall LF, Gautille T, Klauber MR *et al*. The outcome of severe closed head injury. *J Neurosurg* 1991;**75**:S28–S36.

    This study examined 746 patients enrolled in the Traumatic Coma Data Bank. For patients with non-surgical lesions, increased mortality was observed when ICP rose >25 mmHg.

19. Eisenberg HM, Frankowski RF, Contant CF *et al*. High-dose barbiturates control elevated intracranial pressure in patients with severe head injury. *J Neurosurg* 1988;**69**:15–23.

    Prospective multicenter study involving 73 severe head injury patients randomly assigned to a high-dose pentobarbital or placebo-control regimen. Outcomes in patients whose ICP could be kept below 20 mmHg were significantly better than those whose ICP could not be controlled.

20. Ghajar JB, Hariri RJ, Patterson RH. Improved outcome from traumatic coma using only ventricular CSF drainage for ICP control. *Adv Neurosurg* 1993;**21**:173–7.

    Prospective, non-randomized cohort study of 49 severe head injury patients. Patients in group 1 (34) received ICP monitoring and CSF drainage when ICP >15 mmHg; mortality was 12%. Patients in group 2 (15) were not treated for intracranial hypertension and had a mortality of 53%.

21. Rosner MJ, Rosner SD, Johnson AH. Cerebral perfusion pressure: management protocol and clinical results. *J Neurosurg* 1995;**83**:949–62.

    Provocative case series involving 158 patients with GCS of 7 or lower. CPP-based therapy was associated with an unexpectedly low mortality and improved recovery.

22. Clifton GL, Allen S, Barrodale P *et al*. A phase II study of moderate hypothermia in severe brain injury. *J Neurotrauma* 1993;**10**:263–71.

    In this prospective clinical trial of 46 patients, hypothermia was therapeutically induced to maintain CPP >70 mmHg. This regimen resulted in overall mortality of 35% and good neurologic recovery of 45%.

23. Fortune JB, Feustel PJ, Weigle CGM *et al*. Continuous measurement of jugular venous oxygen saturation in response to transient elevations of blood pressure in head-injured patients. *J Neurosurg* 1994;**80**:461–8.

Small series of 14 patients. This study examined the relationship between jugular venous oxygen saturation and outcome. Active maintenance of CPP >70 mmHg achieved a mortality of 14%.

## Class III references

4. Peitropaoli JA, Rogers FB, Shackford SR *et al*. The deleterious effects of intraoperative hypotension on outcome in patients with severe head injury. *J Trauma* 1992;**33**:403–7.

A retrospective review of 53 patients with severe head injury. There were 17 (32%) who developed intraoperative hypotension, with associated mortality of 82%. The 36 (68%) normotensive patients had a mortality of 25%.

15. Dent DL, Croce MA, Menke PG *et al*. Prognostic factors after acute subdural hematoma. *J Trauma* 1995;**39**:36–43.

In this retrospective review of 211 patients, there was a trend toward better neurologic outcome when subdural hematomas were evacuated within four hours after admission.

16. Seelig JM, Becker DP, Miller JD *et al*. Traumatic acute subdural hematoma. Major mortality reduction in comatose patients treated within four hours. *New Engl J Med* 1981;**304**:1511–16.

Involving 82 patients, this important study showed that early surgical decompression of acute subdural hematoma resulted in a mortality of 30%, compared with 90% in patients who underwent surgery more than four hours after injury.

**Management of the comatose patient**

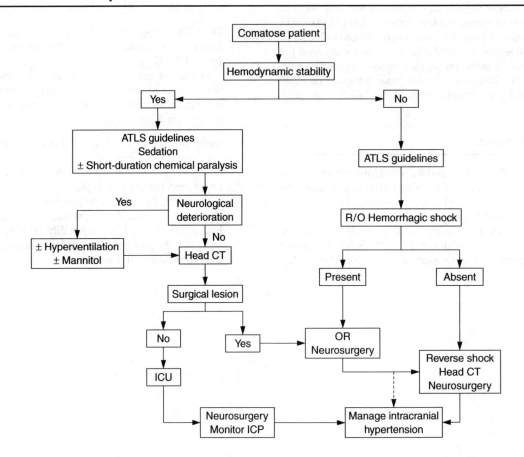

# 21 Mild and moderate traumatic brain injury: Glasgow Coma Scale $\geq 9$

*Philip W Smith, David L Ciraulo*

Approximately 80% of patients presenting following a traumatic injury have some component of traumatic brain injury categorized as mild. Motor vehicle accidents account for 28% of brain injury patients, sport physical activities are responsible for 20%, and assaults for 9%. Over a one-year period, 1.5 million non-institutionalized US civilians sustain non-fatal brain injuries, a rate of 618/100 000 persons per year.[1] Classic presentation is an awake patient who may or may not have amnesia for the events surrounding the injury.[2] These patients may report a brief loss of consciousness but have no focal deficit, earning a Glasgow Coma Scale (GCS) between 14 and 15. Patients presenting with moderate head injuries have GCS of 9–13 and account for approximately 10% of the head-injured patients presenting to trauma centers.[2] These patients can usually follow commands but are confused, somnolent, and may have focal neurological deficit.[2] Patients with mild traumatic brain injury can develop multiple partial seizure-like symptoms. Therefore, a thorough work-up, including EEG and neuropsychological assessment, is often indicated.[3] Three per cent of patients with mild head injuries may progress and deteriorate to the category of severe during the evaluation, whereas approximately 10–20% of patients with moderate head injuries deteriorate and may lapse into coma.[2]

Mild traumatic brain injury is a very common injury resulting in immediate as well as long-term problems. Despite accepted definitions, there exists much controversy over the diagnosis of mild traumatic brain injury resulting in misdiagnosis and failure to provide adequate follow-up care for the injured patient.[4] This creates medicolegal difficulties for the treating physician when cases of vehicular injury or assault progress to litigation.

An accurate and consistent definition of mild traumatic brain injury is important for the initial management and rehabilitation of the patient. The Committee on Head Injury Intradisciplinary Special Interest Group of the American Congress of Rehabilitation Medicine has developed a working definition for mild traumatic brain injury.[5,6] These definitions are based on the presence or absence of mental status changes, amnesia, loss of consciousness, anatomical lesions, and/or neurological deficit.[5,6] Traumatic brain injury significantly impacts upon the morbidity and mortality of the traumatized patient.[7] Approximately 50% of people with mild traumatic brain injury will develop symptomatology and 15% will have permanent disability.[8] TBI is the leading cause of death in patients less than 45 years of age. One hundred thousand deaths per year are attributed to TBI.[7]

Predictors of recovery have been identified for traumatic brain injury. Left brain injury has been associated with longer periods of unconsciousness and a longer time to obeying commands. Premorbid ability is closely tied to eventual recovery.[9] Treatment of the elderly with mild traumatic injury results in 85% returning home after rehabilitation and 54% performing activities of daily living independently.[10]

## Initial evaluation

The initial evaluation of any trauma patient follows the American College of Surgeons Committee on Trauma Advanced Trauma Life Support guidelines with performance of the primary survey.

The American College of Surgeons Committee on Trauma has defined the primary survey to include: ABCDE, with A representing airway maintenance, B breathing and ventilation, C circulation and control of hemorrhage, D disability and assessment of neurological status, and E exposure and controlled environmental variables to prevent hypothermia.[2] Patients should be resuscitated accordingly after placement of IVs in the initial management of blunt traumatic injury. Isotonic crystalloid solution is the fluid of choice although colloid solutions and blood products can be effectively utilized. Hypertonic saline has short-term benefits. Hypotonic solutions have no role in the immediate resuscitation.[11] Favorable outcomes from mild traumatic brain injury and spinal cord injury are dependent upon the rapid initial evaluation and successful hemodynamic resuscitation of the patient.[12]

## Secondary survey

Following the initial evaluation of any trauma patient, the secondary survey is performed in a head-to-toe evaluation.

The secondary survey follows the primary survey once the patient starts to demonstrate normalization of vital functions. This includes a survey and evaluation in a head-to-toe fashion.[2] In this survey, a complete neurological examination is performed including an assessment of GCS.[2] If at any time during the secondary survey the patient's condition deteriorates, the primary survey begins again and the appropriate measures are taken.[2]

## Glasgow Coma Scale

If not completed during the primary survey, Glasgow Coma Scale (GCS) must be addressed prior to completion of the secondary survey. The scale allows for assessment of neurological function. Key components include eye opening, best motor response and best verbal response. GCS below 9 is considered indicative of a severe brain injury. This presentation usually requires aggressive pharmacological intervention and monitoring of intracranial pressure in relation to cerebral perfusion pressure.

The American College of Surgeons recognizes the Glasgow Coma Scale as initial criteria in triage to a trauma center in the prehospital environment.[2] A GSC of <14 warrants transferring the patient to a trauma center with alert of the trauma team.[2] While concussive convulsions have occurred in the presence of mild traumatic brain injury without structural or permanent brain injury, a thorough work-up should be done to rule out a more severe underlying injury.[13]

During the secondary survey, a complete evaluation of the head including the control of hemorrhage, if not already completed in the primary survey, should be performed. An ocular evaluation should be completed to include: visual acuity, pupillary size, hemorrhages

of conjunctiva and fundi, penetrating injuries, contact lenses (to be removed), dislocation of lens, and ocular entrapment.[2]

## Pupillary size and response

Inequality of pupil size and variability in pupillary response is a neurosurgical emergency requiring immediate CT scan for investigation of intracranial injury and neurosurgical consultation with possible operative intervention.

The presence of abnormal pupil reactivity is a strong indicator of significant intraparenchymal injury.[14] Up to a third of patients with unequal or fixed pupil(s) post-trauma have been found to have mass lesions on CT scan of the head[15] and up to a third of patients with mass lesions on CT scan have been found to have pupil inequality.[16]

## Intrahemispheric brain injury

With neurologic deficits but normal pupillary response and size, the question of intrahemispheric brain injury and/or interruption of cerebral blood flow needs to be addressed. Dependent upon presentation of the neurological deficit, spinal cord injury may be implicated in the deficit. CT scan of the brain is mandatory as well as spinal films, with spinal injury level to be determined by clinical presentation. Neurosurgical consultation is advised at this time.

Closed head injury, defined as any loss of consciousness or post-traumatic amnesia, has been shown to occur in 41–49% of spinal cord-injured patients.[17–19] There is no relationship between the incidence of a closed head injury and the level of the spinal cord injury.[17] All spinal cord-injured patients should be thoroughly evaluated for a traumatic brain injury.

## History

If the patient has no pupillary changes and/or neuro deficits, the next step in the evaluation is to perform an assessment of the patient's history for loss of consciousness. It is important to quantify the duration of this period of time with altered mental status as well as an assessment of presence of clinical amnesia.

Any patient with a history of loss of consciousness or posttraumatic amnesia should be considered for CT scan of the brain even if the GCS is 15 on initial presentation. Multiple authors have shown a 2–4% incidence of intracranial lesions requiring surgical intervention in trauma patients who report a history of loss of consciousness or posttraumatic amnesia with an initial GCS of 13–15. Forty-five per cent of these had an initial GCS of 15.[20] Gutman reports a 29% incidence of operable mass lesions for patients with an initial GCS of 13–15, age over 40, and injured in a fall[16] and Schynoll reports that 7% of patients with a GCS of 15 had an abnormal CT scan of the brain.[15] If the practitioner decides not to perform a CT scan on a patient with a history of a minimal loss of consciousness, then a period of close inpatient observation is warranted. Dacey relates one case of a patient injured in a fall with an initial GCS of 15, who developed a rapid decline in his mental state during observation and died five days after urgent craniotomy to decompress a subdural hematoma.[20]

## CT scan

If it is determined that the patient has had no loss of consciousness but GCS assessment is not perfect, the conservative approach to the continued work-up is evaluation of the brain by CT scan. It is entirely possible for a patient to have a GCS between 9 and 14 and have significant intracranial injury. If the CT of the brain is normal but GCS is not 15, an investigation for other mind-altering conditions is warranted.

Alcohol has been a factor in altered consciousness in 28–56% of trauma patients.[21–24] Brickley found 86% of the assault victims in his study were intoxicated.[25] Alcohol has been found to lower the measured GCS on arrival by 2–3 points.[21,25] Other authors have found no significant difference in the measured GCS and the presence of alcohol.[22,23] Alcohol has also been shown to be correlated with higher injury severity scores and mortality rates.[23,25] Schynoll was able to show an abnormal CT scan incidence of 43% in those patients with substance abuse versus 8% for those without substance abuse history following trauma.[15] Cocaine use prior to emergency department presentation has been associated with both metabolic and respiratory acid–base abnormalities and can influence the patient's presentation with an altered mental state.[26,27] Additionally, two widely accepted causes of altered mental status, hypoxia and hypercarbia, must also be investigated.

Patients with a GCS between 9 and 14 with CT scan consistent with intracranial hemorrhage and/or parenchymal bleeding necessitate emergency neurosurgic consultation.

A patient with a GCS of 15 without loss of consciousness is clinically at low risk for having incurred a traumatic brain injury. However, preoperative CT scanning should be considered in the patient who requires general anesthesia and therefore will be clinically unevaluable for a prolonged period of time. The presence of mind-altering drugs, illicit and/or prescription, or the presence of alcohol precludes reliable examination and warrants consideration of CT scan investigation.[8]

## Facial fractures and risks of surgery

The presence of significant facial fractures indicates the transference of significant kinetic energy with rapid deceleration and supports further investigation for intracranial injury. Facial fractures have been associated with a 25% incidence of basilar skull fractures and a 17.5% incidence of closed head injury.[28,29] The location of the fracture had a direct correlation with the severity of the traumatic brain injury, with fractures above the orbital floor having a poorer prognosis.[30] The number of fractures was also directly correlated with the incidence of basilar skull fracture with the presence of one fracture having a 21% incidence, the presence of two fractures a 30.4% incidence, and the presence of three or more fractures a 33.3% incidence.[31]

Patients with a GCS of 15 and no history of loss of consciousness or amnesia but still with a suspicion of traumatic brain injury may be followed by frequent serial clinical neurologic exams. The ability to perform these exams is lost in any patient undergoing sedation for any diagnostic or therapeutic procedure or general anesthesia for surgery. Further risks of surgery unique to the head-injured patient are an elevation of intracerebral pressure with endotracheal intubation, positive pressure ventilation, and/or positive end-expiratory pressure.[32] A patient undergoing massive resuscitation for other injuries can develop dilutional coagulopathies that might exacerbate a previous unrecognized minor intracranial hemorrhage.

## Admission and evaluation

With a history of loss of consciousness, GCS between 9 and 14, and a normal CT scan, it is prudent to admit the patient to the hospital for 24 hours of observation given the possibility of continued deficit in cognitive and/or motor function. Continued work-up should progress as dictated by clinical and radiographic findings. Following discharge or during observation, consideration should be given to neuropsychologic evaluation for cognitive deficits, which potentially can hinder recovery. The sensitivity of CT scans for the detection of subtle injuries to the brain has been recently challenged by the sensitivity of MRI and single photon emission computed tomography (SPECT). The role of these diagnostic modalities is controversial given cost and minimal contribution to changes in the clinical management of the patient.

Elderly patients with mild traumatic brain injury have clinical outcomes comparable to those of the younger population.[34] Repeat CT scans are recommended in patients with initial CT abnormalities if there is no improvement in the patient's condition. The timing of the repeat CT scans depends on the patient's clinical course.

Mild traumatic brain injury and postconcussive syndrome can cause subtle language and cognitive changes. Further evaluation of mild traumatic brain injury should be conducted using neuropsychologic testing.[35] A combination of measurements is valuable in the prediction of postconcussive syndrome and mild or moderate traumatic brain injuries. The Hospital Anxiety and Depression Scale, the posttraumatic amnesia, the short orientation memory and concentration test, and the paced auditory serial addition test are recommended for predictive value in recovery.[36]

Intracranial lesions cannot be completely excluded clinically in head trauma patients who have loss of consciousness or amnesia, even if GCS is 15; therefore, CT scan is warranted.[37] Recent investigation has raised questions regarding normal CT scans of patients suffering mild traumatic brain injuries. The use of MRI may be beneficial to patients with traumatic brain injuries with normal head CT scan, identifying small injuries that are less than clinically apparent on CT scans.[38] The sensitivity of MRI is significantly higher than that of a CT scan in detecting concussion, shearing injury, subdural and epidural injury, and sinus involvement, with an overall rating of 96.4%. The overall sensitivity rating for CT scan was 63.4%.[39] MRI shows diffuse axonal injury in comparison with normal CT scans of patients with mild TBI.[38] The MRI identifies lesions not seen on CT scans but the findings rarely alter clinical management and the cost is significant, approximately $3000 per study.[40]

The technetium-99m SPECT brain scan in mild to moderate TBI has shown very subtle abnormalities in those patients otherwise determined to be normal by CT scan.[41] SPECT scan in mild to moderate TBI is more sensitive for detection of intraparenchymal injury than the CT scan – 87.5% and 37.5% respectively.[42] The use of SPECT scan for mild to moderate TBI is helpful as a predictor of clinical outcome of mild TBI.[43]

## Mild TBI

Patients who have undergone traumatic injury with no history of loss of consciousness, have a GCS of 15, are not intoxicated or under the influence of drugs or medication, and do not require anesthesia can be considered clinically cleared of a traumatic brain injury. Following work-up, these patients can be considered for discharge under the supervision of an adult for 24 hours to prevent morbidity from the rare delayed manifestation of injury.

Mild traumatic brain injury can occur in the absence of any signs or symptoms. In one study, Chambers showed that 32% of patients who presented after blunt trauma with no history of signs or symptoms consistent with traumatic brain injury and no evidence of direct cranial trauma had symptoms of postconcussive syndrome at one month follow-up.[33] None of these patients had imaging studies at the time of presentation due to the lack of suspicion of traumatic brain injury.

## Class II references

2.  American College of Surgeons Committee on Trauma. Head trauma. In: ACS (eds) *Advanced trauma life support for doctors*, 6th edn. Chicago: American College of Surgeons.

3.  Verduyn WH, Hilt J, Roberts MA *et al*. Multiple partial seizure-like symptoms following minor closed head injury. *Brain Injury* 1992;**6**(3):245–60.

    This is a prospective study of 96 posttraumatic patients being followed for mild head injury, who were interviewed by questionnaire to determine their level of cognitive impairment. Seventeen of the 96 self-reported at least 10 of the 41 symptoms. These symptoms were not the classic autonomic motor symptoms of traditional complex partial seizure disorders, but rather symptoms usually associated with postconcussive patients. The patients also underwent extensive neuropsychological testing. The conclusion of the study was that patients with mild closed head trauma frequently develop cognitive deficits that delay their recovery.

15. Schynoll W, Overton D, Krome R *et al*. A prospective study to identify high-yield criteria associated with acute intracranial computed tomography findings in head-injured patients. *Am J Emerg Med* 1993;**11**(4):321–6.

    This prospective study of 264 traumatic head-injured patients describes independent variables that predict the presence of abnormal findings on CT scan of the head. These are alcohol use, amnesia, loss of consciousness, anisocoria, paralysis, GCS <15, and basilar skull fracture.

16. Gutman MB, Moulton RJ, Sullivan I, Hotz G, Tucker WS, Muller PJ. Risk factors predicting operable intracranial hematomas in head injury. *J Neurosurg* 1992;**77**(1):9–14.

This prospective study of 1039 head injury trauma patients evaluated independent variables predictive of operable intracranial lesions. These were GCS, pupillary inequality, and injury by falling.

17. Davidoff G, Thomas P, Johnson M, Berent S, Dijkers M, Doljanac R. Closed head injury in acute traumatic spinal cord injury: incidence and risk factors. *Arch Phys Med Rehabil* 1988;**69**(10):869–72.

A prospective observational study of spinal cord injury patients revealed a 49% incidence of concurrent closed head injury, defined as any posttraumatic amnesia. A significant risk factor is involvement in a traffic accident but not the level of spinal injury.

20. Dacey RG Jr, Alves WM, Rimel RW, Winn HR, Jane JA. Neurosurgical complications after apparent minor head injury. Assessment of risk in a series of 610 patients. *J Neurosurg* 1986;**65**(2):203–10.

A prospective analysis of 610 trauma patients with history of loss of consciousness or other neurologic deficit and GCS ≥13. Eighteen patients required a neurosurgic procedure, with two of these having a GCS of 15.

21. Jagger J, Fife D, Vernberg K, Jane JA. Effect of alcohol intoxication on the diagnosis and apparent severity of brain injury. *Neurosurgery* 1984;**15**(3):303–6.

A prospective study of 257 trauma patients with brain injury that measured the GCS on admission and again 6–10 hours later. The patients were divided on the basis of blood alcohol testing. Patients with a blood alcohol concentration (BAC) greater than 0.20% had a greater improvement in the GCS level than those with a BAC less than 0.20%.

22. Nath FP, Beastal G, Teasdale GM. Alcohol and traumatic brain damage. *Injury* 1986;**17**(3):150–3.

A prospective study of 38 head-injured patients testing the relationship between alcohol intake, GCS, and severity of head injury as measured by serum creatinine kinase (CKBB). No correlation was found between the presence of alcohol in the blood and GCS level or elevation of CKBB. The CKBB level did correlate with outcome. The flaw of this study is that these patients were enrolled in the study upon their transfer to the neurosurgic department (3–48 hours after admission) and an initial alcohol level and GCS evaluation was not available. The level of alcohol is measured as present or absent, not as an absolute level.

24. Holt S, Stewart IC, Dixon JM, Elton RA, Taylor TV, Little K. Alcohol and the emergency service patient. *BMJ.* 1980;**281**(6241):638–40.

This study measured the blood alcohol of 702 consecutive trauma patients; 40% had consumed alcohol and 32% were legally intoxicated. Physical exam to assess intoxication had a false-negative rate of 10%.

25. Brickley MR, Shepherd JP. The relationship between alcohol intoxication, injury severity and Glasgow Coma Score in assault patients. *Injury* 1995;**26**(5):311–14.

This is a prospective study of 242 assault victims comparing their level of intoxication with their severity of injury and Glasgow Coma Scale. There was no correlation between their injury and level of intoxication, but there was a significant correlation between their presenting GCS and level of intoxication. The authors suggest severe intoxication (>240 mg/100 ml) reduces the GCS by 2–3 points.

33. Chambers J, Cohen SS, Hemminger L, Prall JA, Nichols JS. Mild traumatic brain injuries in low-risk trauma patients. *J Trauma* 1996;**41**(6):976–80.

A prospective study of 129 trauma patients discharged from the emergency department after minor trauma without history or physical evidence of traumatic brain injury; 32% of the patients described postconcussive symptoms at one-month follow-up and 17% at 2 months.

34. Cifu DX, Kreutzer JS, Marwitz JH, Rosenthal M, Englander J, High W. Functional outcomes of older adults with traumatic brain injury: a prospective, multicenter analysis. *Arch Phys Med Rehabil* 1996;**77**(9):883–8.

A prospective comparison of older (greater than 55 years of age) trauma patients with younger (younger than 55) with respect to rehabilitation length of stay, charges, and functional change. The study concluded that older patients require longer rehabilitation periods and charges for comparative degrees of functional change.

35. Tucker FM, Hanlon RE. Effects of mild traumatic brain injury on narrative discourse production. *Brain Injury* 1998;**12**(9):783–92.

This prospective study involved a subset of patients from a larger ongoing study. Mild traumatic brain-injured patients were matched with moderate TBI patients and normal controls and asked to interpret a sequence of pictures to measure their ability to process cognitive information with a narrative discourse. Both groups of TBI patients were less likely to provide an accurate narrative description.

36. King NS. Emotional, neuropsychological, and organic factors: their use in the prediction of persisting postconcussion symptoms after moderate and mild head injuries. *J Neurol Neurosurg Psychiatry* 1996;**61**(1):75–81.

A prospective study measuring the incidence of posttraumatic symptoms after mild and moderate head injuries. A questionnaire developed by the study institution is used as both a study subject as well as the control measure. Eight indices are used to predict the occurrence of postconcussive symptoms after injury. Five of the eight are recommended as predictive of postconcussive symptoms; these are the Hospital Anxiety and Depression Scale, posttraumatic amnesia, short orientation and concentration test, the paced auditory serial addition test, and the Rivermead postconcussive symptoms questionnaire.

37. Jeret JS, Mandell M, Anziska B *et al.* Clinical predictors of abnormality disclosed by computed tomography after mild head trauma. *Neurosurgery* 1993;**32**(1):9–15.

A prospective study of 712 trauma patients with GCS of 15 on presentation and history of loss of consciousness or amnesia found that 9.4% had acute intracranial lesions on CT. Two of these patients required operative intervention.

38. Mittl RL, Grossman RI, Hiehle JF *et al.* Prevalence of MR evidence of diffuse axonal injury in patients with mild head injury and normal head CT findings. *Am J Neuroradiol* 1994;**15**(8):1583–9.

This is a prospective study of 20 mild head injury patients with normal posttrauma head CTs who underwent MRI 1–26 days after the initial trauma; 30% had evidence of diffuse axonal injury on MRI. This may illustrate a pathological etiology to the postconcussive syndrome although these patients were not evaluated specifically for this.

42. Nedd K, Sfakianakis G, Ganz W *et al.* 99mTc-HMPAO SPECT of the brain in mild to moderate traumatic brain injury patients: compared with CT – a prospective study. *Brain Injury* 1993;**7**(6):469–79.

This prospective study compares CT scan and SPECT scan with respect to regional cerebral blood flow (rCBF) on 20 mild to moderate head-injured patients. SPECT scans were found to be more sensitive in detecting subtle alterations in rCBF following head injury. However, no additional mass or operable lesions were detected with a SPECT scan and the clinical course and treatment were not affected. The SPECT scan may be best utilized to predict long-term cognitive recovery.

43. Jacobs A, Put E, Ingels M *et al.* Prospective evaluation of technetium-99m-HMPAO SPECT in mild and moderate traumatic brain injury. *J Nucl Med* 1994;**35**(6):942–7.

This prospective study on the utility of technetium-99m-HMPAO SPECT to visualize cerebral flow abnormalities in mild and moderate head injuries demonstrates an advantage over CT. However, the authors present no evidence that it is useful in the immediate posttraumatic period to identify operable lesions. Rather, its use is described as a better predictor of functional outcome.

## Class III references

1. Sosin DM, Sniezek JE, Thurman DJ. Incidence of mild and moderate brain injury in the United States, 1991. *Brain Injury* 1996;**10**(1):47–54.

This retrospective analysis of data from the 1991 National Health Interview Survey describes a rate of brain injury – defined as "head injury resulting in loss of consciousness in the previous 12 months" – of 618 per 100 000 person-years. Of these, 25% did not seek medical care and 25% of those who did were hospitalized.

10. Davis CS, Acton P. Treatment of the elderly brain-injured patient. Experience in a traumatic brain injury unit. *J Am Geriatr Soc* 1988;**36**(3):225–9.

This retrospective review evaluated 26 head-injured trauma patients over the age of 50 with respect to their rehabilitation outcome; 85% returned to home. Of these, only 54% were independent in their activities of daily living.

18. Davidoff G, Roth E, Morris J, Bleiberg J. Assessment of closed head injury in trauma-related spinal cord injury. *Paraplegia* 1986;**24**(2):97–104.

This is a retrospective review of 122 traumatic spinal cord injury patients. 41% had a history of posttraumatic amnesia or loss of consciousness consistent with a closed head injury.

19. Davidoff G, Morris J, Roth E, Bleiberg J. Closed head injury in spinal cord injured patients: retrospective study of loss of consciousness and post-traumatic amnesia. *Arch Phys Med Rehabil* 1985;**66**(1):41–3.

This retrospective review of 101 traumatic spinal cord-injured patients revealed 42% to have a history of loss of consciousness or posttraumatic amnesia consistent with a closed head injury.

23. Pories SE, Gamelli RL, Vacek P, Goodwin G, Shinozaki T, Harris F. Intoxication and injury. *J Trauma* 1992;**32**(1):60–4.

This article describes a mortality rate of 13.3% in trauma patients who are positive for alcohol versus 2.3% in alcohol-negative patients. 427 total patients were studied. It also studied the change in GCS over 24 hours with respect to alcohol consumption and concludes that alcohol does not have a significant influence.

26. Stevens DC, Campbell JP, Carter JE *et al.* Acid–base abnormalities associated with cocaine toxicity in emergency department patients. *J Toxicol Clin Toxicol* 1994;**32**(1):31–9.

This retrospective review measured the blood pH of emergency department patients after cocaine use. Any acidosis or alkalosis was determined to be metabolic or respiratory in origin. Most patients had a normal pH with metabolic acidosis being the second most frequent presentation. The patients' reasons for the visits were cocaine related and not necessarily trauma.

27. Richards CF, Clark RF, Holbrook T *et al.* The effect of cocaine and amphetamines on vital signs in trauma patients. *J Emerg Med* 1995;**13**(1):59–63.

This is a retrospective comparison of trauma patients comparing the effects of sympathomimetics on admission vital signs. While patients who had toxicological evidence of cocaine or amphetamine use had an elevated prehospital respiratory rate, no effect on vital signs on admission was found.

29. Haug RH, Savage JD, Likavec MJ *et al*. A review of 100 closed head injuries associated with facial fractures. *J Oral Maxillofac Surg* 1992;**50**(3):218–22.

This is a retrospective review of 570 trauma patients with facial fractures. One hundred (17.5%) had concomitant closed head injuries (CHI), defined as loss of consciousness or abnormality on head CT. The severity of CHI increased with the number of facial fractures. Mandibular/midface fractures had the largest number of associated CHIs, followed by isolated mandibular fractures.

30. Derdyn C, Persing JA, Broaddus WC *et al*. Craniofacial trauma: an assessment of risk related to timing of surgery. *Plast Reconstr Surg* 1990;**86**(2):238–45.

A retrospective comparison of 49 trauma patients with facial fractures and concurrent intracerebral injury requiring operative intervention or ICP monitoring. The timing of the facial fracture repair was compared with respect to mortality and no significant difference was found.

31. Slupchynskyj OS, Berkower AS, Byrne DW, Cayten CG. Association of skull base and facial fractures. *Laryngoscope* 1992;**102**(11):1247–50.

A retrospective analysis of 268 trauma patients with facial fractures was performed. Review of CT results revealed a 25% incidence of associated basilar skull fractures. The incidence of basilar skull fractures was related to the location and number of facial fractures.

39. Orrison WW, Gentry LR, Stimac GK *et al*. Blinded comparison of cranial CT and MR in closed head injury evaluation. *AJNR Am J Neuroradiology* 1994;**15**(2):351–6.

This retrospective review of 107 head injured patients who had undergone CT and MRI of the head within 48 hours of each other on admission concludes that MRI is more sensitive than CT in detecting intracranial abnormalities, subdural and epidural hematomas, shearing injuries, contusions, and sinus involvement. CT was more sensitive than MRI in detecting fractures. MRI did not alter the acute neurosurgical involvement in any patient although an unsuspected neoplasm was discovered.

40. Fiser SM, Johnson SB, Fortune JB. Resource utilization in traumatic brain injury: the role of magnetic resonance imaging. *Am Surg* 1998;**64**(11):1088–93.

A retrospective review of 40 traumatic brain injury patients who underwent both CT and MRI. While MRI detected small lesions not seen on CT, all lesions requiring surgical intervention or change in management were seen on CT. One case of carotid artery thrombosis was seen on MRA. There was a significant difference in the time to CT versus MRI, 6.3 hours versus 2.9 days. MRI is of limited value in the acute trauma setting.

41. Abdel-Dayem HM, Abu-Judeh H, Kumar M *et al*. SPECT brain perfusion abnormalities in mild or moderate traumatic brain injury. *Clin Nucl Med* 1998;**23**(5):309–17.

This is a retrospective review of SPECT brain perfusion imaging in 228 mild to moderate brain-injured patients. One hundred and sixty-two of the patients had a head CT scan; all were reported as normal. One hundred and seventy-six (77%) of the SPECT scans showed a hypoperfusion abnormality. The basal ganglia and thalami were the most common locations of abnormality. The most common patient complaint was headache, in 139 of 228 (60.9%). Of these, 103 (74%) had an abnormal SPECT. The scans were performed distant to the trauma and were not utilized in the acute setting.

## Technology assessment

28. Gentry LR. Facial trauma and associated brain damage. *Radiol Clin North Am* 1989;**27**(2):435–46.

CT and MRI are compared for their ability to image facial fractures and the associated soft tissue injuries. MRI can better delineate the intraocular and intraorbital injuries as well as intraosseous vascular abnormalities. There is no comparison made of intracerebral imaging.

## Literature review

4. Kibby MY, Long CJ. Minor head injury: attempts at clarifying the confusion. *Brain Injury* 1996;**10**(3):159–86.

This article reviews the various definitions of mild traumatic brain injury that have been proposed. In 1993, the Mild Traumatic Brain Injury Committee of the Head Injury Interdisciplinary Special Interest Group of the American Congress of Rehabilitation Medicine proposed the following definition. A traumatic brain injury with at least one of the following: any loss of consciousness; any posttraumatic amnesia; any alteration in mental state at the time of the trauma; or a focal neurologic deficit that may or may not be transient. The severity of the injury cannot exceed: loss of consciousness of 30 minutes; an initial GCS of 13–15; posttraumatic amnesia of 24 hours. Postconcussion symptoms, defined as headache, dizziness, fatigue, irritability, memory weakness and/or impaired concentration, may be present in up to 90% of mild TBI patients but also may exist after a head injury with the presence of a severe traumatic brain injury.

5. Esselman PC, Uomoto JM. Classification of the spectrum of mild traumatic brain injury. *Brain Injury* 1995;**9**(4):417–24.

This review of the literature compares the various definitions used to describe a mild traumatic brain injury. The criteria used most commonly are: (1) initial Glasgow Coma Score of 13–15 (2) loss of consciousness for less than 20–30 minutes (3) posttraumatic amnesia for less than 24 hours. At least one definition allows for any alteration in mental state at the time of the accident and/or any focal neurologic deficit. These inclusions allow the consideration of a diagnosis of TBI for those without loss of consciousness. The Abbreviated Injury Scale makes allowances for the presence of anatomic lesions when considering the diagnosis.

6. Rosenthal M. Mild traumatic brain injury syndrome. *Ann Emerg Med* 1993;**22**(6):1048–51.

This summary article discusses the complexities involved with diagnosing mild traumatic brain injury. The criteria for definition as adopted by the American Congress of Rehabilitation Medicine are presented: ''A traumatically induced physiologic disruption of brain function, as manifested by one of the following: (1) any period of loss of consciousness; (2) any loss of memory for events immediately before or after the accident; (3) any alteration in mental state at the time of the accident; (4) focal neurologic deficits, which may or may not be transient, but when severity does not exceed the following – loss of consciousness for 30 minutes or less; after 30 minutes, GCS of 13–15; posttraumatic amnesia not greater than 24 hours.'' The author discusses the signs and symptoms of posttraumatic concussive syndrome and the need for further neuropsychological testing if these persist. The majority of traumatic brain injury occurs as a result of vehicular accident, fall or assault and may result in eventual litigation. A well-founded diagnosis and treatment plan is essential.

7. Zink BJ. Traumatic brain injury. *Emerg Med Clin North Am* 1996;**14**(1):115–50.

This rather comprehensive review discusses traumatic brain injury in a systematic and indepth fashion. The pathophysiology section outlines the mechanics and biomolecular aspects of TBI. The physiologic response is reviewed. Initial assessment and treatment to include fluid administration and possible pharmacological interventions as well as early surgical intervention are discussed. The basis for monitoring and radiographic imaging is given.

8. Kushner D. Mild traumatic brain injury: toward understanding manifestations and treatment. *Arch Intern Med* 1998;**158**(15):1617–24.

This article describes the definition, pathophysiology, treatment, and long-term considerations of mild traumatic brain injury.

9. Levin HS. Prediction of recovery from traumatic brain injury. *J Neurotrauma* 1995;**12**(5):913–22.

This review article attempts to correlate the prediction of recovery from traumatic brain injury with physical and radiographic findings at the time of injury. Multiple authors have demonstrated a relationship between left brain injury and increased periods of unconsciousness as compared to right brain

injury. This involvement of the language-dominant hemisphere is also thought to be responsible for an increased time to obey commands due to the language processing. Not surprisingly, the depth of the parenchymal lesion was directly related to the severity and duration of impaired consciousness. Overall, the major predictor of long-term cognitive outcome is the estimated premorbid ability.

11. Zornow MH, Prough DS. Fluid management in patients with traumatic brain injury. *New Horizons* 1995;**3**(3):488–98.

This discussion of the optimal resuscitation fluid for the head-injured patient discusses the pros and cons of lactated Ringer's solution versus 0.9% saline versus colloid (Hetastarch, Pentastarch) versus dextrose solutions versus blood products versus hypertonic saline. Consideration is given to the possible disruption of the blood–brain barrier in head-injured patients. In summary, 0.9% saline appears to be the most effective choice. Hypertonic saline has shown some benefit in short-term stabilization. The most important factor is to resuscitate effectively to prevent hypotension.

12. Marion DW. Head and spinal cord injury. *Neurol Clin* 1998;**16**(2):485–502.

This review discusses the evaluation, work-up, and early treatment for head and spinal cord injuries. Risk factors for delayed neurologic deterioration include loss of consciousness greater than five minutes, posttraumatic amnesia longer than 10 minutes, worsening headache, GCS <15, focal neurologic deficit, and skull fracture. The general management principle in treating traumatic brain injuries is to maintain cerebral blood flow and oxygenation in order to prevent or decrease secondary brain injury.

13. McCrory PR, Berkovic SF. Concussive convulsion. Incidence in sport and treatment recommendations. *Sports Med* 1998;**25**(2):131–6.

This literature review examines the incidence, possible etiologies, and recommendations for treatment for concussive convulsions (CC). CC are infrequent, approximately one out of 70 concussions. The exact etiology is unknown but does not result from, or cause pathologic structural abnormalities. One hypothesis is the causation of a transient functional decerebration that results in the convulsive movements. There is no association with preexisting epilepsy and there is no evidence of resultant posttraumatic epilepsy. Treatment is limited to supportive care and airway management at the time of the injury. No antiseizure treatment or precautions are necessary although medical evaluation to exclude a severe brain injury is needed.

14. Meixensberger J, Roosen K. Clinical and pathophysiological significance of severe neurotrauma in polytraumatized patients. *Langenbecks Arch Surg* 1998; **383**(3–4):214–19.

This review of the literature summarizes the current diagnostic and therapeutic concerns relating to traumatic brain injury. Important prognostic indicators are: injury severity score, Glasgow Coma Score, pupil size and reactivity, coma grade, and primary brain lesion. The potential causes of secondary brain damage include: hypoxia, hypotension, hyperthermia, hyper/hypoglycemia, increased intracranial pressure, decreased cerebral perfusion pressure, seizure activity, vasospasm, and infection.

32. McGrath BJ, Matjasko MJ. Anesthesia and head trauma. *New Horizons* 1995;3(3):523–33.

This review article discusses the concerns of anesthesia in the head-injured patient. Monitoring strategies are delineated. Choice of agents for induction and maintenance of anesthesia is discussed. Consideration is given to the multiply injured patient undergoing a non-neurosurgical procedure in the face of a concomitant head injury. Emphasis is placed on maintaining the cerebral perfusion pressure and limiting the cerebral metabolic rate.

**Mild and moderate traumatic brain injury: Glasgow Coma Scale ≥9**

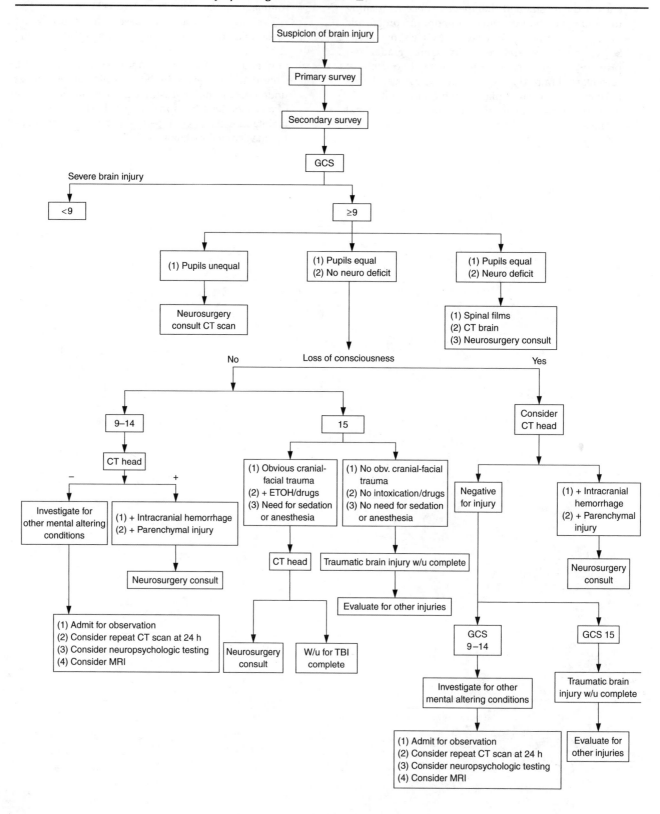

# 22 Maxillofacial trauma

*Bernard J Costello, Keith Silverstein, Patrick M Reilly*

## Primary survey of facial injuries

Blunt or penetrating injuries have the potential to affect structures in the maxillofacial region that must be managed during the *primary* survey of the trauma patient. History and physical findings suggestive of facial injury requiring immediate intervention include:

- history of penetrating or crushing injury and associated trajectory patterns
- history or physical evidence of injury to the laryngeal area
- massive bleeding
- bleeding affecting the airway
- debris in the oropharynx
- stridor
- bilateral parasymphysis mandible fractures may cause an acute airway obstruction (a simple chin lift can alleviate the airway occlusion).

If time permits, a quick facial neurologic exam should be performed prior to paralysis and intubation if facial neurologic injury is suspected from the mechanism or injury pattern.

The C-spine is immobilized if any injury is suspected. Many patients with maxillofacial traumatic injuries have associated cervical spine injuries that require immobilization.[1]

Cervical injuries are discussed elsewhere in this text, but must be considered when evaluating any patient who has sustained a force to the head great enough to cause significant injury. Patients should be immobilized in a cervical collar until an adequate work-up to rule out injury is completed. This may require any operative intervention to proceed with the collar in place.[2]

## Removal of secretions, blood, and/or debris

In attempts to secure a patent airway, physical removal of heavy secretions, blood, and/or debris is essential to avoid aspiration and obstruction. If the patient is obtunded, simple fingersweeping maneuvers may suffice, but suction and retrieval devices should be available. Bronchoscopy may be required for the removal of aspirated bone, soft tissue, and/or teeth.[3,4]

## Surgical airway

Hematoma or active bleeding affecting the airway may require standard emergent intubation under direct laryngoscopy, an emergent fiberoptic intubation or cricothyrotomy. Nasotracheal intubation is contraindicated in the patient with severe midface fractures or suspected base of skull fractures. In the event that severe trauma prohibits visualization for orotracheal or nasotracheal intubation, a surgical airway is obtained. Many studies have shown problems with emergent tracheotomy. Surgical cricothyrotomy is the emergent airway of choice in these situations, since it is more reliable and has fewer complications in the emergent setting. Some authors have suggested the use of, and shown success with, surgical cricothyroidotomy in the field setting by experienced personnel. Gunshot wounds to the face require airway control approximately 30% of the time.[5–7]

## Evaluation and control of bleeding

Because the maxillofacial region is extremely vascular, injury in this region frequently causes significant bleeding. Acute bleeding of a magnitude that compromises the patient's hemodynamics or airway requires emergent treatment with local measures, interventional radiologic treatment or operative exploration and control.[8,9]

- Mild to moderate bleeding in the oral or nasal cavities can usually be controlled with packing or specially designed sponges to tamponade slow bleeding.

- Life-threatening exsanguination from facial vessels is rare and is usually associated with deeper structures rather than superficial facial vessels. While rare, reports of extreme blood loss and even death in patients with facial fractures are present in the literature.[10–12]
- Ligation of the external carotid artery is the preferred method for surgical control of facial bleeding. Many techniques are described, but ligation closer to the source of bleeding diminishes the effect of collateral vessels.[13]

## Secondary survey of facial injuries

After initial resuscitative efforts are complete, a detailed secondary survey of the facial injuries is undertaken.[14] History and physical evidence of facial trauma include the following.

- Mechanism of injury
- Malocclusion
- Facial asymmetry
- Inability to open the mouth fully
- Cranial nerve dysfunction (especially paresthesia or facial nerve weakness)
- Ocular or orbital injury indicated by hematoma, diplopia, enophthalmos, visual changes, and entrapment of musculature. Approximately 65% of patients with facial fractures can be expected to endure some degree of ocular injury[15]
- Step-offs or bony contour irregularities of the craniomaxillofacial skeleton
- Point tenderness of the facial bones
- Depressions over the frontal sinuses
- Nasal deformities, septal hematoma
- Tooth or teeth tenderness
- Soft tissue abrasions, avulsions, laceration or contusions
- Intraoral or intranasal bleeding
- Gingival or mucous membrane lacerations
- Hematoma in the floor of the mouth, posterior auricular space, nasal septum, and conjunctiva indicate probable injury to deeper structures
- Crepitus or emphysema
- TMJ crepitus, dislocation or pain
- Oto- or rhinorrhea
- Parotid gland dysfunction
- Cervical spine injury may occur in a significant number of patients with craniomaxillofacial trauma and a detailed exam should be performed. Immobilization may be required.[16]

## Dentoalveolar injury

Injuries to the teeth and/or alveolus are common in the facial trauma patient. Mandible fractures are associated with dental trauma approximately 30% of the time. All missing teeth or dental appliances should be accounted for at the time of initial assessment. Dental appliances should be saved to help establish the proper occlusion in the patient with facial fractures.[17,18]

- A general dentist or endodontist best handles fractures of the enamel, dentin or roots if no fragments are in danger of immediate displacement. Commercially available calcium hydroxide pastes are available to cover exposed nerve canals until definitive root canal therapy can be performed.
- Intruded teeth should not be repositioned. They may be associated with a high degree of failure when repositioned and devascularized. Subluxed teeth should be repositioned and splinted accordingly.[19,20]
- Time is of the essence and a dental specialist should be consulted as soon as possible when avulsion of a tooth or teeth occurs. If dental or oral and maxillofacial surgical services are not immediately available, replantation of an avulsed tooth should be completed as soon as possible. Teeth replanted within 30 minutes have a greater than 90% chance of retention, but those avulsed for more than two hours generally have a 5% survival rate. Isotonic solution, saliva or milk can be used as a temporary medium for storage.[21,22]
- Although there are no data to support their use definitively, antibiotics are often empirically given to the patient with intraoral injury since these injuries are considered contaminated with oral flora. Penicillin covers the majority of oral bacteria of concern.
- All dental injuries require close follow-up with a general dentist or endodontist.
- Facial, neck, chest, and abdomen radiographs may be required to rule out migration of fragments of teeth and/or bone.
- As mentioned above, fiberoptic bronchoscopy may be required to remove teeth, bone or soft tissue from the brochopulmonary tree.

## Radiology of the facial skeleton

Selective facial radiographs, including PA, lateral, oblique, Towne's view, Water's and exaggerated Water's views, and/or submental vertex views, can be used to evaluate facial injuries that are simple in nature based upon history and physical exam.

Axial and coronal views with 3 mm fine cuts can be used to delineate further facial fracture morphology and diagnose fractures in patients with more severe injuries. Facial swelling and significant soft tissue injury can make examination of the bony skeleton difficult. In the minds of most craniomaxillofacial surgeons CT scanning has become the standard of care for evaluation of moderate to severe facial fractures. Its use is a significant cost burden, but few attempts have been made to evaluate its efficacy and effect upon outcome. At this time no evidence-based data exist regarding the effect upon outcome in these patients. One retrospective review attempted to evaluate the effect of CT scanning and plain radiographs on the treatment of the facial trauma patient. It stated that little benefit was gained from CT scanning or plain films in most facial fractures except those involving the mandible.[23] As a result of inadequate data, there is considerable controversy regarding the indications for CT scanning.

Three-dimensional CT reconstructions are reserved for evaluating only the most severely deforming of injuries. Their effect on outcome has not been evaluated in the literature.

Screening of patients with head injuries for facial fractures is generally not recommended, but evidence is reported of a considerable number of missed facial injuries in patients with depressed mental status.[24] Emphasis should be placed on the tertiary survey of the maxillofacial region rather than relying on CT scanning to make a diagnosis of an occult facial fracture.

## Proximity of injury to neurologic or vascular structures

### Angiography

Both blunt and penetrating injuries can be associated with significant vascular injury that is not immediately apparent. These injuries are often easily diagnosed clinically, but angiography may be used to localize deeper bleeding vessels such as the maxillary artery. Often these injuries can be treated with interventional radiologic techniques such as embolization rather than operative exploration and surgical control.[10–12,25]

### CT brain

Head injury, either closed or open, is discussed elsewhere in this text. Head injuries are associated with facial trauma and should be evaluated accordingly with computed tomography of the brain when indicated. Approximately 20% of patients with closed head injury will exhibit facial fractures. Of those patients with facial fractures admitted to the hospital for management, as many as 55% may have a closed head injury.[26]

### MRI/MRA

These modalities can be used to evaluate neurologic and vascular injury, but few data exist regarding their efficacy in the acute setting when compared with other modalities such as computed tomography and angiography.[27,28]

## Immediate or delayed fracture management

Most facial fractures are best repaired after the initial swelling has resolved to allow for more precise dissection and reduction of delicate fragments.

Procedures in combination with neurosurgery or other subspecialties can be accomplished without increased complications if the patient is going to the operating room for reasons other than facial fracture repair.[29,30]

When possible, gunshot wounds to the face should be reconstructed in the early course of the initial hospital stay to avoid significant scar contracture and loss of soft tissue coverage.[31]

Patients who experience midface fractures that involve the maxillary sinus should be placed on sinus precautions to prevent oral–antral fistula formation:

- no nose blowing
- decongestants and appropriate antibiotics for seven days
- no heavy lifting or Valsalva maneuvers.

A John Rhea Barton bandage can be used to provide stabilization and comfort prior to referring the patient to a maxillofacial specialist.[32]

## Soft tissue injury evaluation

Timing, mechanism, and trajectory of injury are important when deciding the amount of tissue to conservatively debride.

Involvement of the superficial dermis or dermis may require skin care similar to second- or third-degree burns if avulsion or abrasion has occurred.

Orbital and ear trauma may require special reconstructive techniques.

Involvement of the cranial nerves, salivary tissues, and/or the lacrimal system may require immediate or urgent repair as mentioned below.

## Immediate definitive repair of soft tissue injuries

Unlike wounds in other regions of the body, maxillofacial lacerations can be closed even after 24–48 hours after the event, if they have not been extensively contaminated. The length of the "golden period" is variable depending upon host factors. The rich vascular supply allows the surgeon to take significant liberty when deciding which wounds to close.[33]

The need for immediate repair occurs in some specific soft tissue injuries. Patients may be required to go to the operating room immediately or within 24 hours in the event of disruption of cranial nerves, salivary tissues, lacrimal apparatus, orbital tissues, and/or ear avulsion.

The use of tissue adhesive should be considered in dry, superficial wounds. There is some suggestion that time and resources could be saved if superficial wounds not requiring deep layered closure were treated with tissue adhesive rather than fast-absorbing suture or non-resorbable suture materials.[34]

Infection rates after soft tissue injury in the maxillofacial region are believed to be low. Antibiotics are not necessarily needed due to the extensive vascularity of the region. Unfortunately, there are no randomized prospective trials available that thoroughly evaluate this important question in the patient with facial injury.

Since most areas of the face have good elasticity and minimal tension, suture removal should be performed in 4–6 days in most cases. This minimizes the suture-associated reaction and scarring seen with wound repair.

Scalp lacerations can cause significant blood loss. Scalp clips can be used to tamponade the bleeding temporarily if other testing or injury management delays repair.

### Parotid, lacrimal system, and facial nerve injuries

Management of damage to these structures should be considered after all life-threatening injuries have been ruled out. They frequently require long operative repairs and keeping the patient anesthetized for a considerable time. Occult injuries elsewhere can be missed during this time under general anesthesia.

Damage to the parotid duct should be repaired as soon as possible under microscopic guidance. Cannulation of the duct with silastic tubing can be used to encourage healing without stricture, but some authors prefer microsurgical repair without silastic tubing.[35,36]

Injury to the nasolacrimal duct is rare, but should be evaluated by a maxillofacial traumatologist and/or ophthalmologist when a patient sustains nasoorbital-ethmoid (NOE) fractures. The vast majority of patients with NOE fractures do not exhibit injury to the nasolacrimal duct that requires repair or stenting. These injuries can usually wait several days if other injuries demand more attention.[37]

In facial nerve injury, immediate operative repair with or without nerve grafting is essential to achieve acceptable long-term results. Specialists familiar with this procedure should be consulted as soon as possible.[38,39]

### Class II references

14. Hussain K, Wijetunge DB, Grubnic S, Jackson IT. A comprehensive analysis of craniofacial trauma. *J Trauma* 1994;**36**(1):34–47.

    This is one of the few prospective studies dealing with facial trauma patients. The authors prospectively evaluate 950 consecutive patients with any degree of craniofacial trauma. Unlike many of the other retrospective analyses, this study includes the patients treated on an outpatient basis. They report many etiologic and mechanistic aspects of their trauma patients, as well as tabulating the most common types of injury patterns.

22. Andreasen J, Borum M, Jacobsen H, Andreasen H. Replantation of 400 avulsed permanent incisors. Parts 1–4. *Endod Dent Traumatol* 1995;**11**:51–89.

    This is the definitive work available on tooth replantation after avulsion. Andreasen prospectively evaluated 400 patients for an analysis of cellular, physiologic, and clinical aspects of healing after replantation of avulsed incisors. While the work on healing biochemistry is impressive, it does not lend itself to evidence-based protocol construction. Based upon the healing characteristics, they advise immediate replantation with splinting for seven days whenever possible.

27. Lambert DM, Mirvis SE, Shanmuganathan K, Tilghman DL. Computed tomography exclusion of osseous paranasal sinus injury in blunt trauma patients: the "clear sinus" sign. *J Oral Maxillofac Surg* 1997;**55**:1207–11.

    This prospective study evaluates the association of fluid within the paranasal sinuses on CT scan with fractures of the paranasal sinus walls. CT scans were completed on 366 patients to rule out facial fractures. None of the 36 patients without fluid within the paranasal sinuses had maxillary fractures. The authors suggest that unless other areas of the face are suspicious for facial fractures, a quick scan of the sinus region could easily rule out a sinus wall fracture. They suggested that a single Water's view may suffice to rule out fluid within the sinus. The authors admit that further study is needed to say this with any confidence.

28. Rehm CG, Ross SE. Diagnosis of unsuspected facial fractures on routine head CT scans in the unconscious and multiply injured patient. *J Oral Maxillofac Surg* 1995;**53**:522–4.

    This prospective study evaluated all intubated blunt trauma patients who required routine CT scan evaluation of their brains at the time of initial assessment by a trauma surgeon. Of the 116 patients included in the study over one year, there were 19 suspected facial fractures (18 of which required surgical repair). Surprisingly there were 27 unsuspected facial fractures (13 of which required surgical repair).

## Class III references

1. McCabe JB, Angelos MG. Injury to the head and face in patients with cervical spine injury. *Am J Emerg Med* 1984;**2**(4):333–5.

   This retrospective review evaluated 81 patients with acute cervical spine fracture and/or subluxation to determine the incidence of injury to soft tissue or bone in the head or face. Thirty-three patients had injury to the head or face and only five patients had diagnosed fractures of the face or skull.

2. Merritt RM, Williams MF. Cervical spine injury complicating facial trauma: incidence and management. *Am J Otol* 1997;**18**(4):235–8.

   A retrospective chart review was completed over 10 years compiling 1750 patients with facial fractures treated at one institution. Thirty-two patients (1.8%) had associated cervical spine injuries. The concomitant injury did not lengthen the hospital stay of these patients. Immobilization of the neck was continued for the facial fractures treatment phase.

3. Schwarz Y, Bloom Y. Tal-Or E *et al*. Aspirated tooth removal from airway through tracheotomy and flexible bronchoscopy. *J Trauma* 1996;**40**(6):1029–30.

   This is a well-described case report of the technique of retrieval of foreign bodies in the airway after trauma. An interesting use of a Fogarty catheter is described.

4. Fieselmann JF, Zavala DC, Keim LW. Removal of foreign bodies (two teeth) by fiberoptic bronchoscope. *Chest* 1977;**72**:241.

   This is an early report of fiberoptic removal of foreign bodies describing the basic technique and indications.

5. Demetriades D, Chahwan S, Gomez H *et al*. Initial evaluation and management of gunshot wounds to the face. *J Trauma* 1998;**45**(1):39–41.

   This was a well-done retrospective case review of 4139 patients from the Trauma Registry and Trauma Patient Summary database that identifies common features associated with gunshot wounds to the face at a busy urban trauma center. The authors admit to an aggressive protocol for airway management in their trauma patients. They also conclude that most gunshot wounds to the face can be initially managed non-operatively, but they were unable to analyze long-term morbidity and quality of life associated with these injuries that often require further reconstruction.

6. Esses BA, Jafek BW. Cricothyroidotomy: a decade of experience in Denver. *Ann Otol Rhinol Laryngol* 1987;**96**:519–24.

   These authors look critically at the previous literature for and against cricothyroiodotomy and tracheotomy. They also retrospectively analyze 1000 patients for complications and long-term outcome. A 28% complication rate is reported for cricothyroidotomy in this series. Subglottic stenosis occurred in 2.6% of the patients with cricothyroidotomy. This was judged as unacceptable by the authors. They conclude that cricothyrotomy does indeed have a higher incidence of airway stenosis when compared with tracheostomy, but is indicated in emergent situations due to its lower emergent complication rate (especially with respect to acute iatrogenic bleeding).

7. Miklus RM, Elliot C, Snow N. Surgical cricothyroidotomy in the field: experience of a helicopter transport team. *J Trauma* 1989;**29**:506–8.

   Twenty patients were retrospectively evaluated after receiving emergent cricothyroidotomy performed in the field prior to helicopter transport. Seven of the 12 patients with oral and maxillofacial trauma survived with no complications associated with the cricothyroidotomy. Every patient was electively converted to a tracheotomy. Additionally, coroner's reports were reviewed for evaluation of airway complications associated with cricothyroidotomy. No complications were found upon examination of those patients who expired. While this is a small sample size, the effectiveness of this procedure by the field personnel may be a valid consideration.

8. Mokoena T, Abdool-Carrim AT. Haemostasis by angiographic embolization in exsanguinating haemorrhage from facial arteries: a report of two cases. *South Afr Med J* 1991;**80**(11–12):595–7.

   This is one of the few descriptive case reports of angiographic interventional techniques for hemostasis in the facial trauma patient.

9. Sakamoto T, Yagi K, Hiraide A *et al*. Transcatheter embolization in the treatment of massive bleeding due to maxillofacial injury. *J Trauma* 1988;**28**:840–3.

   This study retrospectively evaluated four consecutive patients with massive bleeding in the maxillofacial region that were treated with angiography and embolization. The treatment was successful in all four patients. The authors present their experience with the new technique as well as a comparison with the older techniques of controlling maxillofacial bleeding prior to the development of embolization.

10. Cannell H, Silvester PC, O'Regan MB. Early management of multiply injured patients with maxillofacial injuries transported to hospital by helicopter. *Br J Oral Maxillofac Surg* 1993;**31**:207–12.

    This study evaluates the effectiveness of a helicopter transport system in a trauma center and its effect on treatment of patients with maxillofacial injuries. The authors note that a significant number of patients do present with life-threatening bleeding from the maxillofacial region and require prompt treatment.

11. Murakami WT, Davidson TM, Marshall LF. Fatal epistaxis in craniofacial trauma. *J Trauma* 1983;**23**(1):57–61.

This retrospective case review of two teenage female patients who died from complications associated with severe epistaxis outlines the importance of early diagnosis and treatment of injuries. The authors review the techniques for treating epistaxis and provide a complete algorithm for sequential evaluation and management.

12. Komiyama M, Nishikawa M, Kan M *et al*. Endovascular treatment of intractable oronasal bleeding associated with severe craniofacial injury. *J Trauma* 1998;**44**(2):330–4.

This retrospective case review evaluated nine male patients who underwent angiographic embolization for severe oronasal (mostly nasal) bleeding associated with severe craniofacial traumatic injuries. They reported difficulty with embolization of the ethmoid arteries, but were successful in all other areas. Patient survival was not directly related to oronasal bleeding in this study, but did correlate with presence of intracranial injury.

13. Rosenberg I, Austin JC, Wright PG, King RE. The effect of experimental ligation of the external carotid artery and its major branches on haemorrhage from the maxillary artery. *Int J Oral Surg* 1982;**11**:251–9.

This animal study evaluates the efficacy of surgical ligation of the external carotid and its effect on decreasing bleeding in the maxillofacial region. Higher ligation was found to reduce blood flow more efficiently.

15. Holt GR, Holt JE. Incidence of eye injuries in facial fractures: an analysis of 727 cases. *Otolaryngol Head Neck Surg* 1983;**91**:276.

This retrospective review of 727 patients with facial fractures found that 67% of patients with facial fractures sustained some degree of ocular injury. Most (79%) of these injuries were temporary, 18% were categorized as serious, and 3% caused blindness. The authors recommend documentation of visual acuity and ocular function during a detailed secondary survey.

16. Schultz RC. Facial injuries from automobile accidents: a study of 400 consecutive cases. *Plast Reconstr Surg* 1967;**40**:415–25.

This study is a retrospective review of major craniofacial trauma that documents injuries that are associated with major craniofacial trauma. While somewhat dated, the prevalence of cervical spine injury (approaching 15%) is certainly significant and surprising. Methods of diagnosis of cervical injury were not outlined in detail for this study.

17. Ignatius E, Oikarinen K, Silvennoinen U. Frequency and type of dental traumas in mandibular body and condyle fractures. *Endod Dent Traumatol* 1992;**8**:235.

This retrospective review evaluates the incidence of dental trauma in 207 patients with different types of mandible fractures. Dental injuries were diagnosed in 30% of the patients with mandibular fractures of the body and condyle. The exact classification of the region of the mandible fractures is not well explained in this study.

18. Gassner R, Bosch R, Tuli T, Emshoff R. Prevalence of dental trauma in 6000 patients with facial injuries. *Oral Surg Oral Pathol Oral Radiol Endod* 1999;**87**:27–33.

This was a retrospective review of 6000 admissions for dental trauma, facial trauma or both. The prevalence of dental injuries in patients with facial trauma was 48.25%. The study relies entirely on patients who were admitted to a hospital service for treatment. Presumably, a significant portion of patients were treated on an outpatient basis. Thus, the percentage may be even higher than calculated.

19. Turley PK, Joiner MW, Hellstrom S. The effect of orthodontic extrusion on traumatically intruded teeth. *Am J Orthod* 1984;**85**:47–56.

This study proclaimed a worse outcome in patients with manipulation of traumatically intruded teeth with the aid of orthodontics.

20. Kinirons M. Traumatically intruded permanent incisors: a study of treatment and outcome. *Br Dent J* 1991;**170**:144–7.

This retrospective analysis evaluated 21 consecutive patients with one or more traumatically intruded incisors. The patients were followed for two years and data were collected to evaluate survival and complications. Those teeth that were passively watched did as well as those that were surgically manipulated. Most other authors suggest passively watching the intruded incisor.

21. Hammarstrom L, Pierce A, Blomlof L *et al*. Tooth avulsion and replantation – a review. *Endod J Traumatol* 1986;**2**(1):1–8.

This is a fairly good review of the literature and techniques for management of dentoalveolar injuries, but the paper is mostly opinion and not evidence based. Few outcome data exist on this subject.

22. Thai KN, Hummel RP, Kitzmiller WJ, Luchette A. The role of CT scanning in the management of facial trauma. *J Trauma* 1997;**43**(2):214–18.

This retrospective review attempts to conclude that CT scanning adds little to the management of facial trauma. The authors state that only 18% of patients had management altered by radiographic findings on CT or plain films. This was concluded by reviewing the documentation of a change in treatment plan relative to the presumed evaluation of the radiographic findings. The discussion section of this article points out several difficulties using this method and other issues with this study. Significant selection bias and data recording inconsistencies make this study less than ideal. As a result no management-oriented conclusions can be drawn from this retrospective review.

24. Haug RH, Savage JD, Likavec MJ, Conforti PJ. A review of 100 closed head injuries associated with facial fractures. *J Oral Maxillofac Surg* 1992;**50**:218–22.

   A retrospective review of 100 patients with closed head injury at an urban trauma center was analyzed for associated facial fractures. Of these patients, 17.5% had maxillofacial injuries. Complications in this group were similar to those patients without head injuries from other studies.

25. Chang CJ, Chen YR, Noordhoff MS *et al*. Facial bone fracture associated with carotid-cavernous sinus fistula. *J Trauma* 1990;**30**:1335.

   Patients who were suspected to have a carotid-cavernous sinus fistula by clinical exam or radiographic finding were studied with angiography. Out of 989 facial traumas, 10 patients with carotid-cavernous sinus fistulas were detected. This incidence of 1% is significant considering that other patients in their patient groups may not have been diagnosed or expired prior to evaluation.

26. Davidoff G, Jakebowski M, Thomas D, Alpert M. The spectrum of closed head injury in facial trauma victims: incidence and impact. *Ann Emerg Med* 1988;**17**:6–9.

   This retrospective analysis reviews 200 admissions for acute facial fractures at an urban trauma center. The authors noted a 55% incidence of closed head injury as diagnosed by CT scan and/or history and physical exam. The full spectrum of closed head injury was included in this study.

29. Derdyn C, Persing JA, Broaddus WC *et al*. Craniofacial trauma: an assessment of risk related to timing of surgery. *Plast Reconstr Surg* 1990;**86**(2):238–47.

   This retrospective review of 4000 patients with head injuries identified 49 patients with combined facial fractures and cerebral trauma. No increased incidence of complications was noted when patients were taken for repair of facial fractures in the early (0–3 days), middle (4–7 days) or late (>7 days) time periods. The authors concluded that early surgical repair of facial fractures did not appear to have a negative impact on recovery.

30. Chang C, Chen Y, Noordoff S, Chang C. Maxillary involvement in central craniofacial fractures with associated head injuries. *J Trauma* 1994;**37**(5):807–11.

   This retrospective review evaluates 177 patients with central craniofacial fractures and maxillary components. The authors grouped each of these patients by Glasgow Coma Scale: Group I (13–15); Group II (9–12); and Group III (3–8). They noted that regardless of head injury severity, the fracture repair did not affect the outcomes in each group. Although they have no controls in this study, they do conclude that delaying facial fracture repair because of a more severe head injury is unfounded and possibly flawed in concept. Unnecessary extended hospital stays and prolonged reconstruction may be avoided by treating the maxillofacial fractures early in the course of the patient's initial hospital stay.

31. Gruss JS, Antonyshyn O, Phillips JH. Early definitive bone and soft-tissue reconstruction of major gunshot wounds of the face. *Plast Reconstr Surg* 1991:**87**:436.

   Thirty-seven patients with gunshot wounds to the face were retrospectively evaluated when reconstructed in the early phase of their injury healing. Early bone grafting and soft tissue reconstruction techniques tended to make long-term reconstructive efforts easier to manage. This review is mostly opinion, but illustrates the art of medicine that is difficult to appreciate with prospective studies.

32. Barton JR. A systematic bandage for fractures of the lower jaw. *Am Med Recorder Phila* 1819;**2**:153.

   This is an early report of a bandage used to treat a maxillofacial injury. Variations are still used today to provide comfort and stabilization after a mandible fracture.

33. Berk WA, Osbourne DD, Taylor DD. Evaluation of the "golden period" for wound repair: 204 cases from a third world emergency department. *Ann Emerg Med* 1988;**17**:496–500.

   This retrospective analysis evaluated host factors associated with wound closure success such as diabetes, immune dysfunction, and compliance. Considerable variability was found in patients of different age, immune function, wound location, and comorbid disease state.

34. Osmond MH, Klassen TP, Quinn JV. Economic comparison of a tissue adhesive and suturing in the repair of pediatric facial lacerations. *J Pediatr* 1995;**126**(6);892–5.

   This study uses cost-minimization analysis and a willingness-to-pay survey to evaluate and compare the use of tissue adhesive, resorbable, and non-resorbable suture materials for the treatment of superficial facial lacerations in children under 12. They conclude that it would be less expensive to use the tissue adhesive because the physician treatment time is significantly decreased (including follow-up). The assumption is made that the aesthetic result is the same for each technique when performed by emergency room physicians and staff. This assumption is based upon data from other studies.

35. Epker BN, Brunette JC. Trauma to the parotid gland and duct: primary treatment and management of complications. *J Oral Surg* 1970;**28**:657.

   This is a classic review of the diagnosis and management of injuries to the parotid gland and duct.

Several cases are reported in detail and the literature to date is reviewed. The management of complications is also discussed.

36. Hallock GG. Microsurgical repair of the parotid duct. *Microsurgery* 1992;**13**:243.

    The technique for repair of parotid duct injury is reviewed and a microsurgical technique is discussed. No long-term data are available to assess outcome after attempted repair.

37. Gruss JS, Hurwitz JJ, Nik NA, Kassel EE. The pattern and incidence of nasolacrimal injury in nasoorbital-ethmoid fracture: the role of delayed assessment and dacryocystorhinostomy. *Br J Plast Surg* 1985;**38**:116–21.

    This retrospective review of 46 severe NOE fractures confirms the low incidence of nasolacrimal injuries. Surgical management of nasolacrimal injuries is reviewed.

38. Coker NJ. Management of traumatic injuries to the facial nerve. *Otolaryngol Clin North Am* 1991;**24**:215.

    This article provides an excellent review of the management of facial nerve trauma including intracranial, intratemporal, and extracranial injury management. Outcome data are currently not available to evaluate different treatment strategies. Most of the management techniques are adapted from the neurosurgical literature examining peripheral nerve repair other than the facial nerve.

39. Tachmes L, Woloszyn T, Marini C *et al*. Parotid gland and facial nerve trauma: a retrospective review. *J Trauma* 1990;**30**:1395.

    This is a retrospective analysis of five patients who had facial nerve trauma and repair of their injuries. Because they noted better long-term results in this limited study, the authors advocate primary repair within 24 hours when possible. This recommendation is mostly theoretical in nature, but is supported in the literature that examines repair of other peripheral nerves. The authors also discuss the management of sialoceles, salivary fistulas, and other complications.

## Initial evaluation of traumatic facial injuries

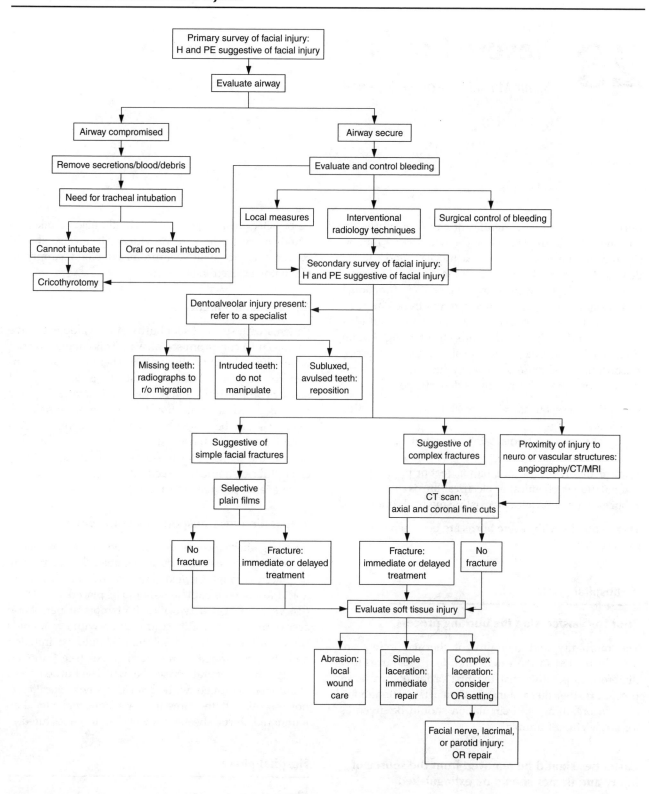

# 23 Severe burns

*Samir M Fakhry, Ronnie S Benoit*

Burn injuries remain a significant cause of morbidity and mortality in the United States, with over 2 million significant thermal injuries each year and 12 000 deaths. Many studies have documented an improvement in survival as well as improvements in functional and cosmetic outcomes following recent trends in treatment. Management of severe burns requires a multidisciplinary and multifaceted approach, utilizing several prehospital, hospital, and posthospital resources. According to the definitions set by the American Burn Association, severe burns can be described as:

- full-thickness burns >10% total body surface area (TBSA)
- partial-thickness burns >25% in adults or 20% at extremes of age
- burns involving the face, hands, feet or perineum
- inhalational, chemical or electrical burns
- burns in patients with preexisting medical conditions.

These patients with severe burns are best managed at a burn center.

## Prehospital phase

### Prior to transfer, stop the burning process

The morbidity and mortality of thermal injury are directly related to the extent and depth of burn. It is therefore imperative that the first order of care is to prevent further thermal injury. Concurrent attention to airway, breathing, and circulation should be given as for any victim of trauma.

### Casualties should be removed from the source of injury and flames should be extinguished

Care should be taken to ensure that smoldering fabric is removed. Liquid chemical burns should be diluted with copious amounts of water. Powdered chemicals should be brushed away. Special care should also be taken to avoid injury to the care provider. All jewelry should be removed to avoid compromised blood supply in edematous extremities.

### Airway management

Patients with severe facial burns can develop extensive edema and a compromised airway. This edema may not be manifested early in the course. Therefore, early intubation should be considered for stridor or other signs of airway compromise. Severe smoke inhalation also may be considered an indication for intubation. Inhalation injury should be suspected in patients confined in a closed space or in those with a history of unconsciousness. If the patient's face is severely burned, endotracheal tubes should be secured using umbilical ties since edema prevents the adherence of tape.

### Preparation for transport to a burn center

Two large-bore intravenous catheters should be placed in non-injured extremities if possible. Catheters may be placed through burned skin if no other site is available. Intraosseous catheters should be placed in children (<6 years of age) if two initial attempts at peripheral access are unsuccessful. Resuscitation with crystalloids (2 l of lactated Ringer's solution) should be initiated and then continued at the burn center (see Parkland formula in "Hospital phase" below). The burned areas should be wrapped with clean dressings. Sterility is not essential. If the dressings are not available, then laundered shirts, sheets or towels can be substituted.

## Hospital phase

### Physical examination

Other than the obvious severe burn, attention should be paid to findings of carbonaceous sputum, singed nasal hair, hoarseness, stridor or wheezing. Fiberoptic laryngoscopy allows differentiation of those patients with inhalation injuries who, while at risk for upper airway obstruction, do not require intubation.[1] Patients with minimal supraglottic mucosal edema, mild pooling of secretions, and mobile vocal folds may not require intubation. In one review of over 1400 patients, the overall mortality for patients with inhalation injury was 31% compared with 4.3% for those without inhalation injury.[2] Nevertheless, the most important factor in predicting mortality was %TBSA burn or a combination of %TBSA burn and patient age.

## Ventilation

Improvement in survival has been linked to improved ventilatory support in severely burned patients.

## Oxygen

The two most common asphyxiants in smoke are carbon monoxide and hydrogen cyanide. Carbon monoxide is tightly bound to hemoglobin and thus impairs oxygen delivery. Symptoms of carbon monoxide poisoning occur at carboxyhemoglobin (COHb) levels >10% and the condition is fatal at levels >60%. With suspected inhalation injury (burns in closed spaces), arterial blood gases (ABGs) with COHb levels should be performed upon arrival at a burn center, but the COHb may be low secondary to previously administered oxygen. High concentrations of oxygen are the essential basis of treatment. The half-life of carboxyhemoglobin is four hours at room air and 40 minutes using 100% oxygen. Initial treatment for hydrogen cyanide toxicity is also 100% oxygen. Utilization of hyperbaric oxygen (HBO) therapy, while attractive, remains controversial in inhalation injury. Some studies suggest some benefit from HBO, while others show no benefit.[3,4] Indeed, some studies suggest a worsened outcome with the use of HBO and do not recommend its use, while others recommend its use in superficial dermal wounds.

## Intravenous fluids

In addition to massive tissue and fluid losses, burn patients suffer from inflammatory changes via cellular mediators that potentiate edema, inflammation, and vasodilatation.[5] Therefore, judicious fluid administration remains the hallmark of burn resuscitation. Fluid requirement is based on the %TBSA. The extent of a burn can be quickly estimated using the Lund–Browder charts (Figures 23.1 and 23.2).[6] These charts are available in burn centers and demonstrate the difference in per cent burns in infants, children, and adults.

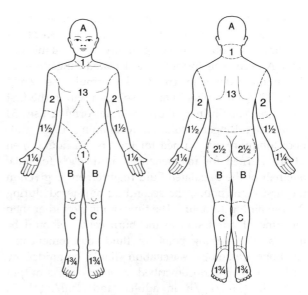

Relative percentages of areas affected by growth

| Area | Age 10 | Age 15 | Adult |
|---|---|---|---|
| A = ½ of head | 5½ | 4½ | 3½ |
| B = ½ of one thigh | 4¼ | 4½ | 4¾ |
| C = ½ of one leg | 3 | 3¼ | 3½ |

**Figure 23.1** Lund–Browder chart to estimate %TBSA in children and adults. Reprinted with permission from reference 6.

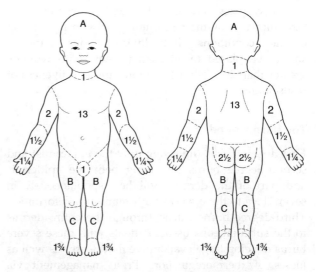

Relative percentages of areas affected by growth

| Area | Age 0 | Age 1 | Age 5 |
|---|---|---|---|
| A = ½ of head | 9½ | 8⅓ | 6½ |
| B = ½ of one thigh | 2¾ | 3¼ | 4 |
| C = ½ of one leg | 2½ | 2½ | 2¾ |

**Figure 23.2** Lund–Browder chart to estimate %TBSA in infants and children. Reprinted with permission from reference 6.

There are several formulas in use in burn resuscitation. The Parkland formula estimates fluid needs for the first 24 hours following injury to be 4 ml/kg/%TBSA burn. This formula uses lactated Ringer's solution without dextrose. The Brooke formula uses 2 ml/kg/%TBSA burn plus 2 l of D5 solution within the first 24 hours. The Shriners Burn Institute formula uses 5 l of lactated Ringer's solution (containing 1.25% salt-poor albumin)/m$^2$ burned for the first 24 hours, then 2 l/m$^2$ burned for maintenance.[5] With each formula, one half of the calculated fluid requirement is given in the first eight hours, the second administered during the remaining 16 hours. The time of injury, rather than the time of admission to the burn center, should be used as the starting point for fluid requirement calculations. Ongoing resuscitation should be guided by end-organ perfusion described as hourly urine output desirable (1 ml/kg/h in adults, and 2 ml/kg/h in children). However, the increased metabolic rate seen in burn patients may cause tissue breakdown and hyperglycaemia, leading to a falsely increased urinary output. Crystalloids (lactated Ringer's solution) should be the primary fluid for burn resuscitation. The use of colloids in burn patients remains controversial and varies among institutions.[7] Colloid administration in a patient with acute inflammation may potentiate fluid losses secondary to increased capillary leaking. Equally controversial is the use of hypertonic saline in resuscitation. Invasive hemodynamic monitoring may be necessary in very severely burned patients unresponsive to "traditional" volume resuscitation or with preexisting cardiac conditions. Indwelling bladder catheters should be placed in all burn patients with wounds greater than 20% TBSA to monitor the effectiveness of resuscitation.

### The burn wound

First-degree burns (involving only the epidermis) and second-degree burns (involving both the epidermis and part of the dermis) will heal spontaneously in seven days to three weeks with minimum deformities. Third-degree burns extend through the entire dermis to the subcutaneous tissue. Patients with these severe burns develop large evaporative fluid losses as well as losses of thermoregulation. Prior management via daily dressing changes and awaiting eschar separation has been changed to aggressive management via early staged excision of the burn wound. Early excision and grafting (within the first week) in an effort to decrease the stress of the prolonged burn wound has been shown in some studies to decrease mortality in young burn victims. These studies also report a reduction in burn wound sepsis and in the length of stay. However,

this treatment algorithm may not be beneficial in the elderly and may even be harmful.[8] A limited approach (e.g. limiting surgery to less than three hours and excising less than 10% TBSA) may improve survival. The patients are returned frequently to the operating room for further debridement until the entire burn wound is excised. Early grafting follows excision.

### Topical antimicrobials

As sepsis and burn wound infections remain major causes of mortality in burn patients, the role of topical antimicrobial agents has increased. The three topical medications commonly utilized to delay the process of wound infection are silver sulfadiazine, mafenide acetate, and silver nitrate. Silver sulfadiazine is probably the most commonly used antimicrobial because it is painless in application and it does not have the potential to cause systemic metabolic derangements. However, its use can lead to leukopenia and thrombocytopenia. Side effects of mafenide include pain on application and metabolic acidosis. Petrolatum jelly can be used on facial burns.

### Systemic burn wound care

All deep burns are considered tetanus prone and require tetanus toxoid if not given in the past five years. If the patient has not been immunized, he/she should receive both tetanus toxoid and passive immunization with tetanus immunoglobulin.

### Analgesia

Significant pain is present in patients with second-degree burns and in patients undergoing burn wound excision. Intravenous narcotics achieve efficient and predictable results.[9] Morphine sulfate (0.1 mg/kg) can be given intravenously every 1–2 hours for pain control. Another method of pain control is topical administration of a local anesthetic such as lidocaine to areas where split-thickness grafts have been harvested.[10] Oral doses of ibuprofen have been mentioned for pain relief, but studies have not been conclusive in burn patients.[11] Also, ibuprofen has been shown to reduce body temperature and metabolic rate in burn patients, but these reductions have not been shown to be beneficial.[12] Additionally, ibuprofen has been shown in some animal studies to reduce the pulmonary and mesenteric vasoconstriction which occur secondary to arachidonic acid metabolism. However, with the lack of randomized clinical trials in the use of this medication, ibuprofen cannot be recommended for routine use in burn patients.

## Gastritis

Patients with burns >25% TBSA are at risk for stress gastritis and should receive prophylaxis with either antacids, sucralfate or $H_2$-blockers. Routine endoscopy is not indicated. A nasogastric tube should be placed in all patients with severe burns since these patients are prone to paralytic ileus.

## Circumferential extremity burns

Patients with deep second-degree or third-degree burns of an extremity run the risk of developing compromise to the circulation of that limb. Coagulated burned tissue, eschar, acts like a constricting band around an extremity. The resultant edema from the injured tissue, as well as that from resuscitation, can cause an increase in the pressure of the subcutaneous tissues of the involved limb and thus impair flow. An early symptom of impaired flow is paresthesia. Early physical exam findings include tense subeschar tissues, numbness or weakness distally (compromised flow to nervous tissue), cyanosis (impaired venous return), and delayed capillary refill (impaired arterial inflow). However, it should be noted that loss of palpable pulses is a late finding and usually indicates necrosis of underlying tissues.

Treatment involves escharotomy. This procedure can be performed at the bedside, under IV sedation, using an electrocautery or a scalpel. The escharotomy is performed through the burned tissue on either the medial or lateral aspects of the involved limb. It is essential that the incision extend through all of the burned tissue. The depth of the incision should extend through the subcutaneous tissue to, but not through, the fascia. Care should be taken not to expose the underlying bone with the escharotomy incision. If there is no evidence of improved perfusion, a second escharotomy should be performed on the opposite side. If there is still no improvement, a fasciotomy should be performed in the operating suite. In legs with impaired circulation, an incision should always be made over the anterior compartment since its small volume renders it at risk for ischemia. The escharotomy wounds should be dressed in saline-soaked dressings and kept moist to avoid desiccation and further destruction of the tissue.

## Infections

These immunocompromised patients are prone to nosocomial pneumonia, line sepsis, and burn wound infections. In many burn centers, it has been the practice to change central lines frequently, e.g. every 48 hours. However, recent data suggest no advantage in changing central line insertion sites every 48 hours.[13] There has been improvement in survival and a decreased incidence of Gram-negative infections with improvements in isolation of burned patients.[14] Burn wound infections remain a significant source of morbidity and mortality. However, routine wound surveillance with biopsy is not indicated. With the suspicion of wound sepsis, a biopsy with determination of quantitative bacterial culture may be performed (considered positive if $>10^5$ CFU/g tissue).

Treatment should be tailored for both Gram-positive and Gram-negative organisms until sensitivity results are available.[15] With the discrepancy in the definition of burn wound infections, a series of proposed burn wound infections have been developed to include burn wound impetigo, open burn-related surgical wound infection, burn wound cellulitis, and invasive infection in unexcised burn wounds. These criteria await further approval.[16]

## Nutrition

Early enteral feeding with decreased use of parenteral hyperalimentation is used by several centers in an effort to decrease bacterial translocation and subsequent nosocomial pneumonias. Studies are being done to assess the optimal nutritional pharmacology for burned patients. Burn patients require high-protein nutritional supplementation. Traditionally, feedings are withheld before, during, and after operative procedures. However, a recent study found enteral nutrition during the operative procedures is associated with fewer calorie deficits and fewer wound infections than in patients who had their feedings withheld.[17] However, there were no differences in sepsis, pneumonia or mortality rate.

## Circumferential chest wall burns

Deep circumferential burns of the chest wall impair ventilation because of loss of thoracic compliance due to the restrictive eschar. Indications for escharotomy include worsening oxygenation and ventilation with an increased arterial carbon dioxide tension and elevations in airway pressures. The lines of incision are along the anterior axillary lines, through all the burned tissue, just past the costal margins. These incisions should be connected inferiorly with a subcostal incision. They should be dressed with saline-soaked dressings and kept continuously moist to prevent desiccation.

## Electrical burns

There are two types of electrical burns: electrical flashover and electrical conduction.

Flashover burns occur when electricity is discharged, encompassing and burning areas of exposed skin. This burn can range from first to third degree. Management is identical to that of thermal injuries mentioned above.

Electrical conduction burns occur when high-voltage current passes through the body. This burn can be the most devastating of all thermal injuries. The electricity travels through the tissue and heat is dissipated from tissues with high resistance such as bone. The injury is frequently underestimated since the skin is typically not involved. The initial injury can cause electrical myocardial standstill, which can progress into ventricular fibrillation. This arrhythmia should be suspected in any unconscious electrical injury patient without a pulse. Care should be guided by the Advanced Cardiac Life Support Protocol. Electrical injury can also cause the development of myoglobinuria from injured muscle, leading to acute tubular necrosis. These patients should receive adequate IV hydration (e.g. 1000–1500 ml/h) to maintain an adequate urine output (2–3 ml/kg/h) until all visible pigment is gone from the urine. The use of sodium bicarbonate or mannitol remains controversial.

Patients suffering electrical injuries should also be observed for the development of compartment syndrome of their extremities. If patients develop tense muscle compartments with paresthesias, then fasciotomies should be performed.

## Posthospital phase

### Outpatient management

Patients can be followed on an outpatient basis with adequate pain medication and education about dressing changes. For a clean wound, a semisynthetic dressing material requiring less frequent changes, such as Biobrane®, may be easier to use than twice-a-day dressing with Silvadene.[18]

### Rehabilitation

Rehabilitation should be initiated early in the patient's hospital course in order to decrease the incidence of contracture. This phase represents the most important phase of care to many patients. Several burn centers have targeted burn rehabilitation (occupational therapy, physical therapy, passive and active range-of-motion exercises) as important adjuncts to the overall management of burn victims. Early and aggressive rehabilitation should be instituted in an effort to improve functional outcome.

## Class I References

3. Scheinkestel CD, Bailey M, Myles PS *et al*. Hyperbaric or normobaric oxygen for acute carbon monoxide poisoning: a randomised controlled clinical trial. *Med J Aust* 1999;**170**:203–10.

   This is a prospective, randomized, double-blind trial that evaluated 191 patients with severe carbon monoxide poisoning to receive hyperbaric (HBO) or normobaric (NBO) oxygen therapy. They found no advantage to HBO therapy and actually, a worsened outcome (measured by neuropsychological testing) with the use of HBO. This was a well-done study, but they excluded burn patients.

10. Jellish WS, Gamelli RL, Furry PA, McGill VL, Fluder EM. Effect of topical local anesthetic application to skin harvest sites for pain management in burn patients undergoing skin-grafting procedures. *Ann Surg* 1999;**229**:115–20.

    This is a randomized, blinded study with 60 patients separated into three arms to receive normal saline, 0.5% bupivacaine or 2% lidocaine (all with 1:200 000 epinephrine and aerosolized) to areas where skin harvest has occurred. They were followed clinically with pain scores and physiologic markers of pain.

11. Petersen KL, Brennum J, Dahl JB. Experimental evaluation of the analgesic effect of ibuprofen on primary and secondary hyperalgesia. *Pain* 1997;**70**:167–74.

    This study evaluated ibuprofen's ability to blunt the response to pain produced by mechanical stimulation and by burn injury. This was a double-blind, randomized, prospective study using 20 healthy male volunteers that discovered that ibuprofen did not reduce the hyperalgesia following burn injury.

12. Wallace BH, Caldwell FT, Cone JB. Ibuprofen lowers body temperature and metabolic rate of humans with burn injury. *J Trauma* 1992;**32**:154–7.

    This study prospectively examined body and rectal temperatures as well as metabolic rates of 15 patients with burn injuries before and after the administration of oral doses of ibuprofen. Patients served as their own controls. There was a significant reduction in temperature and metabolic rate after 72 hours of ibuprofen, but it is not known if this is beneficial.

13. Kealey GP, Chang P, Heinle J, Rosenquist MD, Lewis RW. Prospective comparison of two management strategies of central venous catheters in burn patients. *J Trauma* 1995;**38**:344–9.

    A prospective evaluation of 42 burn patients who underwent central venous catheter changes to either a new site or over a guide wire. Also evaluated were incidence of infection when central lines were placed within and outside of 5 cm of burn wound.

18. Gerding RL, Emerman CL, Effron D *et al*. Outpatient management of partial-thickness burns: Biobrane®

versus 1% silver sulfadiazine. *Ann Emerg Med* 1990;**19**:121–4.

This was a randomized, prospective study comparing the use of Biobrane® (26 patients) with 1% silver sulfadiazine (26 patients) on small wounds. There was improved healing time with burns secondary to grease or tar with Biobrane® but not with contact burns compared to silver sulfadiazine. Patients also experienced less pain with Biobrane® but it was used only on clean wounds.

## Class II references

1. Muehlberger T, Kunar D, Munster A, Couch M. Efficacy of fiberoptic laryngoscopy in the diagnosis of inhalation injuries. *Arch Otolaryngol Head Neck Surg* 1998;**124**:1003–7.

   Six of 11 patients had clinical findings that traditionally would require intubation. Following laryngoscopy, none of the patients was intubated. Patients underwent serial laryngoscopies and criteria for observation were not clear.

2. Smith DL, Cairns BA, Ramadan F *et al.* Effect of inhalation injury, burn size, and age on mortality: a study of 1447 consecutive burn patients. *J Trauma* 1994;**37**:655–9.

   A retrospective review of 1447 patients was performed to assess the relative contribution of burn size, age, and the presence of inhalation injury as predictors of mortality and to identify which combination of these variables provides the best predictive model of outcome. The most important single predictor of mortality was the burn size.

4. Niezgoda JA, Ciani P, Folden BW, Ortega RL, Slade JB, Storrow AB. The effect of hyperbaric oxygen therapy on a burn wound model in human volunteers. *Plast Reconstr Surg* 1997;**99**:1620–5.

   The authors created a burn wound on the volar aspect of the forearm of 12 healthy, non-smoking volunteers and then randomized them to hyperbaric oxygen or sea-level air-breathing equivalent. There were significant reductions in lesion size, wound exudation, and hyperemia on day 2 of treatment with hyperbaric oxygen.

8. Kirn DS, Luce EA. Early excision and grafting versus conservative management of burns in the elderly. *Plast Reconstr Surg* 1998;**102**:1013–17.

   A retrospective review of 73 elderly patients was performed. Patients who underwent early excision and grafting (within seven days) had a greater mortality rate and length of stay than those treated conservatively, though the differences were not statistically significant. This study suffers from being a retrospective chart review with some selection bias.

14. McManus AT, Mason AD, McManus WF, Pruitt BA. A decade of reduced gram-negative infections and mortality associated with improved isolation of burned patients. *Arch Surg* 1994;**129**:1306–9.

    The authors retrospectively looked at the incidence of infection and the mortality rate in two groups of patients over a 20 year period. The patients were divided into an early open ward era (10 years) then an isolated patient ward era (next 10 years). They discovered a greater incidence of Gram-negative infections in the early open ward era.

15. Heggers JP, Villareal C, Edgar P *et al.* Ciprofloxacin as a therapeutic modality in pediatric burn wound infections. *Arch Surg* 1998;**133**:1247–50.

    In this descriptive study, the authors treated 56 pediatric burn patients (average age 8.4 years) with ciprofloxacin and found reductions in bacterial counts and no arthropathy.

17. Jenkins ME, Gottschlich MM, Warden GD. Enteral feeding during operative procedures in thermal injuries. *J Burn Care Rehabil* 1994;**15**:199–205.

    This was a study of 80 patients randomized to receive enteral support during operative procedures or support withheld before, during, and immediately after surgery. Feeding tubes were placed within the duodenum. Unfed patients had a significant calorie deficit and increased wound infections compared to fed patients. However, there were no differences in length of stay, sepsis, pneumonia or mortality.

## Class III references

5. Nguyen TT, Gilpin DA, Meyer NA, Herndon DN. Current treatment of severely burned patients. *Ann Surg* 1996;**1**:14–25.

   A very good review article from the Shriners Burn Institute in Galveston focusing on the physiology and cellular reactions in burn patients.

6. Lund CC, Browder NC. The estimation of areas of burns. *Surg Gynecol Obstet* 1944;**72**:352–8.

   In this widely quoted study, the authors perform their best estimates of the surface proportions to be used in the study of burns. They use estimates based on other estimates and some measurements.

7. Fakhry SM, Alexander J, Smith D, Meyer AA, Peterson HD. Regional and institutional variation in burn care. *J Burn Care Rehabil* 1995;**16**:86–90.

   A survey of burn care was sent to 140 institutions. There was a 60% response rate (83 institutions) submitting answers to questions ranging from choice of fluids, histamine blockers, initiation of tube feeding, and topical antimicrobial use. There was variation in some of the responses.

9. MacLennan N, Heimbach DM, Cullen BF. Anesthesia for major thermal injury. *Anesthesiology* 1998;**3**:749–70.

   A good review article on major thermal injury.

16. Peck MD, Weber J, McManus A, Sheridan R, Heimbach DM. Surveillance of burn wound infections: a proposal for definitions. *J Burn Care Rehabil* 1998;**19**: 386–9.

A working subcommittee of the Committee on the Organization and Delivery of Burn Care (with the approval of the Board of Trustees of the American Burn Association) delineates a set of burn wound definitions.

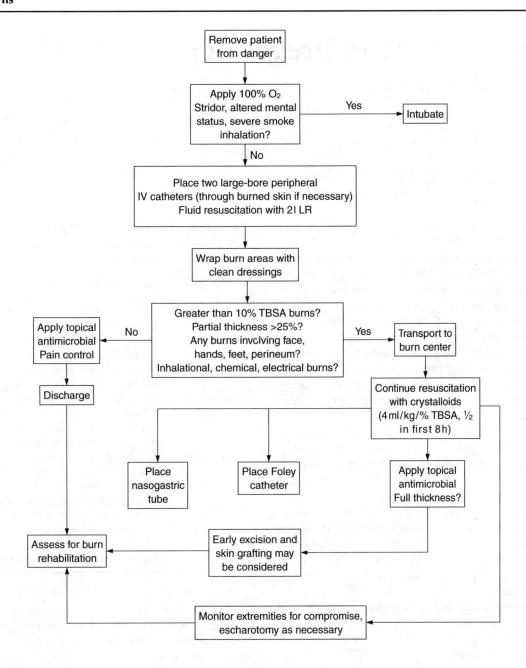

# 24 Trauma in pregnancy

*Glenn K Schemmer*

## Introduction

Trauma is the leading non-obstetric cause of maternal morbidity and mortality.[1] Motor vehicle accidents, violent assaults, and falls are the most common causes of severe maternal trauma.[2,3] Non-fatal trauma has been estimated to occur in 7% of all pregnancies.[4] Fortunately, most injuries are incidental and do not have an impact on pregnancy outcomes. Nonetheless, there is a 9% incidence of pregnancy-related complications in non-catastrophic injuries including preterm labor, placental abruption, fetomaternal hemorrhage, and fetal death.

Optimal maternal and fetal outcomes in the pregnant trauma victim require an informed and organized approach by a team of physicians. A basic understanding of maternal physiologic changes and fetal medicine is helpful to understand the differences between gravid and non-gravid patients. These changes must be taken into consideration during the evaluation and treatment of the injured parturient. As a detailed description of these concepts is beyond the scope of this chapter, Table 24.1 summarizes the major changes pertinent to the trauma patient.

The purpose of this chapter is to provide an overview of trauma in pregnancy. This information will supplement other chapters that address the management of specific types of trauma.

## Maternal assessment

The first steps in caring for a pregnant trauma patient are the evaluation and stabilization of the mother. A concurrent fetal evaluation can be undertaken but it should not delay or interfere with the maternal assessment. Maternal stabilization is a priority and should not be compromised on behalf of the fetus. A cesarean delivery performed prior to maternal stabilization may

**Table 24.1** Physiologic changes of pregnancy

| Organ system | Alteration |
| --- | --- |
| Cardiovascular | Cardiac output: 30–50% increase |
| | Heart rate: 20–30% increase |
| | Systemic vascular resistance: 20–30% decrease |
| Pulmonary | Minute ventilation: 20–50% increase |
| | Tidal volume: 20–45% increase |
| | Functional residual capacity: 20% decrease |
| | $PaCO_2$: decreases to 30 mmHg |
| Hematologic | Blood volume: 50% increase |
| | plasma volume: 30–40% increase |
| | red blood cell volume: 20% increase |
| | Increased coagulation factors |
| Gastrointestinal | Decreased gastric motility |
| | Delayed gastric emptying |
| | Decreased gastric pH |
| | Relaxation of lower esophageal sphincter |
| Genitourinary | Glomerular filtration rate: 50% increase |
| | Ureteral dilatation |
| | Uterine enlargement |
| | Bladder becomes intraabdominal |

further compromise her status. In that certain maternal resuscitative measures may improve fetal testing, such intervention may also be unnecessary.

## General approach to the pregnant trauma patient

The basic principles of general trauma care apply equally well in the obstetric population. The initial approach to the pregnant trauma patient differs little from the non-pregnant state. Still, physicians should be aware that pregnancy can affect the type and severity of injury, as well as alter the presenting signs and symptoms. Several salient features pertinent to the pregnant trauma patient are worthy of comment.

## Different organs of injury

As the pregnancy progresses, the uterus enlarges and displaces the bowel into the upper abdomen. Thus, the uterus and bladder are more prone to blunt and penetrating injuries.[5] At the same time, the risk of intestinal injury is reduced. Conversely, serious retroperitoneal hemorrhage following lower abdominal and pelvic trauma occurs more frequently than in non-pregnant women.

## Obscurement of peritoneal signs

During later pregnancy, as the abdominal wall is stretched, the normal response to peritoneal irritation is altered. Therefore, expected guarding and rebound may be absent even after documented bowel injury. As a result, physical exam may be more misleading with advancing pregnancy.

## Supine hypotension

The pregnant uterus can lead to significant aortocaval compression, resulting in decreased venous return to the heart. Cardiac output and blood pressure can drop dramatically. This physiologic response can be interpreted incorrectly as a sign of early shock. Patients should be positioned appropriately with lateral tilt to avoid supine hypotension and optimize uteroplacental perfusion.

## Risk of aspiration

Pregnancy is associated with a number of variables that place patients at higher risk for regurgitation and aspiration, including relaxation of the lower esophageal sphincter, decrease in gastric motility, and increase in gastric acidity. Use of a non-particulate antacid and placement of a nasogastric tube should be considered, especially in the obtunded patient.

## Less ventilatory reserve

Due to certain pulmonary changes and an increase in oxygen consumption, the pregnant patient has less oxygen reserve and should therefore be treated with supplemental oxygen during her trauma evaluation.

## Hypercoagulability

Pregnancy results in increased levels of fibrinogen and factors VII, VIII, IX, and X. These changes, coupled with vascular stasis and damage, subject the patient to a high risk of thromboembolism. Though rarely a concern in the acute management of the trauma patient, prophylactic use of heparin or pneumatic stockings should be considered in the recovery period.

## Laboratory tests

Complete assessment of the trauma patient should be complemented by appropriate laboratory tests. In addition to the routine studies, one should also obtain the following during the initial evaluation of the pregnant trauma patient: coagulation panel (including PT, PTT, and fibrinogen level), Kleihauer-Betke testing, blood, and Rh typing.

Disseminated intravascular coagulation (DIC) is a common component of severe trauma and, in pregnancy, may occur in association with placental abruption or amniotic fluid embolism.[6] As noted earlier, fibrinogen levels are significantly increased in pregnancy (normal range 350–450 mg/dl). Therefore, levels that would be interpreted as normal in the non-pregnant state may be indicative of early DIC in pregnancy.

Fetomaternal hemorrhage (FMH), fetal bleeding into the maternal circulation, may occur in as many as 28% of cases of severe trauma.[7] This process can result in fetal anemia, distress, and death. The Kleihauer-Betke assay allows for the identification and quantification of FMH. A positive test warrants prolonged fetal heart rate monitoring. Additionally, an appropriate dose of Rh immunoglobulin (300 μg per 30 ml of whole fetal blood) should be administered to all Rh-negative women in whom a FMH is documented. Treatment within 72 hours confers protection from isoimmunization.

## Diagnostic studies

Despite concerns expressed over the use of ionizing radiation during pregnancy, radiographic studies should be performed as necessary for complete maternal assessment. The rates of congenital malformations, intrauterine growth restriction, and childhood cancers are not significantly increased when the fetal radiation dose is less than 10 rads.[8] In general, the fetal exposure from conventional radiographic studies and computed tomography is well below this threshold. Measures such as shielding the uterus during X-rays should be instituted to minimize fetal exposure. Ultimately, such studies should not be avoided when their necessity is clinically indicated.

Diagnostic peritoneal lavage (DPL) can be performed safely in any trimester of pregnancy. A modified open technique has been advocated over blind needle insertion to minimize the risk of injury to the uterus or other displaced organs. Two studies have shown DPL in pregnancy to be sensitive and specific in recognizing intraperitoneal bleeding caused by blunt trauma.[9,10] Alternatively, an ultrasound of the abdomen and pelvis can also be used to evaluate for intraperitoneal injury or hemorrhage.[11] Although reports on the use of computed tomography and magnetic resonance imaging in pregnant trauma patients are limited, these studies may have a role in the evaluation of stable patients or when DPL and ultrasound are indeterminate.

## Hemodynamic status

Hemodynamic stability may be dangerously misleading in the pregnant trauma patient. As noted in Table 22.1, pregnancy is associated with a 50% increase in both cardiac output and blood volume. As a result, alterations in pulse and blood pressure are delayed in onset with hypovolemic pregnant patients. Relying on these parameters to evaluate maternal and fetal well-being may be grossly inadequate.[12] Hemodynamic instability indicating a need for transfusion may not occur until blood loss approaches 1500–2000 ml. Central hemodynamic monitoring may be appropriate to guide blood and fluid replacement in these patients. The use of vasopressors, which may reduce uterine blood flow, is generally discouraged. If there is inadequate response to volume replacement, agents such as dopamine (up to 5 μg/kg min) and ephedrine can improve maternal blood pressure without compromising uterine perfusion. Trauma resulting in maternal shock is associated with an 80% fetal mortality rate, regardless of whether there is direct fetal or placental injury.[13]

## ATLS

Pregnancy should not be the rationale for modifications in the ATLS protocol that might compromise the evaluation and treatment plan for the gravid trauma patient. Although there are two patients to consider, initial treatment priorities are the same as for a non-pregnant patient and are directed to the ABCs of resuscitation. An airway should be secured, adequate breathing ensured, and an adequate circulatory volume maintained. Supplemental oxygen should be administered by whatever means necessary to maintain a hemoglobin oxygen saturation of 95% or greater. Until blood products are available, crystalloid should be given in a volume of 3 ml replacement for each ml of estimated blood loss. If pneumatic antishock trousers are used, the abdominal compartment should not be inflated after the first trimester. If possible, the patient should be placed in the left lateral tilt position to minimize aortocaval compression by the gravid uterus and therefore improve uteroplacental perfusion. Ultimately, it is important to recognize that prompt and effective maternal resuscitation is the best fetal therapy in cases of severe trauma.

## Exploratory laparotomy and/or cesarean delivery

In general, indications for surgical evaluation and treatment of a pregnant trauma patient do not differ from those of a non-pregnant patient. However, one may encounter certain complications that are unique to pregnancy. Although delivery may be warranted in many such circumstances, it is important to recognize that the need to perform a laparotomy is not an indication to proceed with cesarean section. Cesarean delivery should be reserved for uterine rupture, fetal distress, fetal malpresentations in labor, and in laboring patients with unstable pelvic or lumbosacral fractures. On occasion, delivery may be warranted in patients with inadequate exposure at the time of laparotomy for other abdominal trauma.

Perimortem cesarean delivery may be an issue in the context of severe maternal injury. Although there is little information to support this procedure in pregnant trauma patients suffering from hypovolemic cardiac arrest, it should be considered when prompt maternal response to CPR is not evident and the fetus is potentially viable. For other causes of maternal cardiac arrest, there is a favorable chance of neonatal survival if delivery occurs within five minutes of maternal death.[14] Delivery may also improve the effectiveness of the CPR by decreasing both aortocaval compression and oxygen demand from the gravid uterus.[15]

Uterine rupture is uncommon with blunt trauma and occurs in less than 1% of cases. It tends to occur in patients subjected to direct abdominal impact associated with substantial force. Factors that predispose to uterine rupture in labor, such as uterine overdistension and a prior scar, also predispose to traumatic rupture. Due to the significant blood flow to the pregnant uterus, up to 500 ml/min at term, rupture can be associated with catastrophic hemorrhage. Although maternal death only occurs in 10% of such cases, fetal mortality in traumatic uterine rupture approaches 100%.[16] This diagnosis should be considered in pregnant trauma patients with evidence of a hemoperitoneum, fetal death or distress, and shock. Options for surgical management include hysterectomy or, if possible, closure of the uterine defect.[17]

In late pregnancy, the uterus is the most commonly injured organ in gunshot wounds and stabbings to the abdomen.[5] The reported incidence of fetal injury varies from 59% to 75%. A decision to perform a cesarean delivery should consider a number of variables including: gestational age and likelihood of neonatal survival, fetal condition on preoperative ultrasound or fetal heart rate testing, and extent of uterine injury.[18,19] In general, delivery should be avoided in penetrating uterine injuries prior to 24 weeks gestation. Neonatal survival is poor and fetal wounds may heal *in utero*. In such cases of extreme prematurity or fetal death, performing a cesarean delivery should be limited to patients with severe uterine hemorrhage or injury that would preclude labor.

## Fetal assessment

The initial fetal assessment to establish gestational age and presence of fetal heart activity should be undertaken as soon as possible. The clinical implications of this evaluation are ultimately dependent upon the establishment of fetal viability. If the pregnancy is of a non-viable gestational age or a demise is diagnosed, intervention and continuous monitoring on behalf of the fetus are not warranted. In contrast, such measures would be appropriate for a viable pregnancy. Although survival has been reported at earlier gestational ages, most neonatal centers presently consider 24 weeks as the lower limit of viability.[20]

If ultrasound is not readily available, a preliminary assessment can be done quickly and with minimal equipment. A simple fundal height measurement can provide a rapid estimation of gestational age. The fundal height in centimeters, as measured from the symphysis to the top of the fundus, corresponds with the gestational age in weeks in the second half of pregnancy. Fetal heart tones can be detected with a Doppler probe after the first trimester.

## Ultrasound

After maternal stabilization, ultrasound should be performed to establish gestational age and viability and to estimate fetal weight. Sonography is also useful in evaluating fetal presentation and number, as well as placental location. Ultrasound is not sufficiently sensitive to diagnose or exclude placental abruption, though certain findings may support this diagnosis.[21]

## External fetal monitoring

Fetal heart rate and uterine activity monitoring should be instituted in pregnancies after 24 weeks gestation. This may identify non-reassuring fetal testing or raise a suspicion for placental abruption, necessitating further evaluation or intervention. There is no consensus on the appropriate duration of monitoring. Some authors recommend 24–48 hours of continuous monitoring due to the potential for delayed onset of complications.[22] Others suggest that monitoring periods of 2–6 hours are adequate if there is no clinical concern for placental abruption.[23,24]

## Fetal distress

The identification of fetal heart rate accelerations is an indicator of adequate uteroplacental perfusion and fetal well-being. In contrast, late decelerations or fetal bradycardia and tachycardia are indicators of fetal distress. Maternal hypovolemia, fetal anemia, placental abruption or uterine rupture may result in these non-reassuring indications. The identification of these fetal heart rate patterns should not lead to inappropriate delivery. Many such cases improve with institution of certain resuscitative measures including volume replacement, supplemental oxygen, and maternal position change. If the fetal distress persists in a viable fetus and the mother is hemodynamically stable, cesarean delivery may be appropriate.

## Placental abruption

Placental abruption complicates 3% of minor injuries and up to 50% of life-threatening traumas.[25,26] Vaginal bleeding, uterine tenderness, fetal heart rate abnormalities, and fetal death are suggestive common findings. As 20% of cases may occur in the absence of external bleeding, a strong clinical suspicion should be maintained in pregnant trauma patients without these symptoms.[27] Placental abruption usually occurs soon after the traumatic event, though it may be delayed by hours or days in some cases. In contrast with ultrasound, tococardiographic monitoring appears to be quite sensitive in identifying trauma patients with this complication.[24] The clinical management of placental abruption is dependent upon its severity. Deferral of delivery may be appropriate for preterm pregnancies with mild placental abruptions.[28] Cases complicated by fetal distress, heavy vaginal bleeding or coagulopathy should be delivered promptly.

## Class II references

1. Varner MW. Maternal mortality in Iowa from 1952 to 1986. *Surg Gynecol Obstet* 1989;**168**:555–62.
   This retrospective study reviews the 505 maternal deaths occurring in Iowa over a 34-year interval. Cases were classified as direct, indirect or non-obstetric maternal deaths. Trauma was the most common cause of non-obstetric mortality.

2. Dannenberg AL, Carter DM, Lawson HW *et al*. Homicide and other injuries as causes of maternal death in New York City, 1987 through 1991. *Am J Obstet Gynecol* 1995;**172**:1557–64.

This study was undertaken to document the role of trauma as a cause of maternal death in an urban population. The authors reviewed autopsy reports from 115 maternal deaths attributable to injury and found the rates of homicide, motor vehicle accidents, and suicide to be comparable to the non-pregnant population.

3. Williams JK, McClain L, Rosemurgy AS *et al*. Evaluation of blunt abdominal trauma in the third trimester of pregnancy: maternal and fetal considerations. *Obstet Gynecol* 1990;**75**:33–7.

    This retrospective study of 84 pregnant patients with major abdominal trauma identified a 28% risk of preterm labor. The risks for complications such as uterine rupture and placental abruption were less than expected.

4. Peckham CH, King RW. A study of intercurrent conditions observed during pregnancy. *Am J Obstet Gynecol* 1963;**87**:609–24.

    This single-center cohort study followed over 10 000 patients to determine the incidence of intercurrent conditions and complications during their pregnancies. In contrast with other reports suggesting a higher risk for trauma with advancing gestational age, the risk of trauma was similar for each trimester in this study.

5. Awwad JT, Azar GB, Seoud MA *et al*. High-velocity penetrating wounds of the gravid uterus: review of 16 years of civil war. *Obstet Gynecol* 1994;**83**:259–64.

    This retrospective study of 14 patients correlated maternal and fetal injuries with uterine size and site of bullet entry. Maternal visceral injuries were absent in all patients with anterior entry wounds below the uterine fundus. The authors proposed that this information could be used to identify potential candidates for non-operative management.

6. Ali J, Yeo A, Gana TJ *et al*. Predictors of fetal mortality in pregnant patients. *J Trauma* 1997;**42**:782–5.

    This retrospective review of 68 pregnant patients with severe trauma was aimed at identifying factors responsible for fetal mortality. Blood loss, abruptio placentae, and DIC were the most significant predictors of fetal mortality.

7. Rose PG, Strohm PL, Zuspan FP. Fetomaternal hemorrhage following trauma. *Am J Obstet Gynecol* 1985;**153**:844–7.

    The results of this prospective study demonstrated a 28% risk for fetomaternal hemorrhage in the pregnant trauma patient. Due to the adverse perinatal outcome associated with this condition, the authors validate the use of the Kleihauer-Betke analysis in trauma patients to identify fetomaternal hemorrhage.

13. Kissinger DP, Rozycki GS, Morris JA *et al*. Trauma in pregnancy: predicting pregnancy outcome. *Arch Surg* 1991;**126**:1079–86.

    This retrospective review of 93 injured pregnant patients demonstrated that maternal admission physiologic and laboratory parameters failed to accurately predict pregnancy outcome. Fetal death most commonly occurred with direct uteroplacental-fetal injury, maternal shock, pelvic fracture, severe head injury, and hypoxia.

14. Katz VL, Dotters DJ, Droegemuller W. Perimortem cesarean delivery. *Obstet Gynecol* 1986;**68**:571–6.

    Based on their review of 61 reported cases of perimortem cesarean deliveries, the authors recommend that delivery be initiated within four minutes of maternal cardiac arrest to optimize maternal and fetal survival.

16. Rothenberger DA, Quattlebaum FW, Perry JF *et al*. Blunt abdominal trauma: a review of 103 cases. *J Trauma* 1978;**18**:173–9.

    This retrospective analysis of 103 cases of blunt trauma correlated fetal outcomes with severity of maternal injuries. Not surprisingly, worse pregnancy outcomes were associated with the more severe injuries. The authors conclude that the best chance for fetal survival is to assure maternal survival.

20. Morris JA, Rosenbower TJ, Jurkovich GJ *et al*. Infant survival after cesarean section for trauma. *Ann Surg* 1996;**223**:481–91.

    This retrospective study from nine centers reviewed 441 cases of trauma in pregnancy. The authors report a 75% neonatal survival rate after emergency cesarean delivery in viable pregnancies after 26 weeks gestation. Based on their results, the authors present a clinical algorithm for trauma in pregnancy which incorporates fetal monitoring and cesarean section.

21. Nyberg DA, Cyr DR, Mack LA *et al*. Sonographic spectrum of placental abruption. *Am J Roentgenol* 1987;**148**:161–4.

    This retrospective study of 57 cases of placental abruption reviews the spectrum of sonographic findings associated with this condition. The authors outline that these findings can be overlooked or misdiagnosed.

23. Goodwin TM, Breen MT. Pregnancy outcome and fetomaternal hemorrhage after noncatastrophic trauma. *Am J Obstet Gynecol* 1990;**162**:665–71.

    This prospective evaluation reported a 9% pregnancy complication rate in 205 cases of trauma. All such complications, including five cases of placental abruption, were evident on initial patient evaluation. The authors propose that 2–3 hours of fetal monitoring are adequate in patients who lack such complications.

24. Towery R, English TP, Wisner D. Evaluation of pregnant women after blunt injury. *J Trauma* 1993;**35**: 731–6.

    This retrospective review of 125 cases of blunt trauma reported on the usefulness of fetal ultrasound, external fetal monitoring, and Kleihauer-Betke tests in detecting pregnancy-associated complications. All complications occurred within six hours of admission and were identified when these tests were used together.

25. Dahmus MA, Sibai BM. Blunt abdominal trauma: are there any predictive factors for abruptio placentae or maternal-fetal distress? *Am J Obstet Gynecol* 1993;**169**:1054–9.

This retrospective study reported a 3% risk of placental abruption in 233 cases of non-catastrophic blunt abdominal trauma in pregnancy. The authors proposed that hospitalization beyond four hours is only necessary when there is evidence of abruption on initial evaluation with cardiotocographic monitoring.

26. Pearlman MD, Tintinalli JE, Lorenz RP. A prospective controlled study of outcome after trauma during pregnancy. *Am J Obstet Gynecol* 1990;**162**:1502–10.

This prospective cohort study compared pregnancy outcomes in 85 women who suffered trauma during pregnancy with a control group matched for gestational age. Four hours of cardiotocographic monitoring was found to be an extremely sensitive indicator of adverse outcomes, including five cases of abruptio placentae.

28. Sholl JS. Abruptio placentae: clinical management in nonacute cases. *Am J Obstet Gynecol* 1987;**156**:40–51.

This is a retrospective review of 130 cases of abruptio placentae of varying severities and gestational ages. The author advocates measures to defer delivery in preterm pregnancies with non-acute cases.

## Class III references

8. Brent RL. The effect of embryonic and fetal exposure to X-ray, microwaves, and ultrasound: counseling the pregnant and nonpregnant patient about these risks. *Semin Oncol* 1989;**16**:347–68.

An excellent review on the concerns and safety issues regarding radiation exposure in pregnancy. The author provides extensive data and references to support his view.

9. Esposito TJ, Gens DR, Smith LG, Scorpio RS. Evaluation of blunt abdominal trauma occurring during pregnancy. *J Trauma* 1989;**29**:1628–32.

This paper reviews 70 cases of blunt abdominal trauma in pregnancy from a single institution. The authors conclude that suspected intraabdominal injury during pregnancy should be managed no differently than in those who are not pregnant.

10. Rothenberger DA, Quattlebaum FW, Fischer RP. Diagnostic peritoneal lavage for blunt trauma in pregnant women. *Am J Obstet Gynecol* 1977;**129**:479–81.

This paper reports on the safety and accuracy of diagnostic peritoneal lavage in a series of 12 pregnant patients with blunt abdominal trauma.

11. Ma OJ, Mateer JR, DeBehnke DJ. Use of ultrasonography for the evaluation of pregnant trauma patients. *J Trauma* 1996;**40**:665–8.

This report describes the use of ultrasound examination in the management of three pregnant trauma patients and outlines the potential advantages and limitations of the procedure.

12. Biester EM, Tomich PG, Esposito TJ, Weber L. Trauma in pregnancy: Normal Revised Trauma Score in relation to other markers of maternofetal status – a preliminary study. *Am J Obstet Gynecol* 1997;**176**:1206–12.

This retrospective review of 30 pregnant trauma patients demonstrated a poor correlation between the Revised Trauma Score assigned on admission and subsequent pregnancy outcome.

15. DePace NL, Betesh JS, Kotler MN. Postmortem cesarean section with recovery of both mother and offspring. *JAMA* 1982;**248**:971–3.

Based on a single case report, the authors suggest that postmortem cesarean delivery should be considered as part of the resuscitative efforts in pregnant women with cardiac arrest unresponsive to other measures.

17. Smith A, LeMire WA, Hurd WW, Pearlman MD. Repair of the traumatized ruptured gravid uterus: a report of two cases resulting in subsequent viable pregnancies. *J Reprod Med* 1994;**39**:825–8.

This paper describes two cases of uterine rupture that were repaired primarily, with both patients having successful outcomes in subsequent pregnancies.

18. Franger AL, Buchsbaum HJ, Peaceman AM. Abdominal gunshot wounds in pregnancy. *Am J Obstet Gynecol* 1989;**160**:1124–8.

This paper describes three cases of abdominal gunshot wounds in pregnancy and outlines management guidelines.

19. Sakala EP, Kort DD. Management of stab wounds to the pregnant uterus: a case report and review of the literature. *Obstet Gynecol Surv* 1988;**43**:319–24.

Based on their experience and review of the literature, the authors propose an algorithm for management of abdominal stab wounds in pregnancy.

22. Higgins SD, Garite TJ. Late abruptio placenta in trauma patients: implications for monitoring. *Obstet Gynecol* 1984;**63**:10S–12S.

A report of a single case of abruptio placentae occurring five days after trauma. The authors advocate the need for fetal heart rate monitoring for a minimum of 48 hours after an episode of significant trauma.

27. Kettel ML, Branch DW, Scott JR. Occult placental abruption after maternal trauma. *Obstet Gynecol* 1988;**71**:449–53.

This paper presents three cases of occult placental abruption following trauma. The authors recommend maintaining a high index of suspicion for this diagnosis, even in the absence of symptoms.

**Trauma in pregnancy**

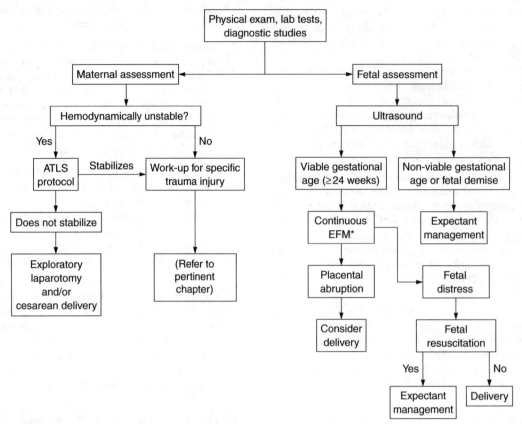

*External fetal monitoring

# 25 Hypothermia

*Christian Tomaszewski*

## Suspect hypothermia

Hypothermia is defined as unintentional lowering of the core body temperature to $\leq 35°C$ (95°F), with severe considered as being below 30°C (86°F).[1] Any patient that appears to be hypothermic with decreased responsiveness deserves an adequate work-up to rule out reversible contributing factors that may cause hypothermia without extreme environmental exposure. These include hypoglycemia and opiate overdose, which can easily be treated with intravenous dextrose and naloxone (2 mg/min), respectively.[2] Most hypothermic cases involve intoxication with ethanol. Factors less likely to be associated with trauma, but still in the differential for hypothermia, include hypothyroidism, adrenal failure, sepsis, and cerebrovascular accident.

## Adequate respirations?

The airway in hypothermic patients is managed aggressively, as in all trauma cases, with for a few caveats. As usual, intubation is indicated in any unresponsive patients who cannot protect their airway and handle their own secretions.[1,3] Although intubation usually does not precipitate dysrhythmias, there is the possibility of prolonged paralysis or sedation because of decreased drug metabolism at lower temperatures. The other difference in hypothermia arises when assessing ventilatory status. Pulse oximetry is of limited value in cold patients who are not perfusing extremities well. Meanwhile, interpretation of arterial blood gases in the presence of hypothermia is controversial. Raw arterial blood gas values result in a depressed pH and elevated oxygen and carbon dioxide levels relative to values corrected to normal body temperature. Most authorities recommend giving the patient 100% oxygen and using uncorrected arterial blood gas, especially with regard to carbon dioxide and pH.[4] This guarantees sufficient ventilation to avoid respiratory acidosis. There is no indication for the administration of bicarbonate, even in the presence of metabolic acidosis. In fact, this may predispose to life-threatening dysrhythmias and further impede delivery of oxygen to tissue.

## Assessment of central pulse

Because of ability to tolerate perfusing rhythms well in spite of hypotension, it is important to spend extra effort assessing for even the faintest pulse. If any rhythm other than ventricular fibrillation, ventricular tachycardia or asystole is seen on the monitor, then a careful palpation of the carotid artery is indicated. If any pulse is found, however weak, then external chest compressions can be avoided. Chest compressions and even movement and central catheterization have all been associated with the precipitation of ventricular tachycardia or fibrillation in severely hypothermic (<30°C/86°F core temperature) patients.[4,5] If bradycardic and hypotensive, transcutaneous pacing may be more useful than medications.[6]

## Warm humidified oxygenation and intravenous fluids

All hypothermic symptomatic patients should receive warm (45°C/113°F) humidified oxygen via either endotracheal tube or face mask.[7] Although of limited thermodynamic contribution, this maneuver will help prevent further loss of core heat.[5,8,9] Most hypothermic patients are dehydrated, which makes them prone to further hypotension as they are rewarmed. Therefore, aggressive fluid resuscitation is indicated, with CVP monitoring as needed.[10] Normal saline is preferred over lactated Ringer's because of the concern with liver metabolism at low temperatures. Fluids can be warmed to 45°C (113°F) using a blood warmer or standard microwave oven (high setting for 1–2 minutes).[11–13]

Unfortunately 1 l of intravenous fluids at such temperature (44°C or 111.2°F) provides approximately half of what one hour of humidified $O_2$ can deliver (17 versus 30 kcal) to a patient with temperature at 28°C (92.4°F).

### Start CPR and check for arrest rhythm

After waiting at least one minute to confirm the absence of any slow carotid pulse, CPR can be initiated. Any ventricular fibrillation or tachycardia seen on the monitor calls for several attempts at electrical defibrillation or conversion. However, such attempts are usually unsuccessful until the heart warms to at least 28°C/82°F. In severe hypothermia with ventricular fibrillation or asystole, external cardiac massage should be continued until definitive rewarming with cardiopulmonary bypass.[3] Until that time, any external rewarming efforts are probably of limited value.

There are not many instances where one would withhold CPR in a hypothermia case. Routine terminal findings such as rigor mortis and dilated fixed pupils are unreliable in severe hypothermia.[3,14] Instead, indications for withholding resuscitation include obvious irreversible injury (e.g. decapitation), frozen stiff body, clotted blood or elevated potassium (>12 mmol/l).[14,15] The last is the least reliable, especially in the presence of crush injury or non-hypothermia related hemolysis. Usually resuscitation is not attempted at core temperatures below 12°C (54°F); however, there is a case of successful resuscitation from 9°C (48°F).

### Defibrillate, consider bretylium, continue CPR

Pharmacological intervention with bretylium is indicated in cases of ventricular tachycardia and fibrillation unresponsive to electrical intervention.[16] This drug has been shown to raise the threshold for fibrillation and even facilitate defibrillation in the presence of hypothermia. All patients in ventricular fibrillation should receive a load of 10 mg/kg IV.

### Check core temperature

After initial stabilization of the patient, it is critical that an accurate core temperature be obtained as soon as possible. For proper measurement of core temperature, continuous monitoring with an esophageal or rectal probe with the ability to measure temperatures below 30°C (86°F) is necessary. The only problem with esophageal probes is that warm humidified oxygen via tracheal tube may falsely elevate core temperature measurements. Bladder monitoring devices are also available

that can be placed with Foley catheterization. One last route proffered for accurate measurement of central core temperature with respect to the brain is tympanic membrane thermometry.[17] Unfortunately, few patients have straight ear canals with unoccluded views of the tympanic membrane, a requisite for tympanic thermometry.

One important aspect of temperature assessment is in distinguishing severe hypothermia from moderate. At core temperatures less than 30°C (86°F), the body loses the ability to promote thermogenesis, particularly through shivering. Furthermore, except for bretylium, chemical and electrical treatments of dysrhythmias are generally ineffective at such low temperatures. As cardiovascular drugs accumulate, due to poor hepatic metabolism in the presence of hypothermia, exaggerated and prolonged effects could lead to life-threatening dysrhythmias upon rewarming.

### Extracorporeal heating

The treatment of choice in severely hypothermic patients with cardiovascular instability or arrest is cardiopulmonary bypass.[3] Rewarming with cardiopulmonary bypass has several advantages including rapidity of response, circulatory support, and rewarming of the heart prior to the periphery. The latter feature theoretically avoids peripheral vasodilatation and core temperature afterdrop (a decrease in core temperature after rewarming has begun), two potential complications of extremity rewarming.

There are other methods of extracorporeal methods for rewarming that may be used in patients that have at least a palpable pulse. The most common is arteriovenous rewarming through a ''fistula'' circuit.[10] This system is relatively easy to set up at the bedside, but does require sufficient blood pressure in the patient for movement of blood through the circuit.[4] Finally, success has been reported with hemodialysis.[18] Hemodialysis not only results in rapid rewarming, but also corrects acid–base abnormalities and can remove certain toxins. The main contraindications to this method include severe hypotension and bleeding due to the need for heparinization. In patients with concern for bleeding from traumatic injuries, heparin-bonded bypass circuits have been designed to avoid systemic anticoagulation.[19,20]

### Suspend resuscitation

The only absolute indication for suspending resuscitation efforts is if the patient is ''warm and dead''. Failure to regain a perfusion rhythm in spite of ACLS drugs (atropine, epinephrine, and defibrillation) with a core temperature >32°C (90°F) is grounds for declaration of death. Other prognostic factors that warrant suspension of efforts at lower temperatures include prolonged asphyxia (i.e. documented submersion of >30 min in a drowning case), severe traumatic injury or extreme hyperkalemia (K >10 mmol/l).[4,15] Such indications would be especially useful in a triage situation with multiple casualties.

## Passive external rewarming

This is an appropriate rewarming method for mild to moderate hypothermic patients with core temperatures above 30°C (86°F).[21] Patients must be able to generate their own heat, usually demonstrated by the presence of shivering.[22] Adding warm blankets insulates the patient and prevents further heat loss. The main advantages of passive external rewarming are ease of application and tendency to avoid core temperature afterdrop and rewarming shock. It is slow, resulting in a rise of body temperature of 0.3–2.0°C (0.5–4.0°F) per hour.[23] Failure to attain this goal should lead to the search for comorbidities (e.g. hypoglycemia or hypothyroidism) and indicates need for more aggressive rewarming, such as active external or extracorporeal.

## Active external rewarming

This is indicated in patients with a core temperature below 30°C (86°F) but who still have a perfusing rhythm. It is also useful in those who have failed to respond to passive rewarming. This process is usually done in addition to heated humidified oxygen and intravenous fluids mentioned previously. External rewarming can be accomplished through either immersion in a 40°C (104°F) bath or forced hot air at 48°C (118°F) over the patient.[2,9,17,23,24] A warming blanket, although not as effective, is probably the easiest to arrange. All external rewarming should be confined to the trunk, thus leaving the extremities vasoconstricted. By placing the emphasis on the trunk, rewarming the core prior to the extremities, one may minimize rewarming shock.

## Active core rewarming

Active core rewarming is reserved for patients who fail to respond to external rewarming or who are severely hypothermic and unstable in the absence of extracorporeal rewarming. This is usually accomplished through

gastric or peritoneal lavage with 45°C (113°F) fluid.[21,25] Although mediastinal and pleural lavage are advocated, they do not offer much more benefit and are more difficult to arrange.[5,26] Patients who have failed these warming strategies or become unstable will probably benefit much more from cardiopulmonary bypass rather than attempting to move large amounts of heated IVF in an invasive fashion through various body cavities.

## Class II references

2. Steele MT, Nelson MJ, Sessler DI *et al*. Forced air speeds rewarming in accidental hypothermia. *Ann Emerg Med* 1996;**27**:479–84.

   This prospective randomized clinical trial examined the rewarming rates of passive insulation with blankets versus convective cover inflated with air at 43°C. All 17 patients received 38°C intravenous fluid and warm humidified oxygen at 40°C by inhalation. The mean initial temperature in both groups was ~28°C. Core temperature (as measured by predominantly tympanic as opposed to rectal) increased faster in the forced air group (2.4°C/h) versus the control blanket group (1.4°C/h). There was no difference in clinical outcome, however. Using forced air appeared to be effective without the traditional feared complications of afterdrop and hypotension that have been reported with warm water immersion. However, the patients were not severely hypothermic and the sample size was small. In addition, only three patients were intubated with no unstable severely hypothermic patients entered in this study. Rewarming appears to be more dependent on the laws of thermodynamics rather than the vagaries of physiological phenomena in these patients. The other unfortunate aspect of this study was the use of tympanic thermometry, although the authors state that in all cases there was a clear non-occluded view of the tympanic membrane.

3. Walpoth BH, Walpoth-Aslan BN, Mattle HP *et al*. Outcome of survivors of accidental deep hypothermia and circulatory arrest treated with extracorporeal blood warming [see comments]. *N Engl J Med* 1997;**337**:1500–5.

   A retrospective series of 15 long-term survivors of deep hypothermia (core temperature <28°C) with circulatory arrest. Rewarming was attempted in 32 patients (of 46) using rewarming with cardiopulmonary bypass. All 15 patients were intubated and on arrival at the emergency department, were in circulatory arrest. Using femoral vessel cannulation and standard cardiopulmonary bypass equipment, 47% of patients were successfully resuscitated as late as 240 minutes after discovery. None of the survivors had long-term neurological disabilities based on neurological exam, EEG, and MRI. The main conclusion of this study is that even patients with fixed dilated pupils in asystole can survive with minimal deficits. Of note, the exceptional success rate was partly due to the fact that these young patients did not have asphyxiating injuries, with few drowning and avalanche victims represented.

5. Otto RJ, Metzler MH. Rewarming from experimental hypothermia: comparison of heated aerosol inhalation, peritoneal lavage, and pleural lavage. *Crit Care Med* 1988;**16**:869–75.

This canine animal model examined the ability to rewarm with a combination of either peritoneal or pleural lavage with or without heated aerosol inhalation. All dogs were cooled to 25°C. Conclusions of this study include the fact that heated aerosol inhalation was not beneficial, with endogenous heat production being much higher. Although aerosol inhalation had little heat contribution, both peritoneal and pleural lavage did well. Limitations of this study include the small sample size of 11 animals with three lost to early ventricular fibrillation. In addition, to sustain temperature increases as seen in this study, flow rates of 350 ml/min must be used for lavage. No details were given of temperatures for the heated fluids or aerosolization. Also of concern is the induction of ventricular fibrillation during manipulation of the animals – two in the pleural, one in the peritoneal group.

6. Dixon RG, Dougherty JM, White LJ, Lombino D, Rusnak RR. Transcutaneous pacing in a hypothermic-dog model. *Ann Emerg Med* 1997;**29**:602–6.

This controlled animal study examined the impact of transcutaneous pacing on external rewarming from a core temperature of 27°C. All 10 dogs in each group were anesthetized with sodium pentobarbital and intubated. Although both groups were rewarmed (to within 2°C of initial baseline core temperature, ~35–36°C) with a warming blanket, only the experimental group received pacing, set at the animal's initial baseline non-hypothermic heart rate. In addition to rewarming more quickly (172 versus 254 min), the paced groups had higher heart rate and cardiac index over the entire rewarming period. There were no malignant dysrhythmias provoked by pacing. This animal model shows that external rewarming can be safely accelerated by providing transcutaneous pacing.

9. Goheen MS, Ducharme MB, Kenny GP *et al.* Efficacy of forced-air and inhalation rewarming by using a human model for severe hypothermia. *J Appl Physiol* 1997;**83**:1635–40.

This is a prospective volunteer study of two women and six men comparing rewarming methods in a severe hypothermia model. Subjects were cooled to ~37°C and then treated sequentially with one of three techniques on separate occasions: (1) spontaneous control rewarming; (2) inhalation warming with warm (43°C) humidified air; or (3) external

rewarming of the trunk with forced air at a temperature to maintain skin temperature at 43°C. Rewarming was significantly greater with external forced air at 2.4°C/h versus inhalation rewarming at 0.23°C and control at 0.41°C. Only the forced air group showed a gain on heat from the environment and resulted in less afterdrop in core esophageal temperature when compared to the other two groups. Of note, rewarming was carried on at −20°C to simulate field conditions. In addition, all patients received meperidine at the time of cooling to prevent shivering. Regardless, this study shows that where shivering is suppressed as in severe hypothermia, inhalational rewarming is not very useful, especially compared to the superior results obtained with active external rewarming with forced hot air.

10. Gentilello LM, Cobean RA, Offner PJ, Soderberg RW, Jurkovich GJ. Continuous arteriovenous rewarming: rapid reversal of hypothermia in critically ill patients. *J Trauma* 1992;**32**:316–25.

This is a collective series of 34 hypothermic patients (<35°C), 16 of whom were treated with continuous arteriovenous rewarming. They were compared to the 18 patients who were treated with standard rewarming alone: heat gas humidifier, circulating blanket, thermal drape, and overhead radiant heater. Although there were 21 cases of major traumatic injury, overall both groups were comparable for Apache II and injury scores. The arteriovenous rewarming group warmed much more quickly than the standard group, attaining 35°C in only 39 min versus 3.23 h. In addition, blood and fluid requirements were reduced by almost half in the continuous arteriovenous rewarming group. Advantages of AV rewarming include ease of administration and the fact that the patient does not require systemic anticoagulation. Limitations of AV rewarming include the requirement for spontaneous circulation (minimum BP was 60 mmHg systolic) in the patient, because flow rate is dependent on adequate blood pressure.

12. Fildes J, Sheaff C, Barrett J. Very hot intravenous fluid in the treatment of hypothermia. *J Trauma* 1993;**35**:683–6.

This animal study examined the safety and warming effectiveness of using intravenous fluids at much higher temperatures than typically advocated. Ten hypothermic dogs (core temp 30°C/86°F) were randomized to either 65°C (149°F) or 40°C (104°F) fluid delivered through a specialized catheter into the superior vena cava. The 65°C group rewarmed much faster than the 40°C group: 3.7°C/h versus 1.75°C/h. There was no evidence of hemolysis or thermal damage to the vena cava. The authors conclude that the use of 65°C centrally administered IVF can improve heating rates without increasing complications.

13. Handrigan MT, Wright RO, Becker BM, Linakis JG, Jay GD. Factors and methodology in achieving ideal

delivery temperatures for intravenous and lavage fluid in hypothermia. *Am J Emerg Med* 1997;**15**:350–3.

There is significant conductive loss of heat as intravenous fluids traverse lengths of tubing. Using thermistor probes, the temperature of 0.9% NaCl was measured along lengths of tubing at various flow rates. To deliver fluid at a temperature of 37°C through standard tubing (230–280 cm length) the fluid must be preheated to 60°C and delivered at 1000 ml/h. Rapid boluses (300 ml/h) through short 50 cm tubing can achieve the same temperature results if one is treating a child. Although delivering warm intravenous fluid to hypothermic patients will not impact core temperature significantly, such maneuvers, combined with high delivery rates, should prevent further heat loss. This avoids infusing room temperature, essentially hypothermic, fluid to a patient.

16. Orts A, Alcaraz C, Delaney KA, Goldfrank LR, Turndorf H, Puig MM. Bretylium tosylate and electrically induced cardiac arrhythmias during hypothermia in dogs. *Am J Emerg Med* 1992;**10**:311–16.

In this prospective animal study, 22 hypothermic dogs were randomized to receive either bretylium (7.5 mg/kg) or an equivalent volume of normal saline. Animals were tested for ventricular arrhythmia threshold (VAT) based on the minimum number of electrical stimuli to the heart necessary to cause such a dysrhythmia prior to and after cooling to 27°C. The control animals had a decrease in VAT from 10.1 to 4.4 as expected. Surprisingly, the bretylium group actually had an increase in VAT from 9.8 to 23.2 impulses. There were no changes in catecholamines to explain this phenomenon. In this anesthetized model of hypothermic dogs, pretreatment with bretylium was shown to be protective of the myocardium against ventricular arrhythmias associated with hypothermia. No human trials on the utility of bretylium in hypothermia are available.

17. Ducharme MB, Frim J, Bourdon L, Giesbrecht GG. Evaluation of infrared tympanic thermometers during normothermia and hypothermia in humans. *Ann NY Acad Sci* 1997;**813**:225–9.

Three commercially available infrared tympanic thermometers (ITT) were evaluated for accuracy in both normothermic and hypothermic patients. In every case, the operator insured that the canal was free of cerumen, but in only 15% of subjects could the entire tympanic membrane (TM) be visualized because of the normal curvature of the canal. In the normothermic group of 95 volunteers, the oral temperature was higher (0.9°C, range −1.0–2.2°C) than that obtained by ITT. In the hypothermia study, 13 subjects were cooled to 33–37°C by esophageal thermometry. The temperature measure by ITT was 1°C lower than that from either esophageal or rectal core measurement. The authors conclude that ITT cannot provide a reliable measure of core temperature,

erring on the low side, usually because of the fact that in most patients there is not a clear view of the entire TM secondary to anatomical considerations.

22. Ducharme MB, Giesbrecht GG, Frim J *et al*. Forced-air rewarming in −20°C simulated field conditions. *Ann NY Acad Sci* 1997;**813**:676–81.

This prospective study looked at forced air rewarming in field conditions. This was tested on 13 subjects who were cooled to either a mean esophageal temperature of 33.9°C (to simulate mild hypothermia) or, on a separate occasion, to 36.7°C with meperidine treatment (to simulate severe hypothermia). Subjects were then placed in a sleeping bag and randomized to one of two rewarming scenarios: forced air rewarming at a torso surface temperature of 48°C or spontaneously without exogenous heat. In the severe hypothermia model, afterdrop was more pronounced in the control group (1.4°C) than in the forced air treatment group (0.9°C). The rate of rewarming was higher in the forced air group (2.4°C/h) than in the control group (0.4°C/h). In the non-meperidine phase, or mild hypothermia phase, of the study, there was no difference in afterdrop (~0.8°C) between both groups. The rate of rewarming, though, was higher in the forced air group (8.1°C/h) than in the control group (7.3°C/h). This study's main conclusion is that in the absence of the ability to shiver, as seen in deep hypothermia, the provision of external heat becomes much more important in the rewarming process. It also results in less afterdrop. Although this study was intended to simulate field conditions, its results have some applicability to hospital rewarming.

23. Collis ML, Steinman AM, Chaney RD. Accidental hypothermia: an experimental study of practical rewarming methods. *Aviat Space Environ Med* 1977; **48**:625–32.

Prospective rewarming of nine subjects whose body temperatures were lowered to 35°C (rectal). Five rewarming methods were tested: (1) inhalation of warm humidified oxygen at 43–48°C; (2) 50°C heating pads over neck, lateral thorax and groin; (3) combination of 1 and 2; (4) whirlpool bath at 26.5–43.5°C over 10 minutes; (5) shivering. The whirlpool bath led to the fastest rewarming to original baseline temperature, at 27 min, with shivering being the slowest, at 63 min.

24. Ledingham IM, Mone JG. Treatment of accidental hypothermia: a prospective clinical study. *BMJ* 1980;**280**:1102.

This is a prospective study over 15 years examining active external rewarming in moderate hypothermia. The 42 patients had core temperatures ranging from 20.0°C to 34.3°C. A radiant heat cradle was applied to the torso to achieve a rewarming rate of 1.13°C/h. The main dysrhythmia seen was atrial fibrillation. In spite of a mean 2 l of fluid infused, 14 patients still had hypotension (systolic blood pressure

<70 mmHg) that showed poor response to various vasoactive agents. Mortality was 27% (12 patients), with two patients dying during the actual rewarming. This is in comparison to a retrospective group of 77 patients, with similar core temperatures, who were rewarmed passively and had a mortality rate of 60%. The study shows that active external rewarming is a safe effective method to treat moderate hypothermia. Of note is that most of the cases (25) were overdoses, which may have resulted in improved outcomes.

25. Levitt MA, Kane V, Henderson J, Dryjski M. A comparative rewarming trial of gastric versus peritoneal lavage in a hypothermic model. *Am J Emerg Med* 1990;**8**:285–8.

   Animal study using rabbits cooled to 25°C based on tympanic membrane probe. They were then randomized, while on ketamine, xylazine, and nembutal, to either gastric or peritoneal lavage (n = 6/group). 40°C dialysate was infused at a rate of 80 ml/min intraperitoneal or 60 ml/min intragastric. Rewarming time was identical, both groups achieving 32°C within 135 min. There were no cardiovascular complications in this study. Limitations of this study include the fact that the gastric lavage group was done as aliquots as opposed to continuous infusion in the peritoneal group. In this study, using a sedated animal model, heating was effective and essentially identical for peritoneal infusion and gastric lavage.

## Class III references

1. Danzl DF, Pozos RS. Multicenter hypothermia survey. *Ann Emerg Med* 1987;**16**:1042–55.

   This prospective multicenter survey collected data on 428 cases of hypothermia from 13 emergency departments. Core temperatures ranged from 35°C to 15.6°C (mean 30.6°C). First hour rewarming rates were 0.5°C/h for passive rewarming to almost 2.0°C/h with active core rewarming. Tracheal intubation was performed without incident in 117 cases. Of the 41 patients requiring CPR, there were 15 (37%) survivors, nine in the prehospital group and six in the ED group. There were 73 fatalities (17%) overall, 62 having an initial core temperature less than 32.2°C. This study stressed the unpredictable nature of survival and how it did not relate to treatment.

4. Mair P, Kornberger E, Furtwaengler W, Balogh D, Antretter H. Prognostic markers in patients with severe accidental hypothermia and cardiocirculatory arrest. *Resuscitation* 1994;**27**:47–54.

   This retrospective series looked at prognostic markers for survival in 22 severe hypothermic patients that were found in cardiopulmonary arrest. They were primarily avalanche victims (n = 12), as well as some drownings (n = 7). All patients were aggressively rewarmed by femoral–femoral cardio-

pulmonary bypass. No patient with initial plasma potassium above 9 mmol/l had circulation restored. Central venous pH of 6.5 or less and activated clotting time above 400 sec were also associated with mortality. Of note, only 10 patients had circulation restored and only two survived to hospital discharge. The authors conclude that laboratory markers, particularly hyperkalemia, can be used to help identify patients that died prior to cooling. This may be especially useful in cases where several hypothermic patients present simultaneously.

7. Miller JW, Danzl DF, Thomas DM. Urban accidental hypothermia. *Ann Emerg Med* 1980;**9**:456–61.

   This retrospective study looked at the outcome of patients admitted to the hospital with hypothermia. Using a heated aerosol mask (40°C) did not change rate of rewarming (0.71°C/h) from that seen in the spontaneously rewarmed group without airway rewarming (0.74°C/h). Of note is that those patients rewarmed through an endotracheal tube rewarmed at the much faster rate of 1.22°C/h. Active external rewarming, using heated blankets or whirlpool but without airway rewarming, was at an intermediate rate of 0.9°C/h. Biases in this study included small numbers (135 patients among four groups) and the fact that treatment was at the discretion of the physician, with the sickest patients getting more aggressive care. In spite of this, mortality was under 10% in all groups except for the active external rewarming group, which did not receive any inhalation rewarming. The only conclusion to be drawn from this study is that for inhalation rewarming to offer any benefit requires delivery through an endotracheal tube.

8. Weinberg AD. The role of inhalation rewarming in the early management of hypothermia. *Resuscitation* 1998;**36**:101–4.

   This Medline collective retrieval sought to determine the effectiveness of inhalation rewarming for hypothermia patients. Letters, reviews, case reports, and original research from the last 10 years were compiled. Inhalation rewarming minimizes further heat loss from the respiratory tract and may in fact assist in core rewarming. Also, it appears to avoid the problems of shivering. To be optimally effective, though, it probably requires delivery via intubation route. There were no blinded controlled studies examining the actual contribution of inhalation rewarming, although overall it appeared safe using temperatures as high as 46°C.

11. Gong V. Microwave warming of IV fluids in management of hypothermia. *Ann Emerg Med* 1984;**13**:645.

   This letter to the editor discusses the use of microwave radiation to warm intravenous fluids for treatment of hypothermic patients. The author found that a routine microwave oven with rotating carousel, set at medium heat for 4 min, can heat 500 ml of normal saline to 37°C safely. Prior studies show that the flexible plastic bags are stable chemically and physically under such conditions. Once the fluid is heated, it can be wrapped in a towel to insulate it during delivery. The major shortcoming of this article is that your results will vary, depending on the particular oven and amount of fluid heated.

14. Ireland AJ, Pathi VL, Crawford R, Colquhoun IW. Back from the dead: extracorporeal rewarming of severe accidental hypothermia victims in accident and emergency. *J Accident Emerg Med* 1997;**14**:255–7.

This is a fascinating case series of revival in three patients from apparent death with rectal temperature as low as 22°C. All had non-perfusing arrest rhythms and there were fixed dilated pupils in one case. In two cases, CPR was initiated and cardiopulmonary bypass was achieved via femoral vessel cutdown and administration of heparin. All patients recovered fully neurologically. Of note, no patient had an abnormal potassium on presentation.

15. Hauty MG, Esrig BC, Hill JG, Long WB. Prognostic factors in severe accidental hypothermia: experience from the Mt Hood tragedy. *J Trauma* 1987;**27**:1107–11.

This is a retrospective case series reviewing the 1986 Mt Hood Oregon disaster. All 10 subjects presented with severe hypothermia after being found exposed during a snowstorm on a mountain. All were treated with cardiopulmonary bypass. There were only two survivors, both of whom were conspicuous in that on presentation, they were not in asystole and unresponsiveness like all the others. Based on this small series, the authors conclude that hyperkalemia (>10 meq/l), as well as elevated ammonia and reduced fibrinogen, were all grave prognostic signs. Of course, limitations of this series include small sample size.

18. Hernandez E, Praga M, Alcazar JM *et al*. Hemodialysis for treatment of accidental hypothermia. *Nephron* 1993;**63**:214–16.

This case study describes a severely hypothermic patient (27°C) treated with hemodialysis. The patient had sustained a barbiturate overdose and was found unresponsive in an open field during winter. Using hemodialysis, the patient was rewarmed successfully at 2°C/h without residual neurologic deficits. This case report shows that hemodialysis may be an alternative for rewarming if cardiopulmonary bypass is not available. In addition, this maneuver can correct electrolyte and acid–base abnormalities while removing certain toxins.

19. Tyndal CM, Rose MW, McFalls RE, Jacks A, Pinson T, Athanasuleas CL. Profound accidental hypothermia in the deep South: clinical experience. *Perfusion* 1996;**11**:57–60.

Two cases are presented of motor vehicle trauma patients that presented in deep hypothermia with core temperatures of 25°C and 27°C. Both were successfully rewarmed with percutaneous femoral-to-femoral cardiopulmonary bypass. Of note, one patient required cardiopulmonary resuscitation and the other had a splenectomy performed during rewarming. These authors show that in severely hypothermic patients who have suffered trauma, cardiopulmonary bypass can be done safely by using a Carmeda-bonded circuit without systemic anticoagulation.

20. von Segesser LK, Garcia E, Turina M. Perfusion without systemic heparinization for rewarming in accidental hypothermia. *Ann Thorac Surg* 1991;**52**:560–l.

This is a case report of a blunt trauma victim found at a core temperature of 24°C in ventricular fibrillation. Because of multiple assaults, he had relative contraindication to heparinization. Using heparin-coated perfusion equipment, he was successfully rewarmed with cardiopulmonary bypass.

21. Kornberger E, Mair P. Important aspects in the treatment of severe accidental hypothermia: the Innsbruck experience. *J Neurosurg Anesthesiol* 1996;**8**:83–7.

Retrospective case series of 55 patients with severe hypothermia (<30°C) who were treated based on initial hemodynamics: (1) stable patients (n = 24) had warmed fluids and oxygen and insulation; (2) unstable patients (n = 7) had peritoneal dialysis; (3) arrest patients (n = 24) had extracorporeal circulation. Survival rates were 100%, 72%, and 13% respectively. The prognosis was good in patients without preceding hypoxic event. The authors conclude that rewarming strategy should be based on the initial hemodynamic status of the patient.

26. Hall KN, Syverud SA. Closed thoracic cavity lavage in the treatment of severe hypothermia in human beings. *Ann Emerg Med* 1990;**19**:204–6.

This case series of two patients who presented with severe hypothermia showed the ability of pleural cavity lavage to raise core temperature quickly. Tap water at 41°C was infused, approximately 40 l over 20 min, via two chest tubes on the left side. Within 20 min, the patients achieved a target temperature of 32°C at a rate of approximately 2°C/h. However, both cases died, one from pulmonary embolism and the second from tricyclic overdose.

**Hypothermia**

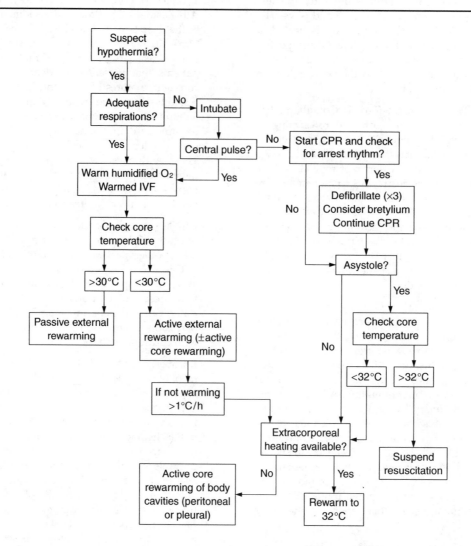

# 26 Evaluation of near drowning
*Andrew D Perron*

## Near-drowning event

"Drowning" was most simply and accurately defined by Modell[1] as death from suffocation by submersion in water; "near drowning" means to survive, at least temporarily, after suffocation by submersion in water. Drowning is the third most common cause of accidental death and the second most common cause of death in persons aged 44 years or less in the United States, exceeded only by motor vehicle accidents. Forty per cent of all drowning deaths are in children less than five years old.[2] Statistics on near drowning are much more difficult to ascertain. Conservative estimates suggest that in the United States, an additional 7000 persons per year experience near drowning that requires medical attention.[3]

Many victims drown due to panic, fatigue or overestimation of skills. Drowning may also be secondary to:

- trauma from boating and diving accidents
- hyperventilating prior to submersion, also called "shallow water blackout"[3]
- underlying medical condition, e.g. individuals with seizure disorders are four times more likely to have a submersion accident regardless of age[3,4]
- alcohol and drug abuse – an estimated 40–50% of adolescent drownings involve alcohol[2]
- hypothermia – predisposes to fatigue, confusion, and cardiac events[5]
- child abuse and neglect – in a recent 10-year review of pediatric bathtub near drownings, an alarming 67% of patients had historic and/or physical findings suggestive of abuse or neglect.[6]

## "Dry" versus "wet" drownings

The final common pathway for submersion in liquid is hypoxemia. Approximately 10–15% of victims of drowning and near drowning have no actual liquid aspiration, due to reflexive laryngospasm.[7] In the remaining victims, a highly variable quantity of liquid enters the lungs, usually 22 cc of fluid or less per kilogram of total body weight.[8]

## Fresh versus salt water

For many years there was controversy regarding the differences in pathophysiology in fresh versus salt water drowning. Different animal model studies showed contradictory results as to whether one or the other is more injurious to the lung. In both cases, surfactant becomes non-functional, the shunt fraction is increased, V/Q mismatch occurs, and hypoxia becomes the common pathophysiologic endpoint.[9] Reported effects of fresh and salt water aspiration on blood volume, electrolyte composition, and hemolysis have recently been refuted.[10] In an autopsy series from 1968, Modell and Davis[8] reported that it is unusual for near-drowning victims to aspirate more than 3–4 ml/kg of body weight. Studies have suggested that aspiration of more than 11 ml/kg must occur before blood volume changes take place and more than 22 ml/kg before electrolyte changes occur.[11]

## Warm versus cold water

A great number of anecdotal cases have been reported of neurologically intact survival after prolonged immersion in cold water. Animal experiments have demonstrated "the diving reflex" where subjects exhibit a marked bradycardia and blood flow is shunted away from non-vital organs to ensure perfusion to the heart and brain.[12] Whether this reflex persists in children is currently the subject of debate.[3] Warm water immersion events carry a more grave prognosis. Reports of neurologically intact survival after prolonged immersion are not found in the literature.

## Cervical spine precautions

Cervical spine radiographs should be performed in all cases where there is evidence of trauma and all unwitnessed drowning/near-drowning events should be considered posttraumatic until proven otherwise. In a small case series, Kewalramani and Taylor reported that 18% of patients with cervical spine injuries admitted to one institution were the result of diving accidents.[13]

## Risk factors for deterioration

In 1980 Modell and coworkers reported a retrospective series indicating that 93% of near-drowning victims who arrived at the hospital with a spontaneous pulse survived without sequelae.[14] Notably, all patients who were alert on emergency department arrival survived neurologically intact.

Pratt and Haynes[15] cite a number of risk factors for deterioration following near drowning from their study. The presence of any *one* of these risk factors places the patient at risk for deterioration following a submersion event.

- CPR at any time
- Cyanosis
- Loss of consciousness
- Significant past medical history
- Extremes of age

## Respiratory distress

Err on the side of early intubation for respiratory difficulties as patients may experience a rapid deterioration in their ability to oxygenate and ventilate. Early intubation is a crucial step in the management of hypoxia unresponsive to supplemental oxygen in the near-drowning patient.

The early use of positive end-expiratory pressure (PEEP) has been extremely helpful in the treatment of all types of near-drowning induced pulmonary injury for the following reasons:[16]

- PEEP shifts interstitial pulmonary water into capillaries
- PEEP increases lung volume by prevention of expiratory air space collapse
- PEEP increases the diameter of large and small airways to improve ventilation distribution.

The end-result is a decrease in intrapulmonary shunting, diminished ventilation-perfusion mismatch, and an increase in the functional residual capacity.

$\beta$-agonists should be used for bronchospasm[3] and no steroids[17] or prophylactic antibiotics[18] should be given. Theoretical benefits have not been proven in clinical trials.

## Observe 4–6 hours, then discharge to home

Older studies warned of the entity called "secondary drowning" where an apparently asymptomatic survivor of a near-drowning event would subsequently suffer a respiratory decompensation. Various reports indicated an incidence of nearly 5% and an "at-risk" period of up to five days,[19] thus necessitating prolonged observation of all near-drowning victims. A later review of these cases by Pratt and Haynes[15] indicated that all patients who later decompensated showed definite early signs and symptoms of respiratory distress.

In their prospective study, Pratt and Haynes demonstrated that all near-drowning victims who ultimately required hospitalization displayed signs of respiratory distress within four hours of their event. A later case series published in 1996 by Noonan and colleagues[20] examined 75 patients hospitalized for near-drowning events. This series demonstrated that 98% developed symptoms by 4.5 hours, with one patient deteriorating after seven hours.

The ability to discharge a victim of near drowning presumes a reliable patient and/or observer and the ability to return to the ED should decompensation occur.

## Abnormal level of consciousness

An abnormal level of consciousness after a near-drowning event is a poor prognostic indicator. In a series by Conn *et al.*,[21] 57% of patients who presented with an altered sensorium either died or were left with a profound neurologic injury. This indicates the need to:

- intubate for airway protection, apnea, obvious respiratory distress, hypoxia despite supplemental oxygen
- screen for other causes of altered mental status with: glucose check, toxicologic/alcohol screen, CT head if trauma suspected, cervical spine evaluation. Administer "coma cocktail".

## Evaluate temperature

Body temperature and the patient's clinical condition guide the management of hypothermia.

## Mild hypothermia (>34°C)

External rewarming, either passive with dry, warm blankets or active with radiant sources.

## Moderate hypothermia (30–34°C)

With stable cardiovascular function, passive warming with active rewarming to truncal areas only (prevent core afterdrop). Can use warm blankets, radiant warmers, hot baths.

## Severe hypothermia (<30°C)

Requires active core rewarming with: warm IV fluids (36–40°C), heated/humidified oxygen, gastric/bladder/pleural warmed lavage, peritoneal dialysis, hemodialysis, extracorporeal circulation.

## Discontinuing resuscitation

Orlowski[22] identified five unfavorable prognostic factors for pediatric near-drowning victims:

(1) Age less than 3 years
(2) Estimated submersion time greater than five minutes
(3) No resuscitation attempts for at least 10 minutes after rescue
(4) Patient "in a coma" on arrival to ED
(5) Arterial blood gas with pH of 7.10 or less

With one or two risk factors present, the victim had a 90% chance of survival. With three or more risk factors present, survival dropped to <5%. One prospective series showed an overall mortality of 48.7%.[23]

Neurologic outcome studies have been contradictory, with rates of neurologic injury following survival reported from 5%[24] to 67%.[25]

Remember the dictum, "You're not dead until you are warm and dead".[26]

## Class III references

1. Modell JH. Drowning vs. near-drowning: a discussion of definitions. *Crit Care Med* 1981;**9**:301–2.

   Editorial comment by Dr Jerome H Modell, who has published more on drowning and near drowning than any other author. Earlier literature was confusing because there was no agreement on the definition of these terms. Drowning is defined to mean death from suffocation by submersion. Near drowning is defined as surviving, at least temporarily, after suffocation by submersion.

2. Fatal injuries to children – United States, 1986. *MMWR* 1990;**39**(26):442–51.

   A standard reference for disease prevalence and incidence. Reports that drowning is the fourth leading cause of death in children <2 years old. Alcohol is associated with 40–50% of drownings and 90% of drownings occur in residential pools.

3. DeNicola LK, Falk JL, Swanson ME *et al*. Submersion injuries in children and adults. *Crit Care Clin* 1997;**13**:477–502.

   The most authoritative and thorough review to date. Very well referenced and organized. Covers all aspects of care for the victim of near drowning.

4. Orlowski JP, Rothner D, Leuders H. Submersion accidents in children with epilepsy. *Am J Dis Child* 1982;**136**:777–80.

   A retrospective review of 100 cases of drowning and near drowning at the authors' institution combined with five other studies purports to show that swimmers with epilepsy have a fourfold increased likelihood of a submersion accident. This is clearly not a metaanalysis but rather a compilation of a number of weak studies on the subject. No firm conclusions can be drawn other than persons who have a seizure while swimming may have a drowning or near-drowning event.

5. Martin TG. Near drowning and cold water immersion. *Ann Emerg Med* 1984;**13**:263–73.

   A review of hypothermia as it relates to drowning and near-drowning events. Has a well-referenced discussion of rewarming techniques and indications.

6. Lavelle JM, Shaw KN, Seidl T *et al*. Ten-year review of pediatric bathtub near drownings: evaluation for child abuse and neglect. *Ann Emerg Med* 1995;**25**:344–8.

   A retrospective review of 21 cases of pediatric bathtub drownings and near drownings, looking for evidence of abuse and/or neglect. The authors find evidence for one or both in a startling 67% of cases, with a mortality of 42%. The article serves as an important reminder to the physician to consider this in the care of the pediatric victim of drowning or near drowning.

7. Modell JH. Drowning. *N Engl J Med* 1993;**328**:253–6.

   A review article that lauds the benefits of PEEP/CPAP and finally buries the issues of corticosteroids, prophylactic antibiotics, and intracranial pressure monitoring in the treatment of the near-drowning victim.

8. Modell JH, Davis JH. Electrolyte changes in human drowning victims. *Anesthesiology* 1969;**304**:14–20.

   A retrospective autopsy series of 110 drowning victims in the 1960s. A pioneering work that showed that the volume of water aspirated by these victims was usually less than 4.1 ml/kg and, therefore, hypoxia rather than electrolyte and blood volume changes was the determining factor in their death.

9. Giammona ST, Modell JH. Drowning by total immersion. *Am J Dis Child* 1967;**114**:612–16.

   A study using a dog model to determine the pathophysiologic changes various liquids cause to the lungs. A total of 20 dogs were subject to aspiration of either normal saline, distilled water, chlorinated distilled water or sea water. The study demonstrated that while distilled water was the most damaging, all liquids damaged the pulmonary surfactant layer and persistent arterial hypoxemia resulted. This helped lay the ground work for Modell's studies in the 1970s.

10. Shaw KH, Briede CA. Submersion injuries: drowning and near-drowning. *Emerg Med Clin North Am* 1989; **7**:355–70.

    A review article most notable for generating the algorithm for the treatment of near drowning that is most commonly referenced to date.

11. Modell JH, Moya F, Newby EJ *et al.* The effects of fluid volume in seawater drowning. *Ann Intern Med* 1967;**67**:68–80.

    Basic science study using controlled aspiration in a dog model demonstrating the large volumes of water that would need to be aspirated to cause a change in blood volume or electrolyte composition. It pointed to hypoxemia as the primary pathological entity.

12. Tisherman S, Chabal C, Safar P *et al.* Resuscitation of dogs from cold water submersion using cardiopulmonary bypass. *Ann Emerg Med* 1985;**14**:389–96.

    A small basic science study using a dog model to determine pathophysiologic changes with cold-water submersion and the maximal period of submersion ending in successful resuscitation using cardiopulmonary bypass. Suggests a 90-minute time window where recovery could be expected in this model . No meaningful neurologic outcome data are presented.

13. Kewalramani LS, Taylor RG. Injuries to the cervical spine from diving accidents. *J Trauma* 1975;**15**:130–42.

    A retrospective case series of 126 patients with spinal injuries admitted to an orthopaedic service, with 23 (18%) coming from diving accidents.

14. Modell JH, Graves SA, Kuck EJ. Near-drowning: correlation of level of consciousness and survival. *Can Anaesth Soc J* 1980;**27**:211–15.

    A retrospective review of 121 cases in both adults and children. Examines outcome based on neurologic examination on arrival. Not surprisingly, it demonstrates that a good neurological level of function on arrival at the emergency department correlates with good outcome.

15. Pratt FD, Haynes BE. Incidence of "secondary drowning" after saltwater submersion. *Ann Emerg Med* 1986;**15**:1084–7.

    A case series of 52 patients prospectively studied using Los Angeles lifeguards to collect data on near-drowning victims. The study followed victims after either beach or emergency department discharge to find cases of secondary drowning. No cases of secondary drowning occurred and all patients who ultimately required hospital admission displayed symptoms by four hours, providing some objective data for the 4-6 hour observation rule.

16. Rutledge RR, Flor RJ. The use of mechanical ventilation with positive end-expiratory pressure in the treatment of near drowning. *Anesthesiology* 1973;**38**: 194–6.

    A case report and discussion of the utility of PEEP to reverse the V/Q abnormalities that accompany near-drowning.

17. Modell JH. Treatment of near-drowning: is there a role for H.Y.P.E.R. therapy? *Crit Care Med* 1986;**14**: 593–4.

    Expert opinion by Modell again calling for the end of steroids, prophylactic antibiotics, and aggressive ICP management in drowning victims, citing the fact that there are no data to support their use.

18. Oakes DD, Sherck JP, Maloney JR. Prognosis and management of victims of near-drowning. *J Trauma* 1982;**22**:544–9.

    A retrospective review of 40 drowning cases at one institution over nine years. Showed a very optimistic recovery rate to normal neurologic status for 20% of victims who came in apparently lifeless, requiring CPR. This series is more optimistic about this population than others published. Significantly, this study also found that 100% of adults were using alcohol at the time of their event.

19. Knopp R. Near-drowning. *J Am Coll Emerg Phys* 1978;**7**:249–54.

    An early review article when it was believed the type of water aspirated played a key role in management and outcome. The syndrome of "secondary drowning" is warned against.

20. Noonan L, Howney R, Ginsburg CM. Freshwater submersion injuries in children: a retrospective review of seventy-five hospitalized patients. *Pediatrics* 1996;**98**:368–71.

    A retrospective review of 75 pediatric patients admitted for near drowning between 1987 and 1994. Ninety-eight per cent of victims who developed symptoms following their event did so within 4½ hours. Confirms the fact that someone who is asymptomatic after 4–6 hours of observation may be safely discharged.

21. Conn AW, Montes JE, Barker GA *et al.* Cerebral salvage in near-drowning following neurological classification by triage. *Can Anaesth Soc J* 1980;**27**:207–10.

    Retrospective case series that examines neurologic outcome in near-drowning victims. Attempts to correlate outcome with presentation neurologic status. Reports 57% dead or neurologically devastated when presenting with altered sensorium. However, 43% had a good or excellent outcome, so it is difficult to know how to use these data in the acute resuscitation setting.

22. Orlowski JP. Prognostic factors in pediatric cases of drowning and near-drowning. *J Am Coll Emerg Phys* 1979;**8**:176–9.

A series of 93 cases of drowning and near drowning that seeks to assign points for certain findings on emergency department arrival in an attempt to prognosticate about outcome. Interesting concept, but hard to apply in the acute setting.

23. Kemp A, Siebert JR. Drowning and near drowning in children in the United Kingdom: lessons for prevention. *BMJ* 1992;**304**:1143–6.

A retrospective population study. Unfortunately only hospitalized patients were included. There are no data on patients discharged from the emergency department. It does report an overall mortality of nearly 49% and a 5.3% incidence of severe neurologic injury in the 306 patients studied.

24. Pearn JH, Bart RD, Yamaoka R. Neurologic sequelae after childhood near-drowning: A total population study from Hawaii. *Pediatrics* 1979;**64**:187–91.

A five-year population study in Oahu. Reviewed 104 children who presented apneic and unconscious to determine neurologic outcome. Excludes children who were "dead on extraction" from the water (i.e. did not have a pulse). Of 75 patients ultimately included in the data set, five died and 70 were "neurologically normal" as defined as "fit and well and functioning normally". The study suffers since it excludes patients needing CPR and never objectively addresses neurologic injury. The authors point out that if a patient presents with a pulse, survival is likely.

25. Peterson B, Morbidity of childhood near-drowning. *Pediatrics* 1977;**59**:364–70.

A small case series that reinforces the belief that if the patient requires ongoing CPR in the emergency department, he/she is unlikely to have a good outcome. Seventy-two patients studied. Of 57 with an ultimate good outcome, none required CPR in the emergency department. Of the 14 with severe anoxic encephalopathy, 13 required CPR in the emergency department.

**Evaluation of near drowning in a patient with *normal* level of consciousness**

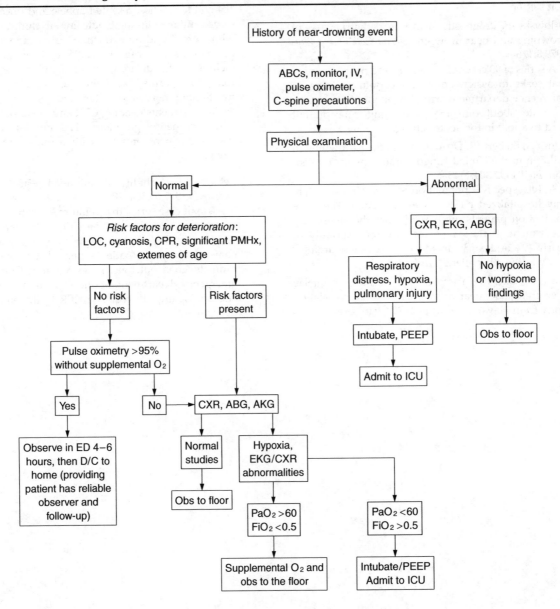

**Evaluation of near drowning in a patient with *altered* level of consciousness**

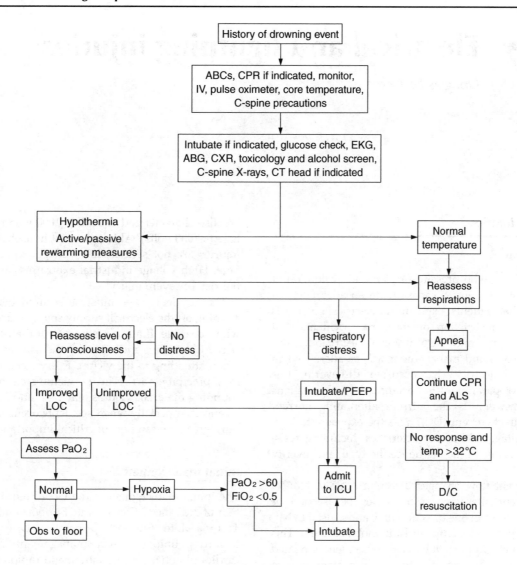

# 27 Electrical and lightning injuries

*Douglas McGee*

## Electrical injuries

### Assessment[1]

Many patients who present for care and evaluation of electrical shock injuries can provide an adequate history. In other patients, exposure to electrical current is less clear. Construction or industrial accidents that involve trauma may also involve electricity. Since injury patterns and management will be altered when exposure to electricity has occurred, discovering this history is of paramount importance. Several questions require answers: Is the current alternating current (AC) or direct current (DC)? Was the exposure to high or low voltage? Other characteristics, including resistance and contact time, influence the type and severity of injury.

AC current flow changes direction rapidly. Household current alternates at 60 cycles per second or 60 Hz. DC flows in one direction only and is used in batteries, electric rail systems, and automobile current. This distinction has important clinical consequences related to the typical duration of exposure, or contact time, to current. Since the amount of tissue destruction is somewhat dependent on contact time, this information is worth collecting from the patient, co-workers or emergency medical service personnel. Contact with DC current often causes singular, tetanic muscular contractions that tend to throw the victim from the electric source, thereby limiting contact time. AC current causes continuous muscular contractions when stimulated at 60 Hz. Because the forearm flexors are stronger than the extensor muscle groups, stimulation of the forearm causes the victim to grasp the source, unable to let go.

Most materials resist electrical flow to some degree. The resistance is dependent primarily on the physical composition of the material, insulation, and amount of moisture. The higher the resistance, the greater the heat generated. Heat generated during resistant flow is responsible for the tissue destruction seen. Injuries are also characterized as high (>1000 volts) or low voltage (<1000 volts). Although most household electrical injuries are not serious, low-voltage exposure can be fatal. High voltage industrial exposures carry substantial risk of severe injury.

The accident scene must be secured before rescue. Turning off the electrical supply source is accomplished when possible. If any question about the power source remains, rescuers must protect themselves from harm when attending to the victim. Every electrical accident may precipitate a fire in the victim's clothing or surrounding material. Victims may be found in precarious locations, especially when accidents occur in industrial settings. Scene safety is of critical importance.

### Initial management

The initial management of the victim requires application of Advanced Cardiac Life Support and Advanced Trauma Life Support principles. Direct attention toward definitive airway management, initiation of cardiopulmonary resuscitation, and rapid correction of life-threatening arrhythmias. Treat victims of serious electrical exposures as trauma patients. Direct attention toward the life threats identified during the primary survey.

Patients are divided into two groups: major electrical injury or minor electrical injury. Patients suffering from major electrical injury experience contact with high-voltage sources or with low-voltage sources while in contact with water, as in a bathtub electrocution. Minor electrical injury is characterized by contact with low-voltage sources without water contact and skin or oral burns.

### Cardiac assessment

Because most serious rhythm disturbances occur in the immediate postexposure period, it is common practice to recommend EKG analysis and rhythm monitoring for as long as 24 hours.[1-3] Recent literature suggests that extended cardiac monitoring is not required for most victims of electrical injuries.[4-11] Several retrospective studies have concluded that victims of minor electrical injury and many victims of major electrical injury are unlikely to develop cardiac dysrhythmias. Rhythm disturbances or cardiac symptoms are often fatal or apparent on the initial evaluation.

## Burn wounds

Patients who sustain burn wounds after low-voltage exposure are managed according to standard burn care. Controversy exists as to the optimal time for surgical debridement. Experimental, low-voltage burns were studied in swine.[12] These authors found that no additional changes were seen in the burn wound 48 hours after the injury. Clinical evaluation could discern between viable and non-viable tissue. In this model, definitive wound coverage was accomplished at 48 hours. Burns to the oral commissure of the mouth, usually sustained after a child chews on an electric cord, require special attention. This type of injury occurs when the electric current arcs through the oral tissues to contact points at the commissure of the mouth. Injury to the lips, tongue, and teeth can occur. Delayed hemorrhage from oral commissure burns has been reported to occur when the burn eschar separates at two days. Recent literature suggests that concern over this complication may be overstated.[13] Twenty-four patients with oral burns due to electrical injury were treated conservatively without oral splinting or early surgery. Reconstructive surgery was performed after burn healing had occurred. No child in this study had delayed hemorrhage.

## Secondary survey

After the primary survey is completed, the secondary survey is performed according to ATLS guidelines. Because victims of electrical injuries are treated as trauma patients, a meticulous search for injury in all systems must be completed. Electrical injuries mandate additional evaluation of the circulatory and musculoskeletal systems. These portions of the secondary survey are discussed below.

## Circulatory system

Major electrical injuries present several threats to the circulatory system. The primary survey will identify life-threatening dysrhythmias that are treated before the secondary survey is started. Most victims of major electrical injuries require cardiac monitoring for many reasons. Associated injuries, massive fluid requirements, and burn wound complications render these patients critically ill. Among patients with high-voltage exposure and minor burns only, cardiac monitoring for 24 hours may be unnecessary according to some authors.[6] Purdue and Hunt reported 11 victims of high-voltage injury. Two patients presented with electrocardiographic evidence of myocardial infarction, confirmed by cardiac enzymes and nuclear scan criteria. Neither patient demonstrated dysrhythmia during their hospitalization. Of the remaining victims of high-voltage injury, none developed cardiac sequelae. All patients were monitored for a minimum of 24 hours.

Significant circulatory compromise can occur due to fluid losses from burns. Hemorrhagic injuries sustained in associated trauma may increase fluid requirements. The modified Parkland formula, 4 ml per kilogram per percentage body surface area burned, may underestimate the fluid requirements for the victim of a major electrical injury. Small entrance and exit wounds often cover large areas of tissue necrosis. Luce and Gottlieb described a group of patients who had sharply demarcated full-thickness burns with obvious entrance and exit wounds.[14] These patients required 7 ml/kg/%BSA burned of Ringer's lactate solution (1.7 times the amount calculated by the Parkland formula) to maintain urine output sufficient to clear urine myoglobin and maintain adequate tissue perfusion. As with all burn patients, the recommended guidelines are designed to maintain adequate urine flow and are tailored to meet the needs of the patient.

Myocardial necrosis has been associated with electrical injuries but the determination of myocardial injury is difficult.[15,16] Many patients demonstrate a wide variety of EKG changes that revert to normal over time and do not result in cardiac symptoms.[3,15,17] Victims of electrical injury often demonstrate elevated levels of creatine kinase (CK) and corresponding elevation of CK-MB fractions suggestive of myocardial necrosis. The role of CK-MB isoenzymes in determining myocardial damage is less clear. In a study of 24 patients with high-voltage electrical injuries, Chandra *et al.* described two groups of patients.[18] Group 1 patients demonstrated elevated CK and CK-MB fraction. Group 2 patients demonstrated CK elevation but without CK-MB present. These authors concluded that presence of CK-MB in group 1 indicated myocardial damage. All the group 1 patients had a vertical pathway of current travel; that is, the current passed between an upper and a lower body segment. Group 1 patients also had a greater body surface area burn than Group 2. Less than half of the Group 2 patients had vertical transmission. This study concluded that vertical transmission of current and percentage body surface area burned were clinical predictors of myocardial damage.

Other authors disagree. Two studies have demonstrated that even when CK-MB fractions are elevated, patients rarely manifest symptoms of myocardial injury or serial EKG tracing consistent with myocardial injury.[3,17] In a study by Housinger, patients with elevated CK-MB fractions all had normal technetium pyrophosphate cardiac scans.[17] CK-MB elevations correlate poorly with EKG abnormalities and, when seen alone, do not indicate myocardial infarction.[3,17] Although cardiac troponin T and cardiac troponin I levels are not generally detected after high-energy DC cardioversion, their role in assessing myocardial injury in victims of electric shock is unclear.[19,21]

### Musculoskeletal system

Fractures resulting from associated trauma may be discovered in victims of electrical injuries. A meticulous search for them is mandated. Fractures caused by tetanic muscle contraction are well documented and have prompted some authors to suggest that radiographs be obtained of bones along the presumed course of current.[22]

Traditional surgical teaching advocated immediate surgery for all victims of high-voltage injuries for the purpose of decompression and debridement.[15,23] The purpose of this practice was to prevent continued ischemia caused by muscle edema and poor tissue perfusion. Fleckenstein *et al.* determined that MRI identified necrotic tissues and distinguished between perfused and non-perfused tissues.[24] These authors suggest that three-phase technetium-99m pyrophosphate scintigraphy delineates transition zones between normal and non-perfused tissue, allowing for better evaluation of muscle viability before surgery. Recent literature advocates a more selective approach. Mann *et al.* published a series of 62 patients who had selective upper extremity decompression and debridement.[23] Patients in this series were operated on based on the presence of peripheral nerve deterioration and signs or symptoms of compartment syndrome. This selective approach yielded an amputation rate of 10%, far below the amputation rate for other series of similar patients. In the opinion of these authors, compartment pressures were not predictive of subsequent amputation.

### Definitive burn care

Because of the unique nature of electrical injuries, patients are evaluated in centers equipped with expertise in the management of traumatic injuries and burn care. After initial stabilization in the receiving hospital, patients are transferred to a tertiary care center. If transfer to a burn center can be made promptly, definitive surgical evaluation of the burn wounds can then take place.

## Lightning injuries

### Suspected lightning strike

Lightning represents a unique electrical phenomenon that is distinctly different from other electrical injuries. Cloud-to-ground lightning strikes occur about 30 million times a year but fatalities from this common environmental event are uncommon. Between 1980 and 1995, 1318 deaths were attributed to lightning. Most patients were males between the ages of 14 and 44 years. In the United States, the greatest number of deaths occur in Florida and Texas.[25] Most victims are engaged in outdoor activities.[26] Because victims are often engaged in outdoor recreational group activities, multiple simultaneous victims are possible.

Emergency medical service workers are trained to focus resources on those patients with the greatest potential for survival when the number of patients overwhelms the resources. Adhering to this dictum would direct EMS personnel to allow those patients without signs of life after lightning strike to remain unattended. Because of the unusual clinical effects of lightning, the opposite is true. In multicasualty incidents, those patients who appear dead are resuscitated first.[25,27,28] Identifying multiple casualties is of paramount importance in a lightning strike.

### Basic and advanced life support protocols

Instantaneous cessation of cardiopulmonary function is the immediate cause of death in lightning injuries. A combination of immediate asystolic cardiac standstill and respiratory failure due to paralysis of the medullary respiratory center causes immediate death. The inherent automaticity of the heart often generates a perfusing cardiac rhythm, enabling many victims to recover. The duration of respiratory paralysis may persist longer than cardiac standstill and precipitate a secondary cardiac arrest caused by hypoxia.[28] Basic and advanced life support protocols are promptly initiated, when available. Trauma may accompany lightning injury. Spinal immobilization, airway stabilization, and the administration of intravenous fluids are initiated by the EMS personnel.

### Complications

Although victims of lightning injuries either die or recover without serious sequelae, many complications are reported.[28] Burns tend to be minor due to the flash of the lightning over the intact skin but serious burns are reported, as are a broad spectrum of neurologic injuries. Most neurologic injuries are transient and include encephalopathy, peripheral neuropathy, spinal cord paralysis, and psychometric impairment.[26–30] Unless a lightning strike occurs directly to the head, axial lesions are uncommon. When focal or persistent abnormalities are present, neuroimaging is indicated. A variety of EKG abnormalities have been described, but myocardial injury is rare.[28] Organ rupture has been reported and may occur as a result of coexistent trauma.[27,28] When hypotension is present, a diligent search for hemorrhage is carried out. Burns tend to be minor, as the brief electrical contact often does not penetrate the skin. Flashover burns can occur, but serious full-thickness burns are also reported.

Because of the potential for serious injury and the need for specialized burn care, trauma or burn center referral is prudent but no literature supports direct triage to specialty centers.

## Class II references

8. Zubair M, Besner GE. Pediatric electrical burns: management strategies. *Burns* 1997;**23**:413–20.

    This retrospective analysis reviewed 127 children over a 25-year period who sustained electrical injuries. These authors conclude that almost every patient who sustained a low-voltage injury could have been cared for as an outpatient.

11. Arrowsmith J, Usgaocar RP, Dickson WA. Electrical injury and the frequency of cardiac complications. *Burns* 1997;**23**:576–8.

    One hundred and forty-five admissions of patients with electrical injuries were reviewed. One hundred and four had an admission EKG, 73 had cardiac monitoring. Three patients developed occasional ectopy that resolved. One patient developed atrial fibrillation that was treated with digoxin. These cardiac complications were greater among patients with high-voltage exposures and with loss of consciousness. The authors conclude that the patient will be unlikely to suffer cardiac complications when the admission EKG is normal and loss of consciousness is not present.

12. Laberge LC, Ballard PA, Daniel RK. Experimental electrical burns: low voltage. *Ann Plast Surg* 1984; **13**:185–90.

    Twenty-five swine received experimental low-voltage injuries. Histological and clinical evaluation of the burns was performed at 48 hours. No further necrosis was seen after 48 hours. Wounds were debrided and covered at 48 hours with good results. These authors conclude that wound necrosis ceases

at 48 hours and debridement and coverage can be safely accomplished at that time.

17. Housinger TA, Green L, Shahangian S, Saffle JR, Warden GD. A prospective study of myocardial damage in electrical injuries. *J Trauma* 1985;**25**:122–4.

    Sixteen victims of non-flash electrical injuries had EKGs performed, CK-MB analysis, and technetium 99m stannous pyrophosphate scans performed prospectively. Although several patients had abnormal EKGs and elevated CK-MB enzyme determinations, no patient had an abnormal technetium study. No patient had clinical evidence of cardiac dysfunction. These authors concluded that CK-MB levels correlated poorly with EKG abnormalities in victims of electrical injury.

18. Chandra NC, Siu CO, Munster AM. Clinical predictors of myocardial damage after high voltage electrical injury. *Crit Care Med* 1990;**18**:293–7.

    CK-MB enzyme determinations were made in 24 victims of high-voltage electrical injury. Myocardial damage was judged to have occurred in 13/24 patients based on elevated CK-MB. The remaining patients had normal CK-MB. The path of current flow in the first group passed between upper and lower body segments in each patient. This group also had larger burns. Less than half of the group with normal CK-MB had a vertical current path. These authors concluded that vertical pathway of current travel and magnitude of burn predicted myocardial injury.

19. Grubb NR, Cuthbert D, Cawwod P, Flapan AD, Fox KA. Effect of DC shock on serum levels of total creatine kinase mass and troponin T. *Resuscitation* 1998;**36**:193–9.

    These authors measured CK-MB and cardiac troponin T in patients undergoing DC cardioversion for atrial fibrillation. CK-MB peaked at 18 hours and correlated with total energy delivered. Total troponin T levels were not elevated after DC cardioversion. They concluded that elevated troponin T seen after out-of-hospital resuscitations was not due to electrical injury.

20. Runsio M, Kallner A, Kallner G, Rosenqvist M, Bergfeldt L. Myocardial injury after electrical therapy for cardiac arrhythmias assessed by troponin T release. *Am J Cardiol* 1997;**79**:1241–5.

    External defibrillation and intracardiac defibrillation give rise to statistically significant elevations of troponin T, CK-MB mass, and S-myoglobin. High-energy DC cardioversion did not cause elevation of these enzyme markers of minor cardiac damage.

21. Bonneyfoy E, Chevalier P, Kirkorian G *et al.* Cardiac troponin I does not increase after cardioversion. *Chest* 1997;**111**:15–18.

    These authors measured various cardiac enzyme markers after elective DC cardioversion for supraventricular tachycardia in 28 patients. No elevation of cardiac troponin I was seen after cardioversion.

24. Fleckenstein JL, Chason DP, Bonte FJ *et al*. High voltage electric injury: assessment of muscle viability with MR imaging and TC-99m pyrophosphate scintigraphy. *Radiology* 1995;**195**:205–10.

These authors compared the clinical findings at surgery with unenhanced and gadolinium-enhanced MRI and with three-phase technetium-99m pyrophosphate scintigraphy on 12 limbs in eight patients with high-voltage injuries. MRI allowed better distinction between perfused and non-perfused edematous muscle. The sensitivity of MRI in non-perfused muscle was low. Scintigraphy increased at the transition zones between normal and non-perfused muscle regions. These authors suggest that these studies may be useful when planning the debridement of high-voltage injuries.

## Class III references

1. Fontanarosa PB. Electrical shock and lightning strike. *Ann Emerg Med* 1993;**22**(pt 2):378–87.

This is a well-written review article with 101 references that discusses the epidemiology of electrical injuries and lightning strikes. The paper reviews the current literature and discusses the physics and pathophysiology of electric shock and lightning injury. Clinical effects and management recommendations are provided. A section discussing myocardial injury in electric shock is extensive and well referenced.

2. Browne BJ, Gaasch WR. Electrical injuries and lightning. *Emerg Med Clin North Am* 1992;**10**:211–29.

This paper is a comprehensive review of electrical and lightning injuries with 105 references. The review discusses the pathophysiology, evaluation, and management of victims of electrical injuries and lightning strikes.

3. McBride JW, Labrosse KR, McCoy HG *et al*. Is serum creatine kinase-MB in electrically injured patients predictive of myocardial injury? *JAMA* 1986;**255**:764–8.

This is a retrospective analysis of 36 victims of high-voltage electrical injury. Total CK elevations were seen in 92% of all patients; CK-MB elevations were seen in 50% yet only two patients had EKG and clinical findings consistent with acute myocardial injury. These authors measured CK-MB activity in normal tissue near the injury site and found increased activity. They conclude that cardiac injury is uncommon and electric current stimulates skeletal muscle to produce and release CK-MB enzyme.

4. Garcia CT, Smith GA, Cohen DM, Fernandez K. Electrical injuries in pediatric emergency department. *Ann Emerg Med* 1995;**26**:604-608.

This retrospective analysis of 78 children divided the patients into major electrical events and minor electrical events. The authors characterized the spectrum of injuries seen. All burns were less than 1% TBSA burned; most were first-degree burns. No adverse sequelae were seen among victims of minor electrical injury. They concluded that hospitalization and laboratory evaluation were not required in this patient population.

5. Bailey B, Gaudreault P, Thivierge RL, Turgeon JP. Cardiac monitoring of children with household electrical injuries. *Ann Emerg Med* 1995;**25**:612–17.

This retrospective analysis of 141 children with electrical injuries evaluated the cohort for cardiac dysrhythmias. Some rhythm disturbances were detected and judged to be benign. Eighty per cent of patients were monitored for a mean of 7.4 hours. No rhythm disturbance was seen. Follow-up was made in 77% of patients; no adverse outcomes were reported. They conclude that ECG analysis and monitoring is unnecessary in most children with household electrical injuries.

6. Purdue GF, Hunt JL. Electrocardiographic monitoring after electrical injury: necessity or luxury? *J Trauma* 1986;**26**:166–7.

Records of 48 consecutive victims of high-voltage electrical injuries were reviewed. An initial EKG was obtained in all patients and sequentially thereafter. All patients were monitored for at least 24 hours. Patients with a normal EKG on admission did not develop serious dysrhythmia. The authors recommend that routine cardiac monitoring be used selectively in victims of high-voltage injuries.

7. Fatovitch DM. Electrocution in Western Australia, 1976–1990. *Med J Aust* 1992;**157**:762–4.

This study reviewed the records of 104 electrocution deaths in Australia. In all cases, the patient developed the lethal dysrhythmia at the time of the accident that uniformly produced death at the scene.

9. Wilson CM, Fatovitch DM. Do children need to be monitored after electric shock? *J Paediatr Child Health* 1998;**34**:474–6.

The records of 40 children exposed to Australian household current were examined. One child had an abnormal EKG on admission, none developed a dysrhythmia, and all survived. These authors concluded that routine cardiac monitoring is not required when the admission EKG is normal.

10. Wallace BH, Cone JB, Vanderpool RD *et al*. Retrospective evaluation of admission criteria for pediatric electrical injuries. *Burns* 1995;**21**:590–3.

Twenty-six cases of exposure to household current and nine cases of exposure to high voltage were reviewed. No child died in either group. No child in the low-voltage group developed dysrhythmia that required treatment. These authors recommended outpatient treatment of healthy children with minor burns exposed to low voltage.

13. Canady JW, Thompson SA, Bardach J. Oral commissure burns in children. *Plast Reconstr Surg* 1996; **97**:738–43.

    This retrospective review of 24 patients with oral commissure burns concluded that conservative treatment without splinting or early surgery was successful. No patient suffered from the feared complication of delayed hemorrhage after eschar separation.

14. Luce EA, Gottlieb SE. "True" high tension electrical injuries. *Ann Plast Surg* 1984;**12**:321–6.

    This retrospective review of 31 patients with characteristic entrance and exit wounds and severe burns analyzed, among other things, the amount of resuscitation fluid required to avoid acute tubular necrosis and clear myoglobin pigment. This group of patients required 1.7 times the usual recommended amount of 4 cc/kg/%BSA burned, or 7 cc/kg/%BSA burned.

15. Carleton SC. Cardiac problems associated with electrical injury. *Cardiol Clin* 1995;**13**:263–6.

    This review paper, written for cardiologists consulted for victims of electrical injury, reviews the pathophysiology, evaluation, and treatment of these injuries. A thorough discussion of the myocardial necrosis possible in electrical injury is presented.

16. Xenopoulus N, Movahed A, Hudson P, Reeves W. Myocardial injury after electrocution. *Am Heart J* 1991;**122**:1481–4.

    This case report discusses the electrocution death of a 19-year-old man. Autopsy findings demonstrated widespread contraction band necrosis, myolysis, coagulative changes, loss of striations, and disappearance of the nuclei, all suggesting ischemic insult. Coronary arteries were normal. These authors postulate that smooth muscle spasm causes coronary artery spasm in victims of electrical injury.

22. Tompkins GS, Henderson RC, Peterson HD. Bilateral simultaneous fractures of the femoral neck: case report. *J Trauma* 1990;**30**:1415–16.

    This case report describes bilateral femoral neck fractures discovered in a 40-year-old male victim of a high-voltage electrical injury. The authors concluded that these injuries resulted from tetanic muscle contraction. They cite several other case reports of fracture associated with electrical injury and recommend that radiographs of bones along the current path be obtained.

23. Mann R, Gibran N, Engrav L, Heimbach D. Is immediate decompression of high voltage electrical injuries to the upper extremity always necessary? *J Trauma* 1996;**40**:584–7.

    This retrospective review of 62 patients and 100 upper extremity, high-voltage injuries was conducted to determine if selective decompression resulted in less operation and amputation than immediate decompression. These authors cite an overall amputation rate of 10% compared with rates 3–4 times that in other series. They suggest that decompression be accomplished in the presence of symptoms of compartment syndrome, rather than immediate decompression as advocated by other authors.

25. Lightning associated deaths – United States 1980–1995. *MMWR* 1998;**47**:391–4.

    This MMWR report summarizes the deaths from lightning during the study period. Data were collected and reported by the National Center for Environmental Health of the Centers for Disease Control.

26. Cherington M, Yarnell PR, London SF. Neurologic complications of lightning injuries. *West J Med* 1995;**162**:413–17.

    This case series is large compared with most reports of lightning injuries. The authors describe 13 cases of lightning injuries and the attendant neurologic complications, which are varied. Most who died of neurologic injury died because of hypoxic encephalopathy caused by prolonged cardiopulmonary arrest.

27. Graber J, Ummenhofer W, Herion H. Lightning accident with eight victims: case report and brief review of the literature. *J Trauma* 1996;**40**:288–90.

    This case series describes eight victims of a simultaneous lightning strike. The series reinforces the idea that most patients suffer prompt cardiopulmonary arrest or only minor injuries that are self-limited. When cardiopulmonary arrest is treated promptly, outcome is generally good.

28. Cooper MA, Andrews CJ. Lightning injuries. In: Auerbach PS, ed. *Wilderness medicine: management of wilderness and environmental emergencies*, 3rd edn. St Louis: Mosby 1995;261–89.

    This chapter is a comprehensive review of lightning injuries. The physics of lightning strike, pathophysiology of lightning injury, injuries from lightning, and treatment of lightning injuries are discussed. One hundred and eighty-seven references are cited.

29. Cherington M, Yarnell P, Lammereste D. Lightning strikes: nature of neurologic damage in patients evaluated in hospital emergency departments. *Ann Emerg Med* 1992;**21**:575–8.

    This case series of six patients describes the neurologic injuries seen after lightning strike. The degree of impairment ranged from mild to severe. No focal intracranial lesions, except for one cerebral infarction, were identified. One patient with spinal cord paralysis had normal MRI but persistent paraplegia one year after the injury. The authors state that spinal cord lesions tend to be permanent but cerebral lesions are likely to show improvement with time.

30. Cherington M, Krider EP, Yarnell PR, Breed DW. A bolt from the blue: lightning strike to the head. *Neurology* 1997;**48**:683–6.

This case report describes a 51-year-old bicyclist who was struck in the head by a bolt of lightning proven to be over 16 kilometers away. The lightning burned a hole in his bicycle helmet and caused a right temporal entrance wound. Cardiopulmonary arrest was immediate. Resuscitative efforts restored a stable rhythm in 19 minutes. The patient survived but suffered permanent neurologic dysfunction.

## Electrical injuries

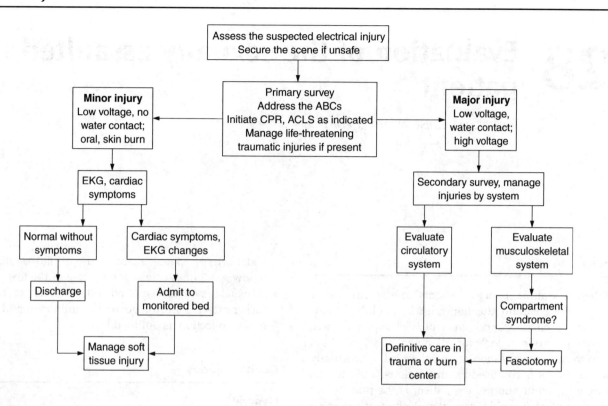

## Lightning strike

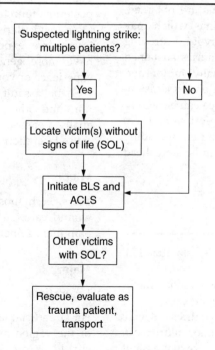

# 28 Evaluation of the sexually assaulted patient

*Barbara M Guise, Marsha Ford*

## Suspicion

When a trauma patient presents to the emergency department, careful attention must be paid to the surrounding circumstances in which the patient was found in order to look for all potential injuries, but also to raise the question of sexual assault, particularly if the patient is confused or unconscious. The medical care and stabilization of the patient is the priority but if the patient is stable, careful collection of materials and specimens, as well as delaying procedures such as bladder catheterization until specimens are obtained, will be helpful in the legal proceedings which may follow.[1] If possible, it is important to avoid destroying potential evidence. The majority of injuries sustained by victims of sexual abuse are usually minor and include bruises, abrasions, and lacerations.[2] Occasionally, injuries sustained to the genital area can be significant and require medical and/or surgical care. There may also be associated non-genital trauma, including strangulation, knife or gunshot wounds, and head injuries.[3]

## Management

- General trauma patient care: ABCs, stabilization, assessment of all injuries.
- Careful history from the patient or emergency medical service (EMS) personnel or police officers.
- First examine the patient for genital injuries if severe injuries are suspected. Otherwise, minor injuries can be examined during the course of the sexual assault examination.
- Non-genital injuries reported in sexually assaulted patients include strangulation, beating, lacerations, ecchymoses, hematomas, head injuries, fractures, and burns.[3,4] Management of these injuries should follow guidelines covered in the rest of the text.
- If sexual assault is suspected and the patient is stable, then proceed with the general examination and evidence collection as outlined below.

## Genital injuries

### General

The most common areas injured in women are the posterior fourchette, labia minora, hymen, and the fossa navicularis.[5–9] Further, women without prior intercourse experience and postmenopausal women have more genital trauma than women with prior experience or younger women.[10,11]

Sexual assault in men involves sodomy, oral penetration, and other sexual acts. Occasionally, victims are anally penetrated with a foreign object, which can cause lacerations and intraperitoneal injuries.[12,13]

### Minor

Tears, ecchymoses, and abrasions require only local wound care, such as sitz baths, tetanus prophylaxis, pain management, and stool softeners.[14]

### Major

#### Lacerations

For superficial lacerations that are in the lower portion of the vagina and perineal area, general wound care should be provided. Large superficial lacerations can be repaired primarily after careful irrigation. Smaller lacerations will often heal spontaneously. These lacerations should be explored to ensure they do not extend into the peritoneal cavity or urethra. The tissue is usually forgiving, but wound edges and mucosal edges should be well approximated.[14]

For wounds in the upper portion of the vagina that require closure, or for vaginal or cervical wounds which are bleeding heavily, a gynecologist should be consulted immediately. For excessively bleeding wounds, the vagina should be packed. Alternatively, a speculum can be opened inside the vagina to provide pressure against the wound.[7] The patient should be monitored closely, as she may become unstable from extensive blood loss.[15] An IV should be placed, serial hematocrits obtained, and appropriate antibiotics, usually a second- or third-generation cephalosporin, given.[7]

Perineal (vaginal, perianal, rectal) injuries should be investigated thoroughly for intraperitoneal, urethral, uterine, bladder, vaginal, and rectal involvement.[7,14]

Periurethral lacerations may also occur from localized trauma. These require primary repair by a gynecologist or urologist.[16] It is important to place a catheter if urethral disruption is not suspected. The catheter will provide a stent to maintain urinary flow and may reveal extension of vaginal lacerations into the urethra.[16] When urethral injury is suspected or found, further examination, including vaginal exam, should be done to determine if there are other injuries.

### *Other*

Rectal prolapse may occur after localized trauma or with intense Valsalva maneuvers. Rectal prolapse will often reduce spontaneously, but may require manual reduction. Prolonged prolapse or prolapse with associated edema may require surgical reduction. All patients should have surgical consultation.[14]

Urethral prolapse in girls or women occurs uncommonly and generally presents with a complaint of "vaginal" bleeding. For mild prolapse, conservative non-operative therapy is appropriate. For moderate or severe cases, operative management is usually required, necessitating urologic or gynecologic consultation.[17]

Victims of sexual assault may suffer from scalding or flame burns to the genitalia or perineal area. Generally, these burns require only local care with topical ointments and antimicrobials. Rarely will the patient require surgical treatment with skin grafts. Urethral catheterization may be necessary depending on the amount of edema.[18]

### The sexual assault examination

Every US state has a sexual assault examination kit or rape kit, which includes documentation forms, swabs, slides, and packets for the collection of evidence. The physician should use this kit if sexual assault is suspected, as it will facilitate accurate evidence collection and examination documentation, as well as maintaining a chain of evidence which is required for legal proceedings.[19] The sexual assault examination can be competently administered after appropriate training and a specialized physician does not need to be consulted.

While rape kits generally recommend collecting specimens from patients whose assault occurred within the previous 72 hours, evidence can still be obtained from patients presenting later, particularly if the patient has not bathed or changed his/her clothes. Regardless of timing or amount of evidence collected, careful documentation of the history and physical is imperative in the care of the patient, particularly with regard to future legal prosecution.

Safety of the patient and reassurance should be emphasized throughout the examination. The patient has experienced an extremely upsetting event and often feels loss of control, as well as embarrassment, guilt, and vulnerability.[20,21] Many emergency departments have special counselors on call to be with the patient during his/her evaluation.

### History

The history should focus on the nature of the assault: where on the body was the patient touched and potentially injured; what were the general circumstances surrounding the assault, i.e. was he/she restrained, the number of assailants, types of instruments used, physical surroundings (dirt, grass or fiber samples found on the patient may be important evidence).[19–21] The history does not need to be detailed beyond what will affect your examination and care of the patient, as too much detail can occasionally conflict with police reports and negatively influence the case.[20]

Events preceding the assault: alcohol or drug use, recent trauma, recent sexual intercourse.[20,21]

Events following the assault: bathing, urination, defecation, douching, location and condition of clothes worn at the time of the assault, time of the last meal.[20,21]

Obtain past medical and surgical history as well as menstrual and sexual history, including time of most recent intercourse prior to the assault and type of birth control used, if any.[20,21]

### Forensic specimens

### *Clothes*

If the patient is wearing the same clothes he/she was assaulted in, then have him/her undress while standing on two pieces of paper, collecting the top piece with the clothes and placing in a paper specimen bag.[19,20]

Save any foreign material found on the clothes, including grass, dirt, and fibers. These can be placed into specimen cups or folded into the paper provided and packaged with the rape kit.[21]

If the patient has a tampon, sanitary napkin or diaper, air-dry the item, then place it in a specimen bag. Clothes should also be allowed to air-dry before placing them into the specimen bag. If placed into the bag wet, mildew can destroy evidence.[22]

Use tape rather than the examiner's saliva to seal the bags. This will avoid contamination.[22]

### Hair and nail scrapings/clippings

Hair samples should be pulled from head and pubic regions to provide the best forensic evidence.[22] Scraping under the nails for dirt, skin, and other debris is also done and the specimens placed in the kit.[19–22]

### Wood's lamp/ultraviolet light examination (UVL)

UVL will reveal non-visible evidence of bodily fluids and trauma to the skin, such as bruises.[23,24] The physician should perform a UVL examination of the patient's entire body. Areas of fluorescence should be documented carefully. A saline-soaked swab should be placed over the area of suspected bodily fluid to collect the specimen which should be air-dried, carefully labeled, and packaged with the rest of the kit.[21] Many types of fluid or debris will fluoresce, including semen, saliva, make-up, and lint. Since the significance of the fluorescing material is unknown, it is best to collect it as customary evidence and let the forensic laboratory delineate its identity and relevance to the legal case.[25]

### Complete physical examination

Examine the entire patient, including under the axillae, for signs of trauma or other evidence, including bruises, abrasions, lacerations, bite marks, ligature marks (from rope restraints), and extraneous hair or fiber samples (save in a specimen cup for the kit).[3,19–22] Any positive findings should be meticulously documented on a drawing, including the location and nature of the injury. Note size and color of markings. Also examine the mouth for bleeding and petechiae, which can occur from repetitive trauma. Areas of dried bodily fluids should be carefully scraped onto paper, the paper folded and collected into an envelope.[21]

Photographs are a useful tool in accurately documenting injuries. Placing a ruler or coin next to the area photographed helps to give an indication of size.[19,20]

Examination of the genitalia and perineum should begin with gross visualization for any obvious injuries. After careful inspection, toluidine blue dye should be placed over the introitus and perianal area, excess dye wiped away with dry cotton swabs, and the area again examined for evidence of lacerations and tears that may have been missed initially.[5] The dye will be taken up by defects in the skin and cannot be wiped away. After external inspection, the vagina should be evaluated with use of a speculum in postpubertal adolescents and women, again assessing for any lacerations, tears, foreign bodies or other injuries. Only use saline or water to lubricate the speculum, as lubricants can alter potential evidence collected.[19,20] Many recommend the use of colposcopy if available as this magnifies the area examined and can show traumatized areas more clearly.[26–29]

Examination of male patients' genitalia can be done while the patient is supine or standing.

Inspection of the perianal area can be done as follows. Position the patient in a left lateral decubitus or knee-chest position, then gently spread the gluteal folds and allow time to pass to see if anal dilatation occurs, which is an indicator of trauma to this area. Also examine for abrasions, swelling, fissures, and lacerations.[30,31]

### Mucosal swab collection

Two swabs should be collected from each site: oral, vaginal, rectal. Even if the patient denies oral or rectal contact, he/she may not recall accurately the events of the assault.[32]

- Oral – under the tongue, behind the tonsillar pillars, and between the lips and the gums
- Vaginal
- Cervical (adolescents and adults only)
- Rectal – swabs should reach ½–1 inch beyond the anus

Swabs need to be air-dried before being placed into packets.

### Diagnostics

Wet prep mounts of vaginal and cervical fluids can be screened to look for sperm. However, some recommend against this practice. Lack of sperm on a wet prep may legally harm a legitimate case of rape.[33]

DNA probe or cultures for sexually transmitted diseases (STDs) should be collected.[19–22]

Obtain a venous blood sample and saliva specimen with 3–4 sterile swabs or a 2 × 2 gauze pad. These will be used to determine and compare secretor status and ABO type of victim and assailant.[21,22,25]

Pregnancy test, urine or serum.

Avoid bladder catheterization until after all specimens are obtained, as this can interfere with potential evidence. Also, if the patient should need to urinate or defecate before swabs can be obtained, save the specimens as part of the kit. Have patient avoid wiping before or after urination or defecation in order to avoid losing evidence.

Draw blood samples for HIV, hepatitis, and syphilis after counseling the patient. These tests provide a baseline status for the patient presenting acutely.[19,20,33]

Collect a urine sample to include in the rape kit. The forensics lab will evaluate it for sperm.[22]

Drug testing for illicit drug use, potential overdose or ethanol is helpful if the patient presents with altered mental status or exhibits signs of amnesia.[21,34,35] Particularly regarding the latter, the examiner should suspect the possibility of the use of flunitrazepam (Rohypnol), a benzodiazepine that may be placed into someone's drink without the victim realizing it. It is odorless, colorless, tasteless, and dissolves rapidly. Testing for Rohypnol is mandated if it is suspected. There are other similar drugs in use, such as gamma-hydroxybutyrate (GHB), which routinely do not show on a drug screen.

## Documentation

Careful documentation of the history and physical findings is imperative for any patient encounter, but more so for victims of sexual abuse, as the medical record will be used as evidence in prosecuting the assailant. Placing patient's words in quotes is useful. Drawing, photographing, and describing injuries are also very helpful.[19–21]

The rape kit is useful in that it provides forms and drawings to document findings easily. However, space may not be adequate and any additional information should be included. Furthermore, the emergency department or hospital record should also be detailed meticulously in case the kit should get lost.

Maintaining the chain of evidence is important and the physician or nurse should be with the kit at all times until it is given to the police. This is necessary to provide confirmation that no one could have tampered with the kit and that the items found in the kit are in fact from the patient examined.[19]

## Treatment

### Injuries

Management as delineated above.

### Sexually transmitted diseases (Table 28.1)

Prophylactic treatment is recommended for STDs, including gonorrhea, chlamydia, and trichomoniasis, at the time of initial evaluation.[19–22] Researchers have found that many rape victims are at a higher risk for having these infections prior to being assaulted, as well as for acquiring these infections from the assault.[36–38]

Recommended therapy is ceftriaxone 250 mg intramuscularly (IM) or spectinomycin 2 g IM or ofloxacin 400 mg po plus doxycycline 100 mg orally twice a day for seven days or azithromycin 1 g orally, single dose plus metronidazole 2 g orally, single dose.[20,39]

HIV management is controversial. The patient needs counseling about HIV, including baseline testing and periodic testing thereafter if the initial test is negative. Prophylaxis can be offered after risks and benefits are discussed. Recommended prophylactic therapy is

**Table 28.1** Treatment of sexually transmitted diseases and pregnancy prevention in the sexually assaulted patient[20,22,39–41]

| Issue | Therapy (adult) | Therapy (child) |
|---|---|---|
| Gonorrhea | Ceftriaxone 250 mg IM<br>or spectinomycin 2 g IM<br>or ofloxacin 400 mg po | Ceftriaxone 50 mg/kg IM |
| Chlamydia | Doxycycline 100 mg po bid × 7 days<br>or azithromycin 1 g po | Erythromycin base 50 mg/kg/day po divided qid × 7 days<br>or azithromycin 10 mg/kg po |
| Trichomoniasis | Metronidazole 2 g po | Metronidazole 40 mg/kg po × 1 dose<br>or 15 mg/kg/day po divided bid × 7 days |
| HIV | (Provide baseline testing and pretest counseling)<br>Zidovudine 600 mg po qd divided bid, tid<br>or six times a day plus lamivudine 150 mg po bid | Consult pediatric infectious disease specialist |
| Pregnancy | 2 tabs (50 μg ethinyl estradiol/0.5 mg norgestrel)<br>or 3 tabs (35 μg ethinyl estradiol). Either dose taken<br>at time of exam and 12 hours later. | Same as for adult if of childbearing age |

zidovudine 600 mg po qd divided bid, tid or six times a day plus lamivudine 150 mg po bid.[40,41]

The risk of hepatitis exists as well. Again, counseling the patient and offering testing are the current recommendations. Immunoglobulin and the hepatitis B vaccine can be offered if the risk was known to be high or the patient desires therapy.[20]

### Pregnancy (Table 28.1)

The risk of becoming pregnant after sexual assault is thought to be low; however, it can occur.[22,23] It is recommended that postcoital estrogens be offered to women of childbearing age who are not already using birth control.

Current therapy recommended is two oral contraceptive tablets (each with 50 µg of ethinyl estradiol and 0.5 mg of norgestrel) taken at the time of the examination and repeated in 12 hours or three oral contraceptive tablets (each containing 35 µg of ethinyl estradiol) taken at the time of the examination and repeated in 12 hours.[19,20,22]

## Children as victims of abuse

### Non-sexual abuse

Each injury should be managed according to current medical standards. If abuse is suspected, appropriate authorities should be notified and measures taken to ensure the child's safety.

### Sexual abuse

It is uncommon for a child to present acutely or within 72 hours of an episode of sexual abuse. When it does occur, a rape kit should be completed as outlined above.[30,31]

The type of medical evaluation the child receives depends on the specific complaint, time of assault, and available resources. Counselors, social workers, and physicians specially trained in child sexual abuse should manage these patients. If a medical condition requires immediate attention, the physician seeing the child primarily should attend to that condition and obtain only enough history from the child and accompanying adult to guide the evaluation.[30,31]

Injuries to the genital and perineal areas should be managed as above. Vaginal or rectal bleeding will need to be evaluated with the child under anesthesia in order to get an adequate exam.[30,31]

A speculum exam is never performed in a young, prepubescent girl unless there is suspicion of vaginal injury. Cervical swabs are not obtained in girls, only vaginal swabs.[42]

- Adequate evidence can be obtained from vaginal swabs.
- Complete penile penetration of young girls' vaginas is rare.
- Sexually transmitted diseases infect the vagina, not the cervix, in a prepubescent girl.
- Speculum examinations required to obtain cervical swabs may cause trauma to the introitus and are difficult to do in an awake child. If deemed necessary, a speculum exam should be done under anesthesia with the guidance of a gynecologist.

Foreign bodies are occasionally found on vaginal exams and are considered an indicator of abuse.[43] If a foreign body is found, this should be collected and saved in a specimen cup as part of the rape kit or handed over to appropriate law enforcement officials.

### General guidelines for interviews and examination[30,31,42]

#### Caregiver/parent

Interview alone. Get as much information as possible: chief complaint, specific events (including what, if any, penetration), specific concerns, past medical history, medical/psychological review of systems (including behavioral changes), social history (how the household is arranged), developmental history.

Counsel the parent/caregiver not to discuss events with the child.

#### Child

Interview alone and establish a good rapport with and comfortable setting for the child. Make the child feel he/she has some control. Explain everything that will happen before it happens.

If other resources are available, the physician's role in interviewing is limited: get enough information to determine if there is reasonable suspicion of abuse and where the child was touched and/or penetrated. Avoid pursuing too much detail and defer to a trained specialist.

If there are no other resources in the community, then obtain as objective and uncoerced a history as possible.

Assess the home situation: who lives there; who visits often; who sleeps where; who bathes, kisses, and hugs the child? Assess discipline: what happens when the child gets in trouble?

Use *open-ended, non-leading* questions: "Has someone ever touched you in a way you didn't like or that made you feel funny? Tell me more about that. What happened? When was the last time that happened?"

If the child doesn't provide information regarding possible abuse, ask the child what he/she would do if someone did do something inappropriate (would child tell someone or not?).

Universalize the child's experience to increase his/her comfort.

Repeated questioning may be harmful and may distort the history. Improper or leading questions can render the child's history inadmissible in court.

Never introduce new information to the child.

*Physical examination*

Have a caretaker of the child's choice and a chaperone (nurse or other) present. Allow the child to lie in the caretaker's lap during the exam if the child so desires. Perform the general examination and evidence collection as above.

Perform the genital-rectal examination as described above. For girls, however, certain positions are used to make evaluation easier and more comfortable for the child.

Genital examination should be performed in the supine frog leg position and knee–chest (prone) position. Inspect the labia majora, labia minora, clitoris, urethra, hymen, vestibule, posterior fourchette, and perineum. Colposcopy or even an otoscope is useful in providing magnification of this smaller anatomy. Again, a speculum is not used except in the postpubertal adolescent.

Labial separation versus traction.

- Allow the child time to relax for better visualization.
- Supine: gently grasp labia between the thumb and forefinger bilaterally and pull downward and outward. It is best to pull labia out straight and gently, as moderate transverse traction can pull and even tear the posterior fourchette.
- Prone: lift labia upward and apart to inspect the posterior hymen, vagina, and anus. This position allows visualization of areas that may have seemed abnormal or normal in the supine position.

Change in position and technique, as well as the amount of relaxation, can alter anal and hymenal configuration.[30]

Note that all girls are born with a hymen and normal hymenal configurations vary according to the age of the child and between girls of the same age.[42,44] It is best for physicians to become familiar with the variations as presented in various texts. Measuring hymenal orifices is not recommended, as the measurements are examiner dependent, as well as dependent on various conditions, such as patient relaxation and amount of tension applied by the patient's position or examiner.[42,44,45]

Injury may be obscured by a fimbriated hymen as found in an older child. One can better visualize hymenal edges by use of a swab or Foley catheter to gently expand the edges to search for tears. To use the catheter, insert the unexpanded catheter into the vagina, then place approximately 3–5 cc of saline into the balloon. Gently pull the catheter out of the vagina with the balloon expanded, noting the hymenal edges spread out against the balloon. Particular attention should be paid to the posterior rim of the hymen, as this is the area most frequently injured by attempted or actual penetration.[42]

Collection of vaginal specimens in girls with vaginal dryness can be improved by using swabs moistened with saline or using a 2 cc saline wash with a dropper or butterfly (needle off) attached to a #12 catheter and syringe. Insert the dropper or butterfly into the vagina and inject saline, then aspirate the fluid. Dip swabs into the collected aspirate and save for analysis. This method can be used to collect swabs as evidence or for STD cultures. Note that this method can cause dilution and lead to false-negative test results.[42]

Examination of the anal area may reveal immediate anal dilatation, fissures, lacerations or thickened tissue or skin tags, which can be indicators of chronic abuse.[30]

Note that often in children, abuse has been ongoing and the tissue heals quickly. Findings on the genital-rectal examination may be minimal or entirely normal.[45]

### Sexually transmitted diseases in children (Table 28.1)[30,42]

The prevalence of STDs in sexually abused preadolescent children is low. Whether or not to test a child is determined by the history and if there are any medical complaints.

- If no history or an unclear history is available, do all tests.
- If there is a reliable history of no penetration or direct contact, then no tests are necessary.
- If symptoms are present, then the child needs to be tested.

Most STD screening tests are inadequate for children.

- Cultures should be used to test for an STD, such as gonorrhea and chlamydia, as the other tests are not specific enough on vaginal and anal specimens.
- Chlamydia also requires use of a special media and swab (dacron, rayon, cotton on plastic), as some swabs are toxic to the chlamydia organism.

Treatment for STDs in children is different from that in adolescents or adults. It is recommended that treatment be given if the child is symptomatic, poor follow-up is expected, the patient or caregiver requests treatment after risks and benefits are discussed, and if the patient is an adolescent. Recommended therapy of chlamydia for children under eight years of age is erythromycin base 50 mg/kg/day orally four times a day for seven days or a single dose of azithromycin 10 mg/kg orally. For gonorrhea, ceftriaxone may be administered with a dose of 50 mg/kg intramuscularly. For trichomoniasis, give metronidazole as a single oral dose of 40 mg/kg or 15 mg/kg/day given as two divided doses for seven days. Adolescents can be treated as adults for STDs, as outlined above.

## Documentation[30,31,42]

The examiner's records must be meticulous and detailed, including noting what position the child is in when remarking on injuries. *Example*: a small defect is noted at 3:00 in the hymen in the supine position which persists in the prone (knee–chest) position.

Note who is with the child, who wanted the child evaluated, who raised the question of abuse, who has provided the history, and who was present during the exam.

Document the child's and adult's mental status and behavior.

## Discharge instructions[30,31]

Notify appropriate authorities, including the police and Department of Social Services, and take measures to ensure the child's safety.

Give appropriate medical instructions, as well as follow-up information, including phone numbers and contacts of appropriate agencies and counselors.

Remind caretakers not to discuss events with the child. A possibly untrue story may become reality to a child.

Counsel the child and caretaker to avoid changing the child's appearance, especially cutting or coloring hair, which can alter evidence that may be needed at a later time.

## Class II references

5. Lauber AA, Souma ML. Use of toluidine blue for documentation of traumatic intercourse. *Obstet Gynecol* 1982;**60**:644–8.

   This prospective study examined 44 women, including women who had been sexually assaulted and women who had engaged in consensual intercourse. Each woman was examined using toluidine blue staining, which revealed that 40% of the sexually assaulted patients had genital lacerations while only 4.5% of the consenting patients had injuries found

by the stain. This study also found that few of the lacerations were found prior to staining, thus making this a useful tool in evaluating victims of rape.

26. Lenahan LC, Ernst A, Johnson B. Colposcopy in evaluation of the adult sexual assault victim. *Am J Emerg Med* 1998;**16**:183–4.

    This prospective study examined 17 sexual assault victims with and without use of colposcopy. The authors found that 53% of the victims had trauma revealed by colposcopy while only 6% revealed trauma by gross visualization.

27. Norvell MK, Benrubi GI, Thompson RJ. Investigation of microtrauma after sexual intercourse. *J Reprod Med* 1984;**29**:269–71.

    This prospective study examined 18 women before and after consensual vaginal intercourse using colposcopy before and after staining with Lugol's solution. Increased vascularity and small abrasions were found in 11% of the women prior to intercourse and 61% after intercourse.

36. Glaser JB, Schachter J, Benes S *et al*. Sexually transmitted disease in postpubertal female rape victims. *J Infect Dis* 1991;**164**:726–30.

    Seventy-six sexually assaulted women were examined and evaluated for sexually transmitted diseases (STD) in this prospective study. The authors found that 20–50% of the women had an STD at the time of the initial exam. They also found poor compliance regarding their follow-up and thus conclude that all sexually assaulted patients should be offered treatment for common STDs (chlamydia, gonorrhea, and trichomoniasis) at the time of their initial examination.

37. Jenny C, Hooton TM, Bowers A *et al*. Sexually transmitted diseases in victims of rape. *N Engl J Med* 1990;**322**:713–16.

    This prospective study examined 204 patients within 72 hours of being assaulted and 109 of them at a follow-up visit; 43% of patients were found to have at least one sexually transmitted disease (STD) on initial exam. The incidence of new disease was lower. The authors concluded that the prevalence of STDs is significant in sexually assaulted patients and the risk of acquiring new disease is lower but substantial.

44. Berenson AB, Heger AH, Hayes JM *et al*. Appearance of the hymen in prepubertal girls. *Pediatrics* 1992;**89**:387–94.

    This prospective study looked at 211 girls without genital injuries or complaints to determine the normal variations in hymenal configurations. The authors found important differences based on age, but not on race. They found that notches, clefts, bumps, and tags can all be normal and measured hymenal openings to find an average size. They argue that physicians need to be familiar with what is normal before they can determine what is abnormal.

## Class III references

1. Aiken MM, Speck PM. Sexual assault and multiple trauma: a sexual assault nurse examiner (SANE) challenge. *J Emerg Nurs* 1995;**21**:466–8.

   This case presentation reviews important aspects in caring for a sexually assaulted patient with multiple injuries.

2. Everett RB, Jimerson GK. The rape victim: a review of 117 consecutive cases. *Obstet Gynecol* 1977;**50**:88–90.

   This chart review looked at various characteristics and injuries of rape victims, including average age and conditions of assault, as well as incidence of sexually transmitted diseases and types of injuries. They found that most patients suffered only minor physical injuries and the average victim was white, single, under age 25, and attacked by a single person.

3. Deming JE, Mittleman RE, Wetli CV. Forensic science aspects of fatal sexual assaults on women. *J For Sci* 1983;**28**:572–6.

   The circumstances surrounding the deaths of 41 rape victims are compared, revealing differences between younger and older victims. Further, mechanical asphyxiation was the most common mode of death, while the use of firearms was unusual.

4. Rambow B, Adkinson C, Frost TH, Peterson GF. Female sexual assault: medical and legal implications. *Ann Emerg Med* 1992;**21**:727–31.

   This retrospective review details injuries, incidence of sexually transmitted diseases (STDs), compliance with follow-up, incidence of pregnancy, and legal outcomes for 182 sexually assaulted women. The authors find that evidence of trauma found during the examination correlated with a successful legal outcome. Further, they conclude that compliance may be poor, particularly in lower socioeconomic groups; therefore, they recommend prophylactic treatment for STDs and pregnancy at the initial visit.

6. Bowyer L, Dalton ME. Female victims of rape and their genital injuries. *Br J Obstet Gynaecol* 1997;**104**: 617–20.

   This retrospective study reviewed case records of women reporting rape to determine if and what type of injuries occurred. The authors concluded that only a minority of patients showed evidence of genital injury, though this did not exclude rape.

7. Geist RF. Sexually related trauma. *Emerg Med Clin North Am* 1988;**6**:439–66.

   The author reviews an extensive list of injuries sustained as the result of sexual activities, consensual and non-consensual, including types, evaluation, and management.

8. O'Brien C. Improved forensic documentation of genital injuries with colposcopy. *J Emerg Nurs* 1997;**23**:460–2.

   This retrospective chart review found that colposcopy improved the examiners' ability to find and evaluate genital injuries. The authors document which areas are injured more frequently when examined by gross visualization alone and compare those data with data collected by colposcopy, finding discrepancies between the two.

9. Slaughter L, Brown CRV, Crowley S, Peck R. Patterns of genital injury in female sexual assault victims. *Am J Obstet Gynecol* 1997;**176**:609–16.

   This is a retrospective review of the colposcopic findings in 311 sexual assault victims, which are then compared with colposcopic evaluations of 75 women examined after consensual intercourse. The authors found that sexually assaulted women had more areas of injury than women who had consensual intercourse and they were able to determine which sites were most frequently injured.

10. Biggs M, Stermac LE, Divinsky M. Genital injuries following sexual assault of women with and without prior sexual intercourse experience. *Can Med Assoc J* 1998;**159**:33–7.

    This retrospective chart review reveals that more women without prior experience had genital injuries than those with experience. It also shows that a significant percentage of all women had injuries, regardless of prior experience.

11. Ramin SM, Satin AJ, Stone IC, Wendel GD. Sexual assault in postmenopausal women. *Obstet Gynecol* 1992;**80**:860–4.

    The records of postmenopausal rape victims (age >50) were compared to those of younger rape victims (ages 14–49), focusing on victim characteristics, circumstances surrounding the rape, and incidence and types of injuries. The authors found injuries to be common in both groups (67% in the postmenopausal group and 71% in the younger group). However, genital injuries were more common in the postmenopausal group, while non-genital trauma occurred more frequently in the younger group.

12. Hillman R, O'Mara N, Tomlinson D, Harris JRW. Adult male victims of sexual assault: an underdiagnosed condition. *Int J STD AIDS* 1991;**2**:22–4.

    This retrospective study reviewed 28 cases of sexually assaulted men, revealing the majority experienced anal intercourse and received a threat of HIV transmission. This has led the authors to recommend encouraging men to seek help, as they may be at significant risk for HIV and other sexually transmitted diseases.

13. Kadish HA, Schunk JE, Britton H. Pediatric male rectal and genital trauma: accidental and nonaccidental injuries. *Pediatr Emerg Care* 1998;**14**:95–8.

    This retrospective study reviewed the charts of male patients presenting with genital and rectal trauma. The authors looked at the mechanism, location, and type of injury, finding that accidental trauma in the perineal region is uncommon, with scrotal injury occurring more frequently than rectal trauma. Male victims of sexual abuse typically have injuries confined to the rectal area.

14. Janicke DM, Pundt MR. Anorectal disorders. *Emerg Med Clin North Am* 1996;**14**:757–88.

   This review of anorectal diseases includes a description of anorectal injuries, types, and management.

15. Smith NC, Van Coeverden de Groot HA, Gunston KD. Coital injuries of the vagina in nonvirginal patients. *S Afr Med J* 1983;**64**:746–7.

   This review of 19 cases of vaginal injuries reminds practitioners to keep coital trauma in mind as an etiology, particularly because the history may be lacking. The presentations of these patients and the management of their injuries are further discussed.

16. Okur H, Kucikaydin M, Kazez A *et al*. Genitourinary tract injuries in girls. *Br J Urol* 1996;**78**:446–9.

   This retrospective chart review describes perineal injuries in girls aged 2–13 years, including injury type, mechanism, and management.

17. Anveden-Hertzberg L, Gauderer MW, Elder JS. Urethral prolapse: an often misdiagnosed cause of urogenital bleeding in girls. *Pediatr Emerg Care* 1995;**11**:212–14.

   This retrospective review looked at 24 patients whose final diagnoses were urethral prolapse, including their initial diagnoses and initial and final management. The authors advocate increasing physician awareness of this condition to improve early recognition and appropriate treatment.

18. Michielsen D, Van Hee R, Neetens C *et al*. Burns to the genitalia and perineum. *J Urol* 1998;**159**:418–19.

   This retrospective study looked at 117 charts of patients with perineal and genital burns to determine the causes, management, and final outcomes. The authors concluded that conservative management provided the most favorable outcome.

19. Beebe DK. Emergency management of the adult female rape victim. *Am Fam Physician* 1991;**43**:2041–6.

   This article reviews the management of a rape victim.

20. Hampton HL. Care of the woman who has been raped. *N Engl J Med* 1995;**332**:234–7.

   The article reviews management of the rape victim, including initial evaluation and follow-up care, as well as statistics on sexual assault and injuries. The author also delineates potential pitfalls in the exam and the importance of careful, but not "excessively detailed", documentation.

21. Ledray LE. Sexual assault evidentiary exam and treatment protocol. *J Emerg Nurs* 1995;**21**:355–9.

   This article presents a detailed protocol for examining rape victims.

22. Sexual Assault. *ACOG Bulletin*, February 1987; number 101.

   This bulletin details the management of a sexually assaulted woman.

23. Barsley RE, West MH, Fair JA. Forensic photography: ultraviolet imaging of wounds on skin. *Am J Forens Med Pathol* 1990;**11**:300–8.

   The authors discuss UV photographic techniques and their application in abuse, rape, and assault cases.

24. Lynnerup N, Hjalgrim H, Eriksen B. Routine use of ultraviolet light in medicolegal examinations to evaluate stains and skin trauma. *Med Sci Law* 1995;**35**:165–8.

   This retrospective review of the use of ultraviolet (UV) light examination of rape cases reveals that stains with saliva and semen, as well as skin trauma, were detected with this method. Some of the skin trauma was not found by gross visualization, thus arguing for the routine use of UV light.

25. Ledray LE, Netzel L. DNA evidence collection. *J Emerg Nurs* 1997;**23**:156–8.

   This article reviews DNA testing, its use in rape cases, and the importance of potential evidence found on the victim, whether it be from stains on her skin or clothing or from vaginal, oral or anorectal swabs.

28. Slaughter L, Brown CRV. Cervical findings in rape victims. *Am J Obstet Gynecol* 1991;**164**:528–9.

   This article provides case reports in which colposcopic examinations revealed cervical injuries as well as their healing when reexamined days or weeks later.

29. Slaughter L, Brown CRV. Colposcopy to establish physical findings in rape victims. *Am J Obstet Gynecol* 1992;**166**:83–6.

   This retrospective review of 131 rape cases which utilized colposcopy as part of their examinations found that physical findings were better characterized and documented as a result of using colposcopy.

30. Hymel KP, Jenny C. Child sexual abuse. *Del Med J* 1997;**69**:415–29.

   This article provides a comprehensive review of sexual abuse in children, providing definitions, epidemiological information, presentations, medical evaluation, and management.

31. Kini N, Brady WJ, Lazoritz S. Evaluating child sexual abuse in the emergency department: clinical and behavioral indicators. *Acad Emerg Med* 1996;**3**:966–75.

   This review of sexual abuse in children delineates particular signs and symptoms of abuse, as well as the physical examination with examples of normal and abnormal findings. The authors provide a differential diagnosis and review the forensic evidence to be collected in these situations.

32. Hook SM, Elliot DA, Harbison SA. Penetration and ejaculation; forensic aspects of rape. *NZ Med J* 1992;**105**:87–9.

The authors conclude after their retrospective review of 104 rape cases that victims may not recall if penetration or ejaculation took place and, therefore, that swabs should be collected from rectal and vaginal areas routinely.

33. Young WW, Bracken AC, Goddard MA *et al*. Sexual assault: review of a national model protocol for forensic and medical evaluation. *Obstet Gynecol* 1992;**80**: 878–83.

    This article reviews aspects of the evaluation of a rape victim and proposes a national protocol that will be used in all states.

34. Anglin D, Spears KL, Hutson HR. Flunitrazepam and its involvement in date or acquaintance rape. *Acad Emerg Med* 1997;**4**:323–6.

    This review reports the increasing use of flunitrazepam (Rohypnol), particularly in association with sexual assault. They recommend screening for it in any rape case where the patient appears intoxicated or has difficulty remembering events.

35. Ledray LE. Date rape drug alert. *J Emerg Nurs* 1996; **22**:80.

    This report warns of the increasing prevalence of flunitrazepam, particularly in relation to sexual assault cases.

38. Irwin KL, Edlin BR, Wong L *et al*. Urban rape survivors: characteristics and prevalence of human immunodeficiency virus and other sexually transmitted infections. *Obstet Gynecol* 1995;**85**:330–6.

    This study presents the results of a survey of 1104 women to determine the prevalence of "recent" rape and characteristics of these women. The authors found that one in seven women admitted to being recently raped. They also found that rape was more common among women who were prostitutes, smoked crack cocaine, and were homeless.

39. Sexual assault and STDs. *MMWR* 1993;**42**:97–102.

    This report presents recommendations regarding initial evaluation, follow-up, and management of sexually transmitted diseases in the rape victim.

40. Gostin LO, Lazzarini JD, Alexander D *et al*. HIV testing, counseling, and prophylaxis after sexual assault. *JAMA* 1994;**271**:1436–44.

    This article reviews the risk of acquiring HIV as a result of sexual assault, and makes recommendations for the counseling, testing, and prophylactic treatment of patients. The authors note that AIDS is more prevalent among prisoners than among the general population; however, it is unclear if this is true of sexual assailants.

41. Public Health Service guidelines for the management of health-care worker exposures to HIV and recommendations for postexposure prophylaxis. *MMWR* 1998;**47**:1–28.

    Reviews current risks of acquiring HIV from exposure in health care workers and provides current guidelines for prophylactic therapy. The report is also referred to when discussing non-occupational exposure.

42. Heger A, Emans SJ, eds. *Evaluation of the sexually abused child: a medical textbook and photographic atlas*. New York: Oxford University Press, 1992.

    This textbook provides a very good review of the care of the sexually abused child, including evaluation and management, with excellent photographs showing normal and abnormal genital findings.

43. Herman-Giddens ME. Vaginal foreign bodies and child sexual abuse. *Arch Pediatr Adolesc Med* 1994; **148**:195–200.

    This retrospective chart review looked at 12 girls who presented with vaginal foreign bodies and found that 11 of them had evidence of sexual abuse. The previous notion that vaginal foreign bodies are an example of "self-exploration" is challenged. The authors recommend investigating for sexual abuse any situation in which a girl presents with a vaginal foreign body.

45. Bays J, Chadwick D. Medical diagnosis of the sexually abused child. *Child Abuse Neglect* 1993;**17**:91–110.

    This comprehensive article reviews sexual abuse in children: physical examination (may often be normal), healing of injuries, conditions which mimic sexual abuse. The authors propose a classification system for physical findings and emphasize the point that the history is the key to diagnosis.

**Evaluation of the sexually assaulted patient**

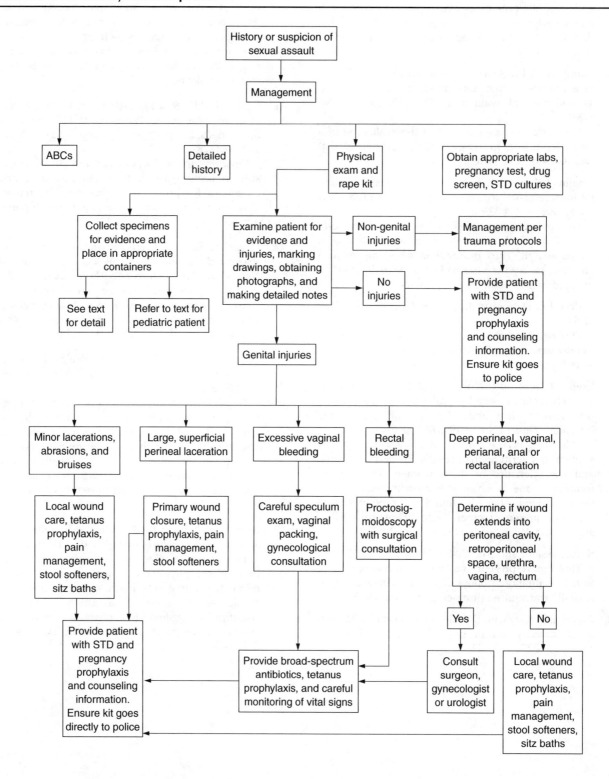

# 29 Mass casualty

*Philip A Visser*

The word disaster is derived from the Latin word *astrum* or *star*. Early mankind believed a calamity was visited upon them when the stars were malaligned. Disasters differ considerably from each other in the needs they generate and the constraints they present.

Every day mass casualty incidents such as transportation and industrial accidents cause comparatively moderate morbidity and mortality. They strain the resources of a small area and can frequently be handled by a single metropolitan hospital. Seldom do they involve more than 100 patients.[1]

Catastrophic disasters involve thousands of casualties. Many catastrophic disasters have never been described in the medical literature. Few, if any, have been fully documented with respect to morbidity, mortality or health care measures taken. Much of the medical care is provided through supplemental medical care facilities staffed by outside disaster relief teams.[2] In general, the worse the disaster, the worse the quality of data available. Many accounts are anecdotal and comprise imprecise estimates. In almost all cases clinical data are available only from hospitalized patients. Minor injuries treated on an outpatient basis are seldom analyzed and frequently overlooked in the injury estimates. Damaged health care systems cannot always provide the volumes of high-quality records they normally produce. Well-developed and undamaged health care facilities may curtail routine record keeping in a disaster in order to devote more attention to patient care.

In large-scale disasters official agencies and the populace look to the local hospital as the appropriate source of emergency medical care.[1] Mobile patients converge there for treatment. Other patients are transported by rescue agencies. Any sizeable event quickly exhausts the capacity of the hospital, whether or not it has been damaged. Further expansion of medical care can only be accomplished in two ways: import more medical care assets or export patients to unaffected areas. In small-scale disasters medical assets are imported through mutual aid mechanisms and patients are exported by transportation to nearby hospitals. In large-scale incidents it is almost impossible to expand the capacity of the local hospital. Supplemental facilities must be established to care for thousands of victims. These must be convenient to the patients and to the rescue workers. They almost always require importation of medical assets from outside.[3]

Finally, local hospital, emergency medical service and rescue and first service responder personnel must be considered. They and their families have been affected by the same catastrophe that has affected the rest of the community. Hospitals and response agencies must contend with the emotional needs and fatigue of their own personnel. They will need periods of rest and relief and time to attend to their personal and family needs. This can best be accomplished by importation of temporary replacement assets. After it is all over, each will need to be given opportunity and permission to go through a formal critical incident stress-debriefing program.[4]

## Preplanning

A disaster is any event which overwhelms the resources and capabilities of local responders.[5] The absolute number of patients is much less important than whether their needs exceed the resources available to care for them. Disaster respects neither jurisdictional nor geographical boundaries. Communications are disrupted. Medical resources normally available may be out of action. Agencies that do not normally interact may have to work together on a common task. Personnel may have to perform tasks outside their normal scope.

Direct medical care to the victims is only a small portion of disaster response.[6–9] There will be need for reliable drinking water, food and shelter, waste management, mortuary services, and vector control.[10,11] Critiques of past disaster experiences, whether large scale or small scale, always conclude with the following recommendations.[12]

Contingency plans are necessary. It is easy to be an ostrich – it will not happen here; there is no money in the budget for this; we do not have time to participate in a drill. Prior training and practice are essential. Paper plans that are written but not tried give a false sense of security. Unpracticed plans are unfamiliar when they need to be put into action. Agencies that need to operate together may have separate and uncoordinated plans.

Dependable communications are critical. Will all responders have radios that operate on the same frequencies? Will towers and repeaters be standing and operational? Can we rely on the telephones? Will cell phones be a viable option? Can a satellite be repositioned? Do our field units have satellite phones?

Command must be clearly established before the incident begins. Who is in command? How is command relinquished/accepted? The incident command system is a standard system used throughout the USA. It provides a flexible command and control structure upon which to organize a response.

The preplanning phase is now, today. It is the most important phase in the management of any mass casualty incident: planning, training, and preparing for a response.[13–18] Unfortunately, planning incurs costs.

## PICE

Koenig and her colleagues have suggested replacing the word disaster with the acronym PICE that stands for potential injury-creating event.[19] A PICE can be static or dynamic. Airline crashes are static events. A finite number of people are known to be injured. Little potential for further harm exists, except perhaps to the rescuers themselves. Dynamic implies evolving. A prolonged ice storm is a dynamic event. When the ice begins to fall it is too soon to know how many people will eventually be affected and what impact the event will have on local responders.

The majority of PICEs can be handled by augmenting a well-rehearsed hospital and EMS response. Most communities have mutual aid agreements with their neighbors. An event such as a hurricane can completely overwhelm capability to mount a normal response. Outside help will be required from state and federal resources.

### Scene survey: number of casualties, mechanism, and scene safety

Once the PICE has occurred the first task is not initiation of patient care but to determine whether there is an ongoing risk to the responders.[20] Building collapses and hazardous chemical spills both present the potential for injuring responders first on the scene. Never risk more than you expect to gain. The second task is to gather and transmit information used to facilitate effective decision making. How many victims are there? What is the medical status of the victims?

### START triage: simple triage and rapid treatment system

Standard hospital-based triage is intended to identify the most severely ill patients to assure they will receive aggressive care rapidly. Delivery of medical care during a catastrophe differs radically from the norm.[21–29] Strict adherence to the doctrine of maximum care for every victim would lead to total paralysis of medical services, resulting in no care for anyone. The philosophy of care no longer centers on the individual patient. Medical resources, personnel, supplies, and facilities are carefully allotted to provide the most good for the greatest number of people. Disaster triage is harsh. Victims who may have been saved by heroic measures under different circumstances may be left unattended.[30–32]

START triage begins with the ability to walk. Those who can walk are directed to a predesignated area for simple first aid and release or transport later. This simple step greatly reduces the number of victims to be considered for immediate transport. As the responder moves through each level of assessment, any condition that is deemed immediate stops the evaluation process. Life-threatening injuries are addressed in simple fashion. The responder may attempt to establish a clear airway by repositioning the victim or by clearing debris from the patient's mouth. Obvious external bleeding may be controlled by pressure. Complete evaluation should take no longer than one minute per patient.[32]

Once triaged, victims may be transported to a casualty collection point which should be safe and have easy access to the flow of incoming victims and to traffic lanes. More definitive triage and stabilization can be performed at the casualty collection point.

### Class II references

1.  Auf der Heide E. Disaster planning part II. Disaster problems, issues and challenges identified in research and literature. *Emerg Med Clin North Am* 1996;**14**:453.

    Analysis of numerous disasters reveals that hospitals are often inadequately prepared for the problems that develop during disasters. Most US disasters are not of extraordinary magnitude. Many of the logistic problems faced in US disasters are not caused by shortages of resources, but by failure to coordinate their distribution.

Domestic civilian disasters are characterized by a predominance of relatively low-severity injuries. Less than 10% of the casualties have conditions that require overnight admission under ordinary circumstances. Approximately twice that many are admitted. Half of those admitted are sent home the next morning.

Proportions of patients admitted to the hospital overnight because of disasters (from Auf der Heide)

| | |
|---|---|
| Loma Prieta Earthquake, San Francisco Bay area | 10% of 325 injured |
| Hurricane Hugo, Charlotte, NC | 4% of 2045 treated |
| Hurricane Andrew | 12% of 17 000 treated |
| Sioux City aircrash | 30% of 193 treated |
| Metrorail crash, Washington DC | 20% of 25 treated |
| Earthquake, Coalinga, CA | 11% of 198 treated |
| Kansas City Hyatt Hotel skywalk collapse | 45% of 200 injured |
| Wichita Falls, TX tornado | 10% of 1700 treated |

Even when disaster medical resources are available in the community, their use frequently is not well coordinated. Typically the majority of casualties are transported to the closest hospital or to the hospital most renowned for its emergency or trauma care. Other hospitals in the area receive few or no victims.

Distribution of casualties in 29 mass casualty disasters (from Auf der Heide)

| Number treated | Hospitals used/ available | Treated at one hospital (%) |
|---|---|---|
| 132 | 8/12 | 41 |
| 34 | 4/11 | 65 |
| 155 | 2/6 | 97 |
| 28 | 2/3 | 89 |
| 103 | 4/4 | 93 |
| 140 | 4/17 | 90 |
| 45 | 3/3 | 60 |
| 94 | 2/7 | 60 |
| 61 | 7/151 | 51 |
| 55 | 4/5 | 55 |
| 398 | 11/105 | 52 |
| 35 | 4/105 | 71 |
| 200 | 13/26 | 42 |
| 51 | 5/12 | 78 |

Few localities have a comprehensive disaster response plan that accounts for government disaster response, civil defense, and disaster medical care. Jurisdictional disputes and competition that exist on a day-to-day basis deter such planning. Hospitals and health care organizations frequently do not participate in planning with other organizations involved in disaster preparedness. Even rarer are plans integrat-

ing local, state, and federal responses. Written disaster plans are frequently not practiced, are frequently not familiar to those participating in the disaster response, and frequently not followed in the actual event. The Disaster Research Center studied 29 domestic disasters. The predesignated communication plan was followed in 21% of the disasters. Less than half transported casualties according to the written plan.

Apathy is the greatest impediment to disaster preparedness. Disasters are low-probability events. Government and public safety agencies struggle to provide expanding service expectations with shrinking budgets. There is a false general perception that disasters are just bigger daily emergencies which can be effectively managed by mobilization of personnel, equipment, and supplies. Nothing overcomes apathy faster than the occurrence of a disaster.

The appendix at the end of the paper provides an excellent bibliography for further readings and lists of resources for disaster training, disaster supplies, and disaster resources on the Internet.

2. Mahoney LE, Whiteside DF, Belue HE *et al*. Disaster medical assistance teams. *Ann Emerg Med* 1987;**16**:354.

The National Disaster Medical System (NDMS) is a voluntary cooperative program carried out by the federal government in partnership with state and local governments and the private sector. It contains three elements: medical response to the affected area in the form of disaster medical assistance teams; patient evacuation to unaffected areas; and definitive care in a national network of participating hospitals. NDMS is most useful for three functions unique to disaster medical care: casualty clearing, medical staging, and field surgical intervention.

Casualty clearing points receive patients from field rescue services, sort them into priority groups for treatment and transport, perform basic and advanced life support, splint fractures and dress wounds, and hold and support patients until they can be evacuated.

In most disasters there will be two queues waiting for available transport. One is at the interface between short-haul transport and the first air transport. The second is at any site that moves patients to longer haul air transport. Medical staging services are necessary at each of the interfaces. Patients are received and retriaged. Those that need immediate attention receive it. The remainder of the patients are sheltered, cared for, and prioritized for outgoing transport. Similar services are required at the receiving airport to screen arriving patients, direct them to receiving hospitals, and provide patient support until they can be transported.

Some patients must be stabilized surgically before transport. Ideally this can be accomplished at surviving local hospitals. In a great disaster the local hospitals may not be available due to damage or overcrowding. Field medical units will receive patients from clearing points and directly from the rescue services. They will provide resuscitative surgery and intensive care to stabilize injured casualties for evacuation, provide pre- and postoperative care for these patients until they can be evacuated, transfer patients to outgoing transport, and shelter and feed both patients and staff.

4. Burkle FM. Triage of disaster related neuropsychiatric casualties. *Emerg Med Clin North Am* 1991;**9**:87.

Disasters by nature are situations involving "massive collective stress". There is significant disruption in the existing social system with a consequent increase in individual stress reaction. Traditional EMS response is geared to victims of physical trauma. Neuropsychiatric casualties are treated as walking wounded.

Most people show signs of emotional disturbance as an immediate reaction to a disaster. There is no such thing as no response. Most reactions are transient and victims recover spontaneously.

Most childhood reactions to a disaster are individually based and influenced by age, developmental level, proximity of family members, losses during and immediately after the disaster, and the secondary effects on how the family and the community at large respond.

Research suggests the elderly may be more resilient than younger victims. Previous life experiences moderate the disaster impact. The elderly frequently get along with less and often function better in a post-disaster, deprived environment. They are more vulnerable to relocation. In a disaster triage situation, the elderly are at risk of being devalued as it may be necessary to triage limited resources away from the elderly. The elderly may elect to refuse treatment offered to ensure resources for the young.

After a major earthquake in Greece, fatal cardiac arrests increased by 50%, peaking on the third day after the earthquake. Sudden stress-related catecholamine-induced ventricular fibrillation, vasovagal syncope, and catecholamine-induced platelet aggregation have been reported.

Rescue personnel, EMS personnel, and medical and nursing staffs represent a specific area of concern. Eighty to 90% of well-trained, experienced first responders cope well at the scene. Debriefing is critical to reduce the risk of posttraumatic stress disorder (PTSD). Symptoms include recurrent dreams, mental flashbacks, intense memories of the event or a sudden feeling that the traumatic event is recurring. At least two of the following symptoms – that were not present before the disaster – must exist to make a diagnosis of PTSD: sleep disturbance, exaggerated startle response, survival guilt, difficulty in concentrating, and avoidance of activities that arouse recollection of the event.

5. Lewis CP, Aghababian RV. Disaster planning part 1. Overview of hospital and emergency department planning for internal and external disasters. *Emerg Med Clin North Am* 1996;**14**:439.

Hospital disaster planners must plan for disasters that pose the greatest potential risk for their specific communities. A clear chain of command and communication is established for each department. The disaster plan should include disaster-related damage to the structural integrity of the hospital.

A hospital command center should be established with key senior management personnel. Department supervisors should receive regular briefings as disaster events unfold. They in turn keep the command center informed about available assets.

The traffic flow pattern for ambulances, employees, visitors, and the press should be predetermined by the disaster plan. Ambulatory and stable patients should be sent to a predesignated area away from the emergency department. Patients who can be discharged but who are unable to leave because of transportation limitations should be evacuated to a Red Cross shelter.

All plans should include the special needs of family, media, volunteers, and hospital staff. Adequate sleeping quarters and sufficient clothing and other linen are required to meet the needs of hospital personnel. Remember the staff and their families have been affected by the same disaster. They need permission to attend to their family needs. Innovative shift scheduling may be required.

6. Mahoney LE, Reutershan TP. Catastrophic disasters and the design of disaster medical care systems. *Ann Emerg Med* 1987;**16**:1085.

The authors focus on catastrophic events with thousands of casualties requiring interstate and international medical assistance. Earthquakes are their major model, though volcanic eruptions and floods are mentioned. The ratio of injuries to deaths approaches 3:1. Critical injuries requiring resuscitative care are conspicuous by their absence. Lacerations are 40–50% of recorded injuries; 18–20% are fractures; 20–25% contusions and abrasions. Most victims have more than one injury; 15–30% have head injuries; up to one third have ocular injuries. Wound infections are common.

Medical needs peak in a few days, then fall rapidly. Persons with minor injuries present rapidly in numbers that may impede care for the more seriously injured. There may not be enough hospital beds in the affected area. Patients may need to be evacuated to hospitals in unaffected areas. Supplemental medical facilities have been used in nearly all large disasters in recent times. A timely response requires a previously organized disaster medical system that can provide needed aid within 24 hours.

7. Noji EK. Disaster epidemiology. *Emerg Med Clin North Am* 1996;**14**:289.

Future catastrophic disasters with the potential for millions of casualties are probable because of increasing population densities in flood plains, in coastal areas, and along faults in the earth's crust. The disaster of today involves loss of property and means of livelihood; famine and population displacements; collapse of basic services, infrastructure, and political structure; and violence ranging from banditry, to civil conflict, to all-out international war.

Specific medical and health problems tend to occur at predictable times. Severe injuries requiring immediate trauma care occur mainly at the time and place of the impact. Priorities then shift to environmental health concerns – safe water, safe food, shelter, sewerage control, and vector control. A second peak of acute injuries occurs as a result of clean-up activities. A major management problem is interruption of medical care to the chronically ill and the elderly.

Of the tons of donated medications and medical supplies frequently arriving at disaster sites, 80–90% are of no value because they expired prior to donation, have already been opened or have labels written in a foreign language.

Immediately after the impact rapid epidemiologic assessments provide information about:

- overall magnitude of the disaster
- geographic extent and estimated duration
- effect on health
- integrity of health services delivery systems
- specific health care needs of survivors
- extent of disruption of public services
- extent of the local response.

This information leads to management decisions about amounts of relief supplies, equipment, and personnel that are required to be moved into the disaster scene. After the disaster, data collected are used to minimize injury and health consequences of future disasters. Future medical and public health responses are preplanned. Caches of supplies and equipment can be prestaged.

8. Noji EK. Natural disasters. *Crit Care Clin* 1991;**7**:271.

Natural disasters arise from the forces of nature such as earthquakes, hurricanes, floods, tsunamis, fire, tornadoes, and extremes of temperature. Increasing population density in flood plains, seismic-prone and hurricane-prone areas points to the probability of catastrophic future disasters with millions of casualties.

Deaths caused by natural disasters in this century (from Noji)

| Disaster type | Range of deaths |
|---|---|
| Earthquake | 900–250 000 |
| Volcanic eruption | 1300–29 000 |
| Hurricane | 56–6000 |
| Tropical cyclone | 10 000–300 000 |
| Tsunami | 1400–3000 |
| Typhoon | 400–10 000 |
| Landslide | 200–10 000 |
| Flood | 1800–57 000 |

Floods are the most common of all natural disasters: 50% of disasters and 50% of deaths. Mortality is the result of drowning, exposure, and trauma from fast-moving debris. A high proportion of victims of US flash floods die in their automobiles. Only 0.2–2.0% of survivors require medical attention.

Hurricanes generally cause few deaths. Nine out of 10 hurricane fatalities are caused by drowning associated with the storm surge. Most injuries occur in the post-storm clean-up. Crowding in shelters increases the probability of communicable disease outbreaks.

Tornadoes are the most violent and most lethal of all natural atmospheric phenomena. Approximately 4% of all injuries sustained are fatal. The leading causes of death are head trauma, followed by crushing injuries to the chest and abdomen. Fractures are the most frequent non-fatal injuries. For every person injured or killed, approximately 44 others will require some type of emergency medical attention.

Volcano-related deaths occur in approximately 5% of all eruptions. The immediate life-threatening effects are through suffocation due to inhalation of ash, scalding due to blasts of superheated steam, and surges of lethal gases. Mudflows account for 10% of all volcano-related deaths. Weight of accumulated ash can collapse buildings, resulting in trauma and entrapment of occupants. Ash is irritating to the eyes and mucous membranes of the respiratory system.

Earthquakes can be one of the most destructive events of nature. The primary cause of death and injuries is building collapse. Most injuries in survivors are minor. Approximately 2–3% of survivors require hospitalization. Some entrapped victims have been found alive after 48 hours but most die within the first 2–6 hours. Rapid response and rescue are essential.

| Effect | Earthquake | High winds | Tidal waves/ flash floods | Floods |
|---|---|---|---|---|
| Deaths | Many | Few | Many | Few |
| Severe injury | Overwhelming | Moderate | Few | Few |
| Increased risk of communicable disease | Yes | Yes | Yes | Yes |
| Food scarcity | Rare | Rare | Common | Common |
| Major population movements | Rare | Rare | Common | Common |

12. Cowley RA, Myers RAM, Gretes AJ. EMS response to mass casualties. *Emerg Med Clin North Am* 1984;**2**:687.

Review of the literature critiquing responses to disasters reveals five common recommendations.

(1) Contingency plans are necessary.
(2) Prior training of personnel is essential.
(3) Dependable communications are critical.
(4) Specific attention must be directed to control.
(5) Command must be clarified in advance.

Three phases of disaster (from Cowley)

| Phase | Time postincident | Goals |
|---|---|---|
| Primary (immediate) | 0–6 hours | Neutralize hostile environment<br>Salvage life/EMS-augmented response<br>Establish perimeter security:<br>traffic control<br>crowd control |
| Secondary (follow-up) | 6–24 hours | Maintain perimeter security<br>Organize hazard/debris removal<br>Establish public health:<br>sanitation<br>immunization<br>prescription maintenance |
| Tertiary (clean-up) | 48 hours to 60 days | Provide survivor assistance:<br>food, clothing, shelter<br>Provide human/social services:<br>relocation, employment, benefits,<br>insurance claims, loans |

13. Doyle CJ. Mass casualty incident. Integration with prehospital care. *Emerg Med Clin North Am* 1990;**8**:163.

Prehospital providers are usually more comfortable with field care than physicians. They are used to working in the cold, heat, rain or snow and to starting IVs by headlight.

Many hospitals have an in-house system of providing resources and personnel according to a phased plan based on the number of victims the hospital is expecting. General standing orders may be issued in advance to non-physician personnel: oxygen for all dyspneic patients, IV lines for all who are bleeding, etc.

Traffic patterns must be kept as simple as possible. One-way direction traffic must be maintained, at the scene and at the hospital, so vehicles do not become congested and ingress and egress are possible.

Communication problems are common in multi-casualty incidents. Radios may not all be on the same frequency. Telephone lines may be damaged or overwhelmed. Dedicated, buried landlines are a must. Cellular phones can be valuable if the system is not overwhelmed. They can be fixed or moving. Using a small computer with a modem or fax machine can expand cell phone capabilities. Sometimes messengers and runners are the most reliable forms of communication.

Disaster communication is most successfully accomplished by preplanning. Who needs to communicate with whom? What type and how much traffic volume are anticipated? Which hardware and software will fulfill these needs? The plan must include a back-up system in case the primary system fails.

Mutual aid agreements among jurisdictions should be established before a disaster incident. Hospitals should have written mutual aid agreements with hospitals outside their local community. When the

hospital itself is damaged or destroyed a triage system must be available to prioritize which patients should be evacuated first. Those who can should be discharged to home or to a shelter. Patient transport should be part of the preplan.

14. Binder S, Sanderson LM. The role of the epidemiologist in natural disasters. *Ann Emerg Med* 1987; **16**:1081.

Natural disasters are caused by subterranean stress (volcanoes and earthquakes), surface instability (landslides and avalanches), high winds (hurricanes and tornadoes) or by abnormal precipitation or temperature (floods, blizzards, heat waves, and droughts). Natural disasters that require international assistance to the affected population occur weekly.

Man-made disasters include famines, fires, explosions, chemical and radioactive material releases, major transportation accidents, and war.

Epidemiologists study past disasters to aid in planning the response to future disasters. Earthquakes in industrialized areas will destroy pipelines and release hazardous materials stored in underground containers. Knowledge and planning lead to ordinances that regulate the storage and handling of toxic materials. Some disasters such as hurricanes can be predicted. Preestablished evacuation routes save lives.

15. Waecherle JF. Disaster planning and response. *N Engl J Med* 1991;**324**:815.

Planning must be based on valid assumptions derived from the study of past disasters. Most disasters of moderate size produce 100–200 casualties. Approximately 15% of these will be seriously injured.

Disasters are classified according to the level of resources needed to meet the demands adequately.

- Level I    Escalated response by local EMS in cooperation with community agencies
- Level II   More regional response
  Local medical resources are exceeded
  Mutual aid agreements allow quick recruitment of crucial resources
  Protocols must provide for special equipment and skilled personnel that may be available only in the private sector
- Level III  State and federal involvement to cope with massive, widespread destruction

After a disaster, aid is usually not available for 24–48 hours. Communities must prepare to manage the incident on their own during the early stages. Experience is the key to success. Community drills, whether desktop or full field with simulated patients, provide a good alternative to first-hand experience with a real disaster.

The first wave of victims usually arrives within 30 minutes of the incident. They usually arrive by their own transportation and have minor injuries. These walking wounded can quickly overwhelm a hospital's capacity, impeding care of the soon-to-arrive seriously injured patients. A hospital's disaster plan must incorporate areas to treat the walking wounded located away from the emergency department. Planners must also make arrangements for fatalities with temporary morgues, near casualty collecting points but in a separate location well protected from the public view. The surviving population will require food, water, shelter, clothing, and sanitation.

Involved personnel should evaluate each disaster response. What went well? What did not go well? How can the response be changed for the better?

16. Eisner ME, Waxman K, Mason GR. Evaluation of possible patient survival in a mock airplane disaster. *Am J Surg* 1985;**150**:321.

The authors report on a mock airplane crash of a DC Super 80 jet at Orange County's John Wayne Airport involving 200 patients. They tracked 27 mock patients triaged to the University of California Irvine Medical Center. Nine of 10 "fair to good" mock patients arrived within 1.5 hours. Nine of 17 mock patients with "life-threatening, severe, or critical injuries" arrived later than 1.5 hours post-crash. Twenty-three of the 27 were admitted to the hospital. Four were sent home from the emergency department. The trauma center is 15 minutes away from the airport. The authors concluded that the ability to triage critically injured patients in a timely fashion was only slightly better than chance routing.

19. Koenig KL, Dinerman N, Kuehl AE. Disaster nomenclature – a functional impact approach; the PICE system. *Acad Emerg Med* 1996;**3**(7):723.

This article describes a model system to characterize disasters more precisely. It begins with the acronym 'PICE', which stands for potential injury-creating event. Descriptive modifiers are added to account for different scenarios. Modifiers predict the potential for additional casualties. Following this model allows those in command to predict the probability that their own resources will be overwhelmed and whether or not outside aid sources should be put on alert or brought into the scene.

20. Bissell RA, Becker BM, Burkle FM. Health care personnel in disaster response. Reversible roles or territorial imperatives? *Emerg Med Clin North Am* 1996;**14**:267.

This paper begins with a description of the chaos associated with large-scale disasters. The basic sequence to follow is:

- scene assessment
- initiation of the incident management system
- search and rescue of victims
- primary assessment and triage
- secondary assessment and stabilization
- transport
- definitive care
- address public health needs
- infectious disease control
- reestablishment of primary care services
- postevent stress debriefing and management.

Specific skills and usual roles of EMS, nursing, and physician personnel are discussed with reference to their usual place of employment. The discussion of flexibility and interchangeability ends with the following rules.

(1) Medics should perform initial assessment and triage, stabilization and transport to the triage/treatment area and on to definitive care if no physicians are available at the treatment area. The earliest point of physician intervention should be at the triage/treatment area.
(2) Only physicians and nurses specially trained to work in the field environment should do so.
(3) Only if physicians are in surplus in the hospital/clinic environment should they be sent to the field as care providers.
(4) Medics are poorly prepared to replace nurses in the hospital.
(5) Physicians are better prepared than medics to meet the public health needs of a disaster-affected population.

21. Gans L, Kennedy T. Management of unique clinical entities in disaster medicine. *Emerg Med Clin North Am* 1996;**14**:301.

Review of the disaster literature shows that triage frequently does not occur on the scene. The authors recommend that separate triage and treatment areas should be established early to prevent the initial extraction and transportation of casualties by bystanders.

Explosives are commonly used for commercial and terrorist purposes. Approximately 5% of the victims will receive a significant blast injury, but presentation may be delayed for hours. In a study of 5600 blast incidents including 495 deaths, the five injuries most commonly seen in fatalities (excluding soft tissue injuries) were:

- brain (subarachnoid hemorrhage) – 66%
- skull fracture – 51%
- diffuse lung contusion – 47%
- tympanic membrane rupture – 45%
- liver laceration – 34%.

In survivors, 1/3 will have leg injuries and 1/3 will have injuries involving the head and face. Only 15% will be sufficiently injured to require hospitalization.

Entrapment of people under collapsed buildings for four hours or longer may lead to crush injuries.

A rough estimate is 3–5% of victims, but this can be as high as 40%. Myoglobinemia/myoglobinuria leads to acute renal failure in 50%. Prevention involves beginning volume expansion before extraction.

Increased particulate matter in the air may become a health hazard following volcano eruptions, earthquakes, wildfires, and individuals trapped in collapsed buildings. Exacerbation of COPD and asthma are common. Many patients with no previous disease will present with wheezing and rales. Treatment is symptomatic, including supplemental oxygen.

22. Nancekievil DG. Disaster management. Practice makes perfect. *BMJ* 1989;**298**:477.

Recent disasters in Britain have required severely injured victims to be treated on site. Large numbers of casualties made it impossible to transport everyone to the hospital immediately. A mobile team of six physicians and nurses is recommended. White coats provide no protection; each team member should be properly equipped with distinctive protective overalls, clearly labeled "doctor" and "nurse". Gloves and eye protection are recommended. All members of the medical team should regularly practice resuscitation wearing gloves, goggles, and overalls.

23. Butler FR, Hagemann J, Butler, EG. Tactical combat casualty in special combat operations. *Military Med* 1996;**161**(suppl 1):3.

The paper discusses triage and care under enemy fire. At the tactical field care level the authors recommend the nasopharyngeal airway as the least likely device to be dislodged during patient transport. Needle decompression is adequate for tension pneumothorax. Direct pressure and tourniquet control external blood loss. IV fluids are recommended for hypotension secondary to external wounds, once the bleeding has been controlled. The authors recommend against IV fluid resuscitation for uncontrolled hemorrhage caused by penetrating abdominal and thoracic wounds. They review the literature to support their recommendations.

32. Benson M, Koenig KL, Schultz CH. Disaster triage: START, then SAVE – a new method of dynamic triage for victims of a catastrophic earthquake. *Prehospital Disaster Med* 1996;**11**(2):117.

Most triage systems in use today assume a short transport time to definitive care or a long time to initial triage. Mass casualty incidents frequently involve multiple scenes, which are widely dispersed. Infrastructure is commonly damaged. Available local medical resources are limited, frequently damaged, and are usually overwhelmed. Significant outside help cannot realistically be expected to arrive for at least 48–72 hours. Early evacuation is not possible. Time to definitive care is uncertain. Only limited, austere, field-type advanced life support equipment is available. This scenario requires a dynamic triage system, one that permits evolution

over hours and over days. Limited resources must be used efficiently to maximize benefit to the majority of patients. 'Simple Triage and Rapid Treatment' (START) uses ability to walk, respirations, presence of a radial pulse, and ability to follow commands to sort victims into expectant, delayed, and urgent categories. Evaluation of one victim should take less than one minute. 'Secondary Assessment of Victim Endpoint' (SAVE) assesses patient survivability based on the victim's injuries compared against known trauma statistics. Pre-existing disease and age are factored into the decision process. By comparing expected benefits to resources consumed, limited medical resources can be directed to those patients expected to benefit most from their use.

## Class III references

3. Roth PB, Vogel A, Key G *et al*. The St Croix disaster and the national disaster medical system. *Ann Emerg Med* 1991;**20**:391.

The National Disaster Medical System was designed to respond to a catastrophic disaster by creating a group of specifically trained civilian disaster medical assistance teams. The teams are designed to be self-sufficient with adequate supplies of food, water, and medications. The team is transported to the periphery of the catastrophic event to triage, stabilize, and prepare victims for evacuation. This paper describes the New Mexico Disaster Medical Assistance Team's experience in St Croix following Hurricane Hugo.

9. Leonard RB, Teitelman U. Manmade disasters. *Crit Care Clin* 1991;**7**:293.

Dealing with a disaster cannot begin when the first patient arrives at the door. Disasters are community and regional events of great complexity. How well they are handled depends on preplanning and an understanding of the unique circumstances presented by a disaster. Man-made disasters are transportation crashes, building collapses, releases of hazardous materials, terrorist activities, fires, and explosions.

Disasters produce three categories of patients: surgical, medical, and psychiatric. Surgical patients will have either mechanical trauma (head, chest, abdomen or extremity) or burns (thermal or chemical). Medical patients will primarily have toxic inhalation causing pulmonary damage, systemic toxicity from absorbed chemicals or radiation injuries.

Hazardous materials disasters may produce injuries unfamiliar to physicians; pulmonary and systemic injuries of bewildering variety. Corrosive chemicals may also produce skin burns. Trucks, barges, and pipelines ship many of these chemicals daily. Victims whose skin, clothing or both are contaminated with chemicals must have their clothing removed and be decontaminated by washing with water. Contaminated patients who arrive at the hospital are untreated essentially and are potentially dangerous to hospital personnel. The authors present a concise discussion of chemical burns, toxic inhalation, agricultural poisons, radiation accidents, terrorism, and chemical warfare agents.

10. Klein JS, Weigelt JA. Disaster management. Lessons learned. *Surg Clin North Am* 1991;**71**:257.

Disasters are a mixture of four variables: injury to human beings, destruction of property, overwhelming of local response resources, and disruption of organized societal mechanisms. Successful management requires planning and practice. All of us believe we will never experience a disaster or we will be only a limited participant. We believe disaster drills are a waste of time because medical care in disasters is merely an extension of normal everyday activity. The authors share some lessons learned from three aircraft crashes in Dallas.

There was difficulty obtaining reliable information from the field. City, county, and airport disaster plans had minor differences regarding communication and chain of command. It was unclear which plan was operational. No communication devices were available for field triage teams or medical staging areas. The command post was unable to obtain information about numbers and severity of casualties.

The ability of the command post to communicate with hospitals was limited by personnel and by access to appropriate communication lines. Phone lines were all tied up with internal communication.

Media control was a major problem. Media personnel wandered through the emergency department and the operating rooms, interfering with patient care. Crowd control became an extra burden when 491 people arrived at the hospital to donate blood in response to a media broadcast.

The first crash site was never secured. Onlookers and media wandered in and out at will. Similarly, ambulances had to pass through a crowd of onlookers at the emergency department door. For the second and third crashes, field security was resolved by the disaster plan clearly identifying who was responsible for field and hospital security. Color-coded name badges identified those who were authorized to be in the field. Hospital traffic lanes were predetermined and secured by hospital security personnel.

Triage never occurred at the first plane crash because the triage team never went to the crash site. Ambulances rushed to the site in response to public media announcements of the crash. Each ambulance immediately transported the first victims they came across to their own hospital. Ambulance gridlock was resolved by defining response and traffic patterns in the revised disaster plan.

At the first crash there were too many physicians at the hospital trying to take care of too few patients.

Most of the physicians present had no understanding of mass casualty protocols. Creating teams consisting of a senior surgeon, two resident surgeons, two nurses, and a respiratory therapist solved the problem. Each team was admitted to the emergency department as a group and was responsible for caring for one patient from start to finish. Extra physicians were assigned to treatment areas specifically set up to handle minimally injured patients.

Honest critiques were held after each disaster. Debriefing of acute care areas was accomplished within 24 hours. A hospital-wide debriefing was held within 72 hours. Psychological support and debriefing are essential not only for victims and their families, but also for first responders and hospital personnel.

11. Noji EK, Kelen GD, Armenian HK *et al*. The 1988 earthquake in Soviet Armenia. A case study. *Ann Emerg Med* 1990;**19**:891.

Collapsed buildings trapped 40 000 people; 15 000 were rescued; 25 000 bodies were recovered. Another 31 000 people were injured, of whom 12 200 required hospitalization. The death rate was 81.4% for trapped individuals and 1.2% for those not trapped. Every single trapped individual was injured in some manner. Only 8.8% of those not trapped were injured.

All hospitals in the region were severely damaged and 80% of the local medical personnel were killed or injured. Three hundred and eleven people were transported to hospitals outside the region. Ten per cent of the transfers were due to crush syndrome, half of whom developed acute renal insufficiency secondary to the crush injury.

Rescue response time was critical. Ninety-three percent of those who were trapped and survived were rescued in the first 24 hours. Within the first 2–6 hours less than 50% of those who were buried were still alive. Any significant reduction in earthquake mortality can only be achieved by attention to search and rescue within the first 24 hours. The major problem with extraction of the trapped victim is lack of adequate equipment and trained rescue personnel.

17. Lewis FR, Trunkey DD, Steele MR. Autopsy of a disaster. The Martinez bus accident. *J Trauma* 1980;**20**:861.

A charter bus with 50 passengers rolled over a highway railing, turned upside down, and fell 22 feet. It became impossible to maintain a secure perimeter. The scene became chaotic with a large group of people milling around the bus undirected. Communication proved almost non-existent. Ambulances took patients to hospitals of the driver's choice, sometimes bypassing closer hospitals. Twenty-four victims reached the hospital alive. One subsequently died of an irreversible head injury. Two died en route to the hospital and 24 were dead at the time of evacuation from the bus. Reviews of autopsies suggest 10 of the

24 who died at the scene might have survived if extraction had been more rapid.

The fire department functioned effectively in the rescue and emergency treatment role since their intrinsic organization and hierarchy provided order at the scene. In addition, they had previously held disaster drills and had some expectation of the problems to be encountered. Police services were less effective because of functional uncertainties about jurisdiction. The result was lack of perimeter control. Ambulance services were least coordinated. Lack of a centralized communication resulted in bypassing well-equipped hospitals because of lack of knowledge about them. Physicians at the scene performed poorly. They were not easy to identify because they were in civilian clothing. The physicians remained oriented to a detailed evaluation of individual patients rather than to triage of victims as they were extricated.

The authors make the following recommendations to all communities. Have a plan to handle predictable "mini-disasters". Identify resources within the community. Methods of coordinating public and private agencies are essential. Responsibilities should be clearly defined in the plan to fully utilize each agency's strengths. Disaster drills are essential to identify weaknesses in actual field practice.

18. Nicholas RA, Oberheide JE. EMS response to a ski lift disaster in the Colorado mountains. *J Trauma* 1988;**28**:672.

The main support wheel on a ski lift broke, catapulting 50–60 skiers from their chairs 40–50 feet to the ground. Forty-nine patients were triaged, stabilized, and treated by two family physicians in a small office at the base of the mountain. There were 12 critically injured skiers, 10 seriously injured, and 27 with moderate to minor injuries.

The preexisting disaster plan designated a command post, incident commander, defined roles for county and state EMS systems, and communication with defined radios and defined frequencies. Location of the command post in the medical facility serving as the triage collection point provided instant communication between the medical triage officer and the incident commander. A ground ambulance staging area two miles away from the triage collection point prevented congestion. The authors believe implementation of the preconceived plan ensured smooth and efficient patient care in a setting that could have been chaotic.

24. Anonymous. Disaster epidemiology. *Lancet* 1990;**336**:845.

Contemporary disaster relief has been described as a crisis-dominated convergence of unsolicited donations of mobile hospitals, time-expired drugs, medical students volunteering for disaster safaris, and vaccines for diseases with zero incidence.

In acute disasters such as earthquakes and cyclones most deaths occur within hours of the precipitating event. Postdisaster morbidity is generally low. Large-scale epidemics and disease outbreaks are uncommon.

Chronic disasters such as droughts, famines, and exodus of refugees are characterized by a period of migration, followed by congregation in relief camps. High disease risk and high mortality characterize migration. Crude mortality rates for refugee camps may be 20–30 times higher than the local "normal" population. Diarrheal diseases, measles, acute respiratory diseases, and malaria are the most common causes of death. Malnutrition contributes to mortality. The greatest number of deaths is due to infections in individuals who are not severely malnourished.

25. Buerk CA, Batdorf JW, Cammack KV *et al*. The MGM Grand Hotel fire. Lessons learned from a major disaster. *Arch Surg* 1982;**117**:641.

There were 6000 persons in the 26-story MGM Grand Hotel at the time of the fire. EMS processed 3000 persons in five hours; 1700 were referred to the secondary triage-refuge center in the community center; 720 were referred to four local hospitals; 320 were admitted to the hospital. Eighty-four persons died in the fire from burns, related trauma or smoke inhalation.

Initially a primary triage station was established near the secondary main entrance to the hotel. As the flood of evacuees overwhelmed this station, two additional triage sites were established. Each triage station used one base hospital, which accepted its patients, restocked its ambulances, and sent basic information with the ambulance drivers. The secondary triage-refuge center alleviated pressure at the scene by accepting the minimally injured, the displaced, and the bewildered. The refuge center also functioned as a clearing house and data center.

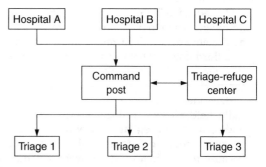

Flow of information (from Buerk).

Las Vegas had an established and practiced disaster plan sufficiently flexible to allow for innovative responses to unforeseen problems.

Lessons learned were as follows.

• Disasters affecting thousands of people can happen.

- Such disasters include large numbers of medical injuries. Medical personnel and support facilities should receive more consideration in disaster planning.
- Multiple triage stations should be considered when perimeter control is not feasible.
- In a major disaster, "loading and transferring" should be the primary response of EMS, rather than diagnosis, categorizing, and treating.
- Helicopter evacuation should be controlled by strict protocol.
- Disaster planning should provide for evacuating minimally injured and displaced persons away from the disaster site.

26. Hull D, Grindlinger GA, Hirsch EF *et al*. The clinical consequences of an industrial aerosol plant explosion. *J Trauma* 1985;**25**:303.

   Twenty-four workers were inside a plant for filling aerosol cans with commonly found household products and their pressurization with a flammable isobutane gas mixture as a propellant. A flash explosion occurred, without fire, but with sufficient energy to knock out walls of the plant.

   All 24 victims were taken by ambulance to nine area hospitals. Eighteen were hospitalized. Five eventually died of burn complications. Some workers were thrown to the ground by the blast, but none sustained traumatic injuries other than burns.

   Proximity to the explosion was correlated with increased body surface area per cent burns. Partitions, crates stacked on skids, and other objects present in the path of the explosion protected workers. Those behind these protective barriers sustained only minor injuries and did not require hospitalization. Victims wearing garments made of synthetic fabrics sustained larger and deeper burns than their co-workers wearing clothing made of natural fibers. All patients had face and hand burns. Clothing does not normally cover the face and hands.

27. Leibovici D, Gofrit O, Stein M *et al*. Blast injuries: bus vs open-air bombings – a comparative study of injuries in survivors of open-air and confined-space explosions. *J Trauma* 1996;**41**:1030.

   Four suicidal bombings resulted in a total of 297 casualties. Two bombings were in the open air, one in a bus station and one near a crowded trade center. The other two occurred inside public buses. All four terrorists used similar explosive devices. Victim density at a close range around the suicidal terrorist was similar in all four attacks.

   A larger number of casualties resulted from explosions in the open air. Fragments can travel a considerable distance from the detonation focus and injure more people. Closed compartments contain much of the energy of the explosion, accounting for the more severe injuries and higher mortality in this group.

|                    | Open air   | Closed space |
|--------------------|------------|--------------|
| Total              | 204        | 93           |
| Admitted           | 73 (36%)   | 40 (43%)     |
| Mortality          | 15 (7.8%)  | 46 (49.5%)   |
| Primary blast injury | 25 (43.2%) | 31 (77.5%)  |
| Penetrating trauma | 22 (30.1%) | 7 (17.5%)    |

From Leibovici

28. Mallonee S, Shariat S, Stennies G *et al*. Physical injuries and fatalities resulting from the Oklahoma City bombing. *JAMA* 1996;**276**:382.

   Detonation of a vehicle bomb containing 4000 lb of ammonium nitrate soaked in fuel oil resulted in the partial collapse of a nine-story office building. There were 759 people injured, 592 survived and 167 (22%) died. Of the 592 survivors, 83 (14%) were hospitalized, 351 (59%) were treated in the emergency department and released, and 158 (27%) were treated by their private physician. Many patients had more than one injury.

Injuries in survivors of the Oklahoma City bombing (from Mallonee)

| Injuries        | Patients |
|-----------------|----------|
| Head            | 80       |
| Pulmonary       | 13       |
| Abdominal       | 4        |
| Ear             | 210      |
| Eye             | 59       |
| Burns           | 9        |
| Musculoskeletal | 210      |
| Soft tissue     | 506      |

29. Nania J, Bruva TE. In the wake of Mount St Helens. *Ann Emerg Med* 1982;**11**:184.

   A cascade of steam, gas, and pumice was responsible for 31 people dead and 34 missing and presumed dead. Autopsies performed on 22 recovered bodies showed the cause of death to be ash inhalation and suffocation in 16, thermal burns in three, and head injury in three. People falling off their roofs during clean-up and repair caused five injuries and one death.

   Hospital admissions decreased 17% due to postponement of elective surgeries. Emergency department visits increased from 10% to 35%. There was a striking increase in the number of respiratory cases seen in the ED, along with conjunctivitis, nasopharyngitis, and bronchitis secondary to volcanic ash.

30. Rosemurgy AS, Norris PA, Olson SM *et al*. Pre-hospital cardiac arrest: the cost of futility. *J Trauma* 1993;**35**:468.

   This is a retrospective review of 12 462 trauma patient ambulance run sheets for October 1 1989 through March 31 1991. There were 410 patients who suffered traumatic cardiopulmonary arrest. Two hundred and seventy-two were not transported to the hospital because they had injuries incompatible with life. The trauma center received 183 patients who arrested at the scene or in the ambulance. Injuries were caused by blunt trauma in 70% and penetrating trauma in 30%. None survived. Eleven (8%) sets of corneas were procured for transplantation. Death nearly always resulted from blood loss, inability to ventilate, closed head injury or a combination of these processes.

The authors conclude that patients without vital signs but with signs of life such as electrocardiographic activity, purposeless eye movement, swallowing activity or brainstem reflexes should be transported. Non-reactive pupils indicate a critical hypoxic insult to the cerebral cortex. If hypoxia persists, the brainstem becomes involved and the respiratory center ceases to drive. Survival is inconceivable. Five minutes of CPR prior to arrival indicate a hopeless cause. Patients without vital signs and without signs of life at the scene have no chance of surviving and returning to their premorbid lifestyle.

31. Washington B, Wilson RF, Steiger Z *et al*. Emergency thoracotomy: a four-year review. *Ann Thoracic Surg* 1985;**40**:188.

The authors retrospectively reviewed the records of 200 patients who underwent emergency department thoracotomy for penetrating trauma. There were 12 patients who had no signs of life at the scene and received CPR en route. None survived. Nineteen patients had signs of life in the field and arrested in the ambulance. After emergency department resuscitative thoracotomy, 15 of 19 had return of a spontaneous heartbeat and were taken to the operating room; three of 15 survived to discharge. Mattox pointed out in his critique that cardiac arrest after penetrating trauma, plus five minutes or more of CPR prior to arrival in the emergency department is irreversibly fatal.

**Potential injury-creating event: dynamic triage**

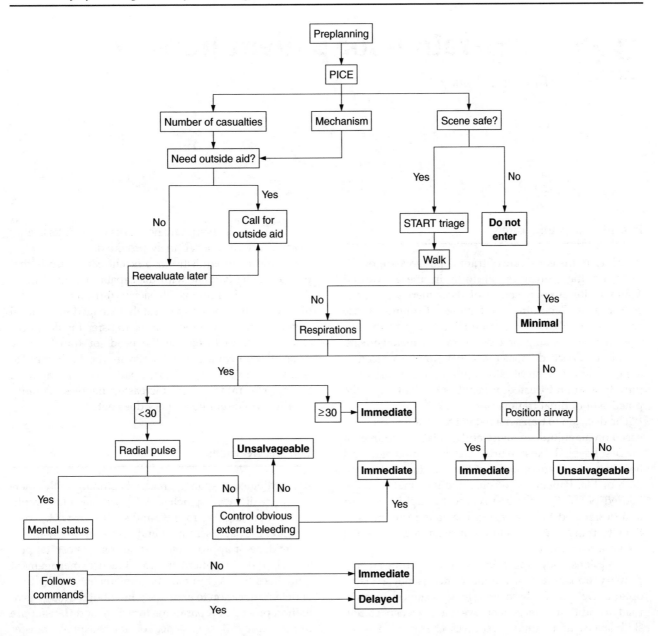

# 30 Preparation for patient transfer

*Thomas V Clancy*

## Priorities in trauma care

Priorities in the early care of trauma patients are predicated on the principles set forth in the Advanced Trauma Life Support course of the American College of Surgeons Committee on Trauma.[1] Common sense and clinical judgment are essential to the early and critical decision-making process in trauma management. Ample evidence demonstrates that trauma outcomes are enhanced when critically injured patients are carefully triaged and treated in facilities committed to the practice of optimal trauma care.[2–5]

The decision to transfer a patient to a trauma center is based on magnitude of injury and available resources at the first hospital. Most injuries may be treated at a local hospital as they are of low severity and do not threaten limb or life. Patients who constitute the smaller, more injured population are best served by rapid transport to a designated trauma center. Previous recommendations to transfer patients to the nearest larger hospital are no longer valid.

Exceptions may apply in the rural setting where primary transport to a trauma center is not a viable option. Delays in discovery, long distances, unsafe road conditions, inclement weather, transportation skill levels, and limited resources characterize some rural environments and may justify patient transfers to the nearest larger hospital.[6]

New to triage, particularly in rural areas, is the application of telemedicine, a modality which enables interhospital on-line image transmission. Direct observation of the patient and visualization of radiographs by the receiving physician may now begin in the first hospital during the patient assessment phase. Decisions regarding diagnostic interventions, initial therapy, mode and staffing of transportation, and medical control may be more rationally established through employment of this technology. As cost and technical obstacles are reduced, telemedical techniques will be employed by all health care networks where interfacility referral services are routinely provided.[7–9]

A critical prerequisite for efficient early care is that physicians be familiar with the capabilities and limitations of their institutions. Physicians must readily recognize which patients may be safely managed in the local hospital and those who require transfer for definitive care. Failure to recognize the need for transfer may jeopardize outcome through delay in care. Early transfer is cost effective. Hospital costs, particularly in the rural setting, rise rapidly with increasing degrees of injury severity while reimbursement does not.[10]

## Transfer decisions

A coordinated response process beginning with emergency medicine dispatch (EMD) will facilitate rapid "patient packaging" for safe and swift transport. Accurate prehospital assessment and communication allows assemblage of appropriate and necessary hospital personnel prior to patient arrival. Practice management guidelines (i.e. ATLS) may be implemented at the time of field notification to expedite a brief but thorough evaluation process. Preparations for triage and transfer are facilitated by the existence of interhospital transfer agreements.[11]

The timing of interhospital transport varies based on the distance of transfer, available skill levels for transport, and circumstances within the local hospital. Diagnostic testing should be limited only to measures essential for ruling out life-threatening injuries. Intervention prior to transfer is a surgical decision. Procedures for life-threatening injuries should be performed prior to transport if possible.

Multiple clinical and non-clinical factors may influence decisions regarding whether or not to transfer a patient. Standard interhospital transport criteria include the presence of high-risk clinical factors and injuries

**Box 30.1 Criteria for consideration of transfer**

**High-risk clinical factors**
Age >55
Children
Pregnancy
Morbid obesity
Immunosuppression
Insulin-dependent diabetes
Cardiac or respiratory disease

**Multisystem injury**
Head injury with face, chest, abdominal or pelvic injury
Injury to more than two body regions
Major burns or burns with associated injuries
Multiple, proximal long bone fractures

**Secondary deterioration (late sequelae)**
Mechanical ventilation requirement
Single or multiple organ system failure (deterioration in central nervous, cardiac, pulmonary, hepatic, renal or coagulation systems)
Major tissue necrosis/sepsis

**Central nervous system**
Head injury
    Penetrating injury or depressed skull fracture
    Open injury with or without CSF leak
    GCS score <14 or GCS deterioration
    Lateralizing signs
Spinal cord injury or major vertebral injury

**Chest**
Cardiac injury
Major chest wall injury or pulmonary contusion
Patients who may require prolonged ventilation
Widened mediastinum or signs of great vessel injury

**Pelvis/abdomen**
Open pelvic fracture
Unstable pelvic ring disruption
Pelvic ring disruption with shock and evidence of continuing hemorrhage

**Extremity**
Ischemia
Major crush injury
Severe open fracture
Complex articular fractures
Traumatic amputation

requiring specialty or subspecialty management not available at the referring hospital[11] (Box 30.1).

Mode of transfer is based upon the premise that time to definitive care and quality of care are critical to survival. Ground vehicles are the most frequently used means of transportation for interhospital transfers. Distance, injury severity, road conditions, and traffic patterns serve as basic criteria for determining the choice between air or ground. The skill levels required for safe transport are determined by the responsible physician, availability of local resources, and magnitude of problem. Air medical dispatch guidelines have been developed by the National Association of EMS Physicians.[12] Careful attention must be paid to the medical indications and other variables employed in the decision to use helicopter transportation.[13,14]

It is the responsibility of the transferring physician to identify the need for transfer, initiate the transfer process by direct contact with the receiving surgeon, institute resuscitative measures within the capability of the facility, determine the mode of transfer in consultation with the receiving physician, and transfer all records, including ambulance call reports, laboratory results, and radiographs.

## Optimal transfer information

Information pertinent to management should accompany the patient in the transfer process. The nature of the injury event, time of occurrence, and prehospital/hospital interventions are most relevant to the continuing diagnostic and resuscitative phases of care. Patient demographic data, names and phone numbers of next of kin, and facts relative to the patient's past medical history, to include medications and allergies, immunizations, previous surgery, and personal habits (alcohol and tobacco consumption), represent valuable information to physicians in the receiving hospital. A general rule of thumb for transfer is that the more relevant information that can be transmitted with the patient, the better. Information relative to advance directives, living wills, and code status should be documented and shared with receiving physicians.

A readily available and legible summary of the patient's condition including vital signs, nature and volume of fluids, urinary output, medications (i.e. steroids, tetanus, antibiotics) and all invasive procedures should be on the chart and clearly communicated by the transferring to the receiving physician.

## Packaging the patient

Diagnostic, resuscitative, and interventional measures are performed in accordance with recommended ATLS standards. Unique to the trauma patient is the requirement to initiate therapy without benefit of a comprehensive history, physical and radiographic evaluation.

Diagnostic measures should not delay transport. Preliminary radiographic examination optimally includes the cervical spine (AP, lateral, oblique views), chest, pelvis, and injured extremities. Laboratory evaluation includes hemoglobin or hematocrit, electrolytes, arterial blood gas, type and crossmatch, and pregnancy test on all females of childbearing age. Alcohol and drug testing are recommended in select patients, indications for which may include clinical suspicion for positivity, brain injury, and penetrating trauma. Additional testing is performed at the discretion of the attending physician. The goal of "packaging" is to have the patient securely immobilized and medically prepared for continuing resuscitative care and vehicle transfer.

Clinical priorities are based on whether the patient is stable or unstable, hemodynamically and neurologically, and whether or not the patient can be stabilized. Physical examination and initial management are focused on five areas.

## Airway

Is the airway patent and protected? Does the patient need a mechanical airway?

### *Initial therapy*

- Administer 100% oxygen by rebreather face mask.
- Remove dentures.
- Intubate if hypoxic, hypercarbic, unable to maintain patent airway, or unconscious. If unsuccessful, perform surgical airway.
- Confirm tube placement by auscultation of both hemithoraces and epigastrium. Suction oral cavity and trachea as necessary.
- Insert gastric tube to reduce risk of aspiration.
- Apply $O_2$ saturation monitor with goal of 90% or greater.

## Breathing

Is the patient breathing comfortably and symmetrically?

### *Initial therapy*

- Determine rate, rhythm, and manner.
- Apply mechanical ventilation as indicated and adjust as indicated.

- Insert chest tubes as needed (fifth interspace/between anterior and midaxillary line).
- Autotransfuse from container as indicated.
- Apply EKG leads.

## Circulation

Is the patient in shock? Are the neck veins distended? Is it pump failure? Consider tension pneumothorax, pericardial tamponade, air embolism or myocardial infarction. Are the neck veins flat? Is it a volume problem? If no evidence of external or thoracic hemorrhage, pelvic fracture or extremity trauma, consider peritoneum or retroperitoneum as potential sites of blood loss.

### *Initial therapy*

- Insert two large bore (16 gauge or greater) intravenous lines in each upper extremity; other venous sites (i.e. femoral, subclavian) may be used as necessary.
- Utilize crystalloid solution (i.e. Ringer's lactate) to establish adequate perfusion.
- Transfuse packed cells if hypotension and poor perfusion persist after 2–3 liters of crystalloid; consider response to early resuscitation as a diagnostic measure to assist in further decision making.
- Insert urinary catheter to monitor urine output.
- Monitor temperature, cardiac rate and rhythm, respiratory rate, and pattern. Assessment of perfusion status is based on mental status, skin color, temperature, capillary refill, venous filling in the hands and feet, blood pressure, pulse and respiratory rates, distal pulse status, urinary output.

## Central nervous system

Does the patient have a brain or spinal cord injury? Is there a mass lesion? Is there evidence of cerebral edema, diffuse axonal injury or contusion?

### *Initial therapy*

- Full immobilization of head, neck, thoracic, and/or lumbar spine.
- Use mechanical ventilation when possible in the unconscious patient (GCS <9).
- Use steroids as indicated (spinal cord injury causing neurologic deficit: solumedrol (loading dose 30 mg/kg, maintenance dose 5.4 mg/kg for 24 hours if begun within three hours of injury, and 48 hours if started between three and eight hours of injury).[15]
- Avoid hyperventilation, hypotension, and hypoxia (secondary injuries).[16] Cervical spine X-rays are unnecessary in alert, oriented patients with no associated drug or alcohol use who do not have neck

pain or tenderness or major distracting injuries (e.g. femur fracture).

## Wound care

- Control external hemorrhage. Direct pressure, tourniquet (if applicable) or clamp and suture (if vessel is clearly visualized) are all acceptable techniques in the appropriate setting.
- Administer tetanus prophylaxis.
- Antibiotics as indicated.
- Examine carefully and document findings, with particular attention to sensory-motor findings and pulse status.
- Debride, irrigate, close or cover as appropriate and as soon as possible.
- Remove rings and other constricting paraphernalia.
- Explore vascular wound in the OR.
- Splint fractures.

## Transporting the patient

Medical control must be established prior to departure. Options include the transferring physician, the receiving physician, the medical director of the transport service or a shared responsibility, often based on regional protocols and distance-based communication capabilities. Patient status, diagnoses, and potential for problems in transport dictate the level of personnel attending the patient. It is expected that the same level of care provided in the first hospital will be continued in transport within the limitations imposed by the vehicle. Monitoring of vital signs, cardiac rate, and rhythm must continue throughout transport at appropriate intervals. Blood replacement and cardiopulmonary resuscitation capability are prerequisites for safe transfer of critically ill patients. Standing order protocols should match transport team capability when physicians do not serve on the transport team.

## Class I Reference

15. Bracken MB, Shepard MJ, Holford TR *et al.* Methylprednisolone or tirilazad mesylate administration after acute spinal cord injury: 1-year follow up. Results of the third National Acute Spinal Cord Injury randomized controlled trial. *J Neurosurg* 1998;**89**(5):699–706.

## Class II References

3. Sampalis JS, Lavoie A, Boukas S *et al.* Trauma center designation: initial impact on trauma-related mortality. *J Trauma* 1995;**39**(2):232–9.

13. Arfken CL, Shapiro MJ, Bessey PQ *et al.* Effectiveness of helicopter versus ground ambulance services for interfacility transport. *J Trauma* 1998;**45**(4):785–9.

## Class III References

2. Shackford SR, Hollingworth-Fridlund P, Cooper GF *et al.* The effect of regionalization upon the quality of trauma care as assessed by concurrent audit before and after institution of a trauma system: a preliminary report. *J Trauma* 1986;**26**(9):812–20.
4. Thompson CT, Bickell WH, Siemens RA *et al.* Community hospital level II trauma center outcome. *J Trauma* 1992;**32**(3):336–43.
5. Mullins RJ, Veum-Stone J, Hedges JR *et al.* Influence of a statewide trauma system on location of hospitalization and outcome of injured patients. *J Trauma* 1996;**40**(4):536–46.
6. Young JS, Bassam D, Cephas GA *et al.* Interhospital versus direct scene transfer of major trauma patients in a rural trauma system. *Am Surg* 1998;**64**:88–92.
7. Reid JG, McGowan JJ, Ricci MA *et al.* Desktop teleradiology in support of rural orthopaedic trauma care. Proc. AMIA Annual Fall Symp. 1997:403–7.
8. Burdick AE, Mahmud D, Jenkins DP *et al.* Telemedicine: caring for patients across boundaries. *Ostomy Wound Manage* 1996;**42**(9):26–30, 32–4, 36–7.
9. Lambrecht CJ. Emergency physicians' roles in a clinical telemedicine network (see comments). *Ann Emerg Med* 1997;**30**(5):667–9, 682–7. Comment in: *Ann Emerg Med* 1998;**30**(6):790–1 and *Ann Emerg Med* 1997; **30**(5):670–4.
10. Rutledge R, Shaffer VD, Ridky J. Trauma care reimbursement in rural hospitals: implications for triage and trauma system design. *J Trauma* 1996; **40**(6):1002–8.
14. Cunningham PR, Rutledge R, Baker CC, Clancy TV. A comparison of the association of helicopter and ground ambulance transport with the outcome of injury in trauma patients transported from the scene. *J Trauma* 1997;**43**(6):940–6.
16. *Severe head injury: guidelines for the management of severe head injury.* The Brain Trauma Foundation, 1995.

## Further reading

1. American College of Surgeons Committee on Trauma. *Advanced trauma life support for doctors: student manual,* 6th edn. Chicago: First Impression, 1997.
11. American College of Surgeons Committee on Trauma. *Advanced Trauma Life Support: Program for doctors,* 6th edn. Chicago: ACS, 1997.
12. Air Medical Dispatch. Guidelines for trauma scene response. National Association of EMS Physicians. *Prehospital Disaster Med* 1992;**7**:77–8.

**Preparation for patient transfer**

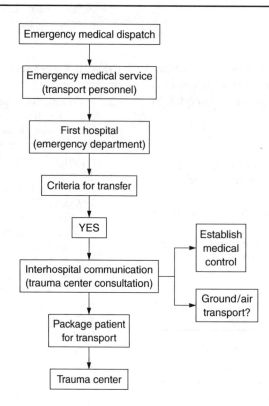

# Index